Activists and Advocates

Toronto's Health Department, 1883-1983

Heather MacDougall

Toronto and Oxford
Dundurn Press
1990

Editor: Leslie Derbecker
Printing and Binding: Gagné Printing Ltd., Louiseville, Quebec, Canada

The writing of this manuscript and the publication of this book were made possible by support from several sources. The publisher wishes to acknowledge the generous assistance and ongoing support of **The Canada Council, The Book Publishing Industry Development Programme** of the **Department of Communications,** and **The Ontario Arts Council.**

In addition, the author and publisher are particularly grateful to **Associated Medical Services, Inc.** and **The Hannah Institute for the History of Medicine,** for a publications grant.

J. Kirk Howard, Publisher

Canadian Cataloguing in Publication Data

MacDougall, Heather Anne
Activists and advocates

ISBN 1-55002-072-2

1. Toronto (Ont.). Dept. of Public Health - History. 2. Public health - Ontario - Toronto - History. I. Title.

RA186.T6M22 1990 362.1'09713'541 C90-094638-5

Dundurn Press Limited
2181 Queen Street East, Suite 301
Toronto, Canada
M4E 1E5

Dundurn Distribution Limited
73 Lime Walk
Headington, Oxford
England
OX3 7AD

Activists and Advocates

Toronto's Health Department, 1883-1983

Heather MacDougall

CONTENTS

Foreword

"A STORY THAT SHOULD BE TOLD" was my reaction to the history of the City of Toronto's Department of Public Health when I first looked into it early in the 1980s. It seemed to me that Toronto's prentive health efforts had all the components of a good novel, with the central theme of dedication to the initial removal of the major causes of infectious disease and later to the prevention of non-communicable diseases.

Since relatively few histories of municipal public health departments have been written, a study of Toronto's experience fills a gap in our knowledge of the past. By examining the changing focus of the staff's educational backgrounds and the services and programs that they provided, we can begin to assess Toronto's role as a leader in public health work in English-speaking Canada and the international impact of some of its activities such as the generalized system of public health nursing and the diphtheria toxoid campaign of the 1930s and 1940s. In the modern era, the Department's Family Planning Services Division, its Health Advocacy Unit, and its public championing of health and advocacy have once again focused national and international attention on the city. How could this story be explained?

In Canada, as elsewhere, there is a dearth of trained historians and historical researchers with an interest in health generally but especially public health. Fortunately from within the ranks of the University of Toronto (now from the University of Waterloo) emerged such a person; Heather MacDougall, an individual whose research interests were in the area of public health (primarily pre–1890), who knew the general history of Toronto and who had lived through the modern era of this community.

Dr. MacDougall readily agreed to research the history of public health in the City of Toronto within certain parameters. The major parameter being the time of study. The uninterrupted one hundred years (1883 to 1983) of the Health Department seemed to be the most logical and important time and certainly would take the reader from the appointment of the first permanent medical officer to a major modern reorganization of the Department.

Late in the 1970s the Toronto Board of Health embarked upon the most far-reaching reorganization of the Department of Public Health since the era of Dr. Charles Hastings, the second and third decade of the twentieth century. The 1970s became a period of reflection on the many issues that emerged during the transformation decade of the 1960s. Governments became more accountable, economic growth without long term health and environmental planning became an issue and the need for a resetting of priorities within the health field generally, and public health specifically, became a necessity. Through the appearance of the Lalonde report, Canadians identified the new problems, classified the issues and developed the basis for a national strategy for reducing non-communicable diseases.

By the end of the 1970s, the Toronto Board of Health produced *Public Health in the 1980's*. A document that provided a blueprint for the future by highlighting the need for greater emphasis on non-communicable diseases and their associated risk factors, conditions and behaviour, using the strategies of education, promotion and advocacy. This document demanded a recognition of the new ethnic demographics in Toronto and refocussed attention on both communicable and non-communicable diseases among the lower socio-economic population. It directed the Department to reorganize to get closer to the people, become an advocacy group for the disadvantaged and disenfranchised, place greater emphasis on planning and become accountable through greater emphasis on evaluation. It led to the development of a decentralized Department with a new focus and a new formula for addressing old, emerging, and new issues.

By 1982 the department, after 100 years of uninterrupted existence, had restructured itself to better address the health needs of the people of Toronto with an expanded management, an inventory of reemphasised strategies and an enlarged mandate. It will be interesting to see how the author of the history of the second one hundred years reflects on this moment in time.

Dr. MacDougall's work has, in a very professional manner, provided substantiation for my first impression. The public health history of Toronto is positive and progressive and the story should be told. I think you will agree.

William J. Shannon, B.A., M.A., Ed.D.
Director
Health Education
Ministry of Health
Province of British Columbia

(formerly Manager
Community Health Promotion and Advocacy Section
Department of Public Health
City of Toronto)

Acknowledgments

Since this study began in the summer of 1982, many individuals and institutions have contributed to its completion. First and foremost, Dr. Bill Shannon, of the Toronto Health Department, deserves credit for initiating the project and obtaining funding for our summer researchers from the Department of the Secretary of State in 1982, and the City of Toronto in 1986. Both Bill and his support staff, particularly Ms. Sylvia Dyson, devoted much time and energy to ensuring that the technical aspects progressed smoothly. Their continuing interest and encouragement have been invaluable.

During the summer of 1982, Mary Beth Mills, Jim Williamson and Hamish Stewart researched the Health Department's records, its annual reports and the local board of health minutes. Their activities were assisted by the staffs of the City of Toronto Archives, the Toronto Academy of Medicine, the Provincial Archives of Ontario, and the University of Toronto Science and Medicine Library. The Metropolitan Toronto Reference Library was a good source of photographs, and the University of Victoria College Archives and the Toronto Board of Education Archives also provided illustrative material.

To flesh out the official record, I interviewed Mrs. Audrey Williams, Charles Hastings's daughter, in June 1984, and my research assistant, Anne Marie Hagan, conducted a lengthy series of interviews with current and former employees, and members of the local board of health, all of whose recollections add a human dimension to the story. Bud Connery, Alex McDonald and James Flaherty, offered insights into the evolution of public health inspection, while Mary Willett, Madeline Smillie, Betty Davidson, Nancy Cuyler and Michael Davis provided a fascinating overview of public health nursing in the city. Linda Latchford and Elizabeth Parker described their respective experiences as a city nutritionist and a member of the Family Planning Services Division. Carrie Moore and Nancy Laing's recollections vividly recalled the work that secretarial staff performed, while Ted Tennant and Marcia Moss's interviews highlighted contemporary management practices. Drs. Mavis Rampersaud, Edgar Wong, Bill Frank and Arthur Steurmann discussed the challenges facing health professionals providing medical services, mental health counselling, district medical care, communicable disease control and public health dentistry. And Dr. George Moss, Toronto's Medical Officer of Health from 1972 to 1981, commented on the trials and tribulations of directing such a complex organization in tumultuous times. Former alderman and board of health chairman, Anne Johnston, and former Board of Education trustee, Dan Leckie, both offered trenchant observations on the process of decentralization; their recollections added greatly to my understanding of the reformers' strategy and objectives. And finally, Dr. Charles Sheard of Stamford, Connecticut, and his brother Matthew of Limehouse, Ontario, shared memories of their grandfather and provided his picture for this study.

Scholarly books are not published without significant financial support, and I would like to thank Associated Medical Services Inc., and the Hannah Institute for the History of Medicine, for their generous contribution to the publication costs. The comments of their anonymous assessment committee were also appreciated.

This book could not have been completed without the support of colleagues, friends and my family. Professor Margaret Andrews, of Washington State University, read an early draft and made helpful suggestions for improvement. Mrs. Gail Heideman of the University of Waterloo History Department cheerfully typed the reference notes. Ian and Ella Stewart did yeoman service reading the manuscript, and provided illuminating insights on the changes that they have seen in the city, during their years of teaching at Woodsworth College at the University of Toronto, and for the Toronto Board of Education in inner city schools. And Roger Riendeau, of Innis College, helped me to maintain my focus by asking why this study is important. For all their advice and support my thanks; any errors are mine alone.

This book is for my grandparents — three Torontonians by adoption, one by birth.

Dougal Peter MacDougall (1888–1971)
Helen Wright MacDougall (1892–1975)
George Harris White (1900–1941)
Daisy Newton White (1902–1989)

Introduction

"What does public health mean to you?" In 1954, when the national magazine *Health* asked its readers this question, most Torontonians would immediately have answered that it meant the public health nurses, who visited their homes and worked in the schools and child health centres, the inspectors, who protected the city's sanitation standards and food supply, and the medical officer and his senior staff, who administered the Health Department. Today we would reply that it means health promotion through anti-smoking campaigns, and health advocacy on contentious social and environmental issues, by all the staff, including health educators and community workers. Both responses would have surprised citizens in 1883.

Prior to the creation of the Medical Health Department, the city's response to its emerging sanitation problems and epidemics of cholera, typhus, and smallpox, had been limited because of lack of money, political will, and public interest in long-term solutions.[1] By 1883, however, circumstances had changed. After expanding by 30,000 inhabitants during the 1870s, Toronto had become a bustling commercial city of over 86,000, second only to Montreal in terms of population and economic importance. With its mixture of native born and British immigrants, the city was proudly Tory and Protestant: a bastion of Empire in the New World. Its rail links and business connections with the United States tied Toronto to the North American way of life. As the capital of Ontario, the Queen City of the West was a focal point for government, education and cultural institutions.[2] Since urban-industrial growth was occurring throughout the new Canadian nation, federal and provincial governments began to introduce permissive legislation and funding which made municipalities responsible for protecting and promoting the health of their citizens. All of these factors produced demands for a more sustained and effective approach to burgeoning urban health problems such as slums, polluted water supplies, and waste disposal. In 1883 the city's aldermen responded to these concerns by appointing Toronto's first permanent medical health officer , to fulfil the conditions of a federal government grant to collect mortality statistics. From this small beginning, the city's present Health Department evolved.

By making the new appointment permanent, Toronto, in fact, joined a trend that was part of the modernization of municipal government in the English-speaking world. As acknowledged experts, medical health officers were at the forefront of the drive to professionalize the civil service in Britain, the United States and Canada. Many of them were prominent participants in the progressive reform movement which flourished from 1880 to 1920. Strongly humanitarian in outlook, these men argued that their training fitted them to promote public health concerns at all levels of government.[3] In all three countries, however, local health officers discovered that municipal politics determined the extent of their success, because in general, the solutions which they proposed either threatened individual civil liberties or required significant funding. Until provincial legislation was changed in 1909 to ensure a solid financial base for preventive work, Toronto's health officers, like their counterparts elsewhere in Ontario, had to rely on their powers of persuasion to increase their staff and expand the services which the Health Department provided.

Many of the arguments which the city's medical health officers used were drawn from similar campaigns waged by their British colleagues because each of the first four medical officers had done post-graduate study in London and other centres. As well, the continuous arrival of British immigrants prior to 1913 strengthened the links between the two countries. The provincial government also modelled its public health legislation on that in operation in the mother country, and fostered the development of professional identity by funding the Association of Executive Health Officers of Ontario, which in turn had its intellectual roots in the British Society of Medical Officers of Health, founded in 1856.[4]

But the most significant British contribution lay in the transfer of the "sanitary idea" to the United States and Canada. Based on the erroneous belief that rotting human and animal waste produced noxious vapours or miasma, which caused disease, the "sanitary idea" emerged, as a result of the rising death rate that accompanied rapid industrial and urban growth during the 1830s and 1840s. Most clearly presented by reformers such as Edwin Chadwick, the first component of the international public health movement focused on cleaning up the urban environment, providing pure water supplies, and ending citizens' dependence on privies and cesspools to remove waste.[5] The concept gave birth to the science of vital statistics, promoted the development of engineering and technology, and led to the creation of two new municipal positions: medical officers and sanitary inspectors.[6] The apparent success of British cities in lowering their death rates from enteric diseases as a result of the work of the new appointees, supportive local councils and sanitary engineers,[7] encouraged reformers in New York, Milwaukee, Newark, Hamilton, Ottawa, Montreal[8] and finally Toronto to imitate the British model.

As a result, the "sanitary idea," with its stress on eliminating premodern waste disposal practices and environmental "nuisances" was introduced in North American cities during the latter half of the nineteenth century. To educate the public in its sanitary responsibilities, Toronto's health officers slowly persuaded the city council to appoint sanitation and food inspectors. But even these enthusiastic new appointees had great difficulty in persuading ratepayers to support their efforts to improve the quality of urban life because of the uncertain economic climate of the 1890s. Prior to 1911 when the census indicated that Toronto had grown by nearly 81% in the preceding decade to a population of 376,538, only reform politicians had backed trunk sewer projects and by-laws which restricted businesses and homeowners from causing sanitation problems. Nevertheless, the inspection system which Toronto's health officers devised, and the annual reports which they presented to the local board of health between 1883 and 1910, gradually educated citizens and politicians to improve their households' waste disposal practices, and to expect basic urban amenities including pure water. With this essential foundation in place, the twentieth century medical officers, like their colleagues in other centres, expanded the Department's activities into new areas.

In large measure, the change occurred in response to the bacteriological revolution which began in the 1880s, and to the introduction of health education after 1900. These two developments represented the second and third phases of the international public health movement. As scientists in Louis Pasteur and Robert Koch's laboratories uncovered the microbiological origins of many communicable diseases, the public health movement used these discoveries to hone its disease control procedures. By 1900, diagnostic testing had become the norm in large urban health departments, and medical officers in Britain, the United States, and Canada were awaiting the discovery of vaccines to prevent many of the diseases which took such a toll on the children of the nations' rapidly growing cities.[9]

They were not disappointed. In 1895, the antitoxin treatment for diphtheria became the first of many advances which have made childhood diseases such as whooping cough, measles, polio and scarlet fever, relics of the past. The international research community made a vital contribution to this work, and Toronto was fortunate to be the site of the University of Toronto Medical Faculty, the School of Hygiene, and the Connaught Laboratories. Basic research in biochemistry, virology and immunology resulted in the discovery and production of vaccines, which city medical officers and their staffs could use to combat epidemics of contagious disease, and to prevent further outbreaks.[10] From the 1910s onward, Toronto's Health Department had a close relationship with researchers in the city and the international community, and was the site of clinical trials of diphtheria toxoid and poliomyelitis vaccines. By 1940, the city's success in virtually eradicating diphtheria had earned it an international reputation. This success entrenched the medical research model as one of the dominant features of the Department's work culture.

The Department's role in disease prevention, however, was not without controversy. In the same way that establishing basic sanitation standards infringed on individual liberty, creating disease control and prevention procedures required citizens and local practitioners to surrender some of their civil rights to ensure "the greatest good for the greatest number." Toronto's medical officers and their communicable disease inspectors, district medical officers and public health nurses, experienced the same type of opposition and frustration that their colleagues in other large cities faced. Education, persuasion, and only as a last resort, prosecution, were the stages that municipal staff went through as they attempted to control or prevent widespread epidemics. Although the provincial authorities passed legislation defining standard disease control procedures and organized regulations for notification by practitioners and householders, they limited their activity to providing free biological products and assisting local boards who requested help. In many instances, the members of the Provincial Board of Health and its successor, the Ontario Health Department, relied on Toronto for supplies of serum, and cited the city as a model of effective public health administration in this field. By the 1940s, the communicable diseases which had been the leading causes of death at the beginning of the twentieth century had been superseded by chronic diseases, accidents, suicide and lifestyle diseases, as the major killers. Although Canadian and American public health leaders argued in favour of shifting attention to these new concerns, the continuing presence of contagious diseases among the refugees from war-torn Europe, and their successors who arrived in Toronto from Third World countries beginning in the 1960s meant that the Department was not able to dismantle its disease-fighting apparatus quickly.

Both the "sanitary idea" and the bacteriological revolution, contributed to the evolution of the public health movement by providing the infrastructure on which further development could take place. After 1900, Canadian and American public health enthusiasts in city, provincial and state health departments, and voluntary groups, such as the Canadian and American Public Health Associations, joined the progressive reformers who were agitating to create a better world by redefining the public health crusade. The "New Public Health" condemned the continuing emphasis on sanitation work as a city health department function, stressed the importance of scientific research and laboratory facilities at the local level, urged improved professional education for public health doctors and nurses, and shifted attention to "educating" women and children in their health duties.[11]

To achieve these goals, city health departments had to hire new staff and adopt new strategies. Underlying their efforts was strong faith in the perfectibility of human beings, and the effectiveness of expert intervention. Helping immigrants and rural migrants adjust to the demands of urban life was one of the greatest challenges that American and Canadian public health workers faced prior to 1914. To make health education an effective aspect of its work, Toronto pioneered the generalized system of district public health nursing. Each nurse was assigned a specific area within her district and developed a variety of contacts with women, school children, TB victims, and others who required city services. Many of the nurses and the district medical officers were frustrated because they found that some citizens were unable to adopt modern health practices because they were poor. To deal with this problem, Toronto's nurses also became part of the network of charitable organizations in the community. This broadened the Department's focus but also moved it away from the reform impulse, which had dominated since the 1880s. By the 1930s, social work methods had replaced the Christian zeal which characterized early reformers, as the Health Department staff professionalized.

The process of professionalization included training in administrative practices. Within the municipal system, trying to achieve the high standard of performance and expert impartiality that the scientific management system presupposed was tempered by political realities. Lack of money was a continual problem because health departments, generally, were not revenue-producing agencies. The combination of this feature and the restrictions which disease control procedures and sanitation standards imposed made Toronto's Health Department a focal point for conflict during the Great Depression. Even post-war prosperity did not entirely ease the situation, because the arrival of the second large wave of non-English-speaking immigrants meant that essential services had to be explained once again and a new group persuaded to accept them.

By 1951, Toronto's population had grown to 675,754, and its senior Health Department administrators, like their colleagues in Britain and the United States, were trying to redefine their staff's activities. With the assistance of national health grants from the federal government, and increased interest in local matters by the province, Toronto, like New York and Oxford, moved into adult health services. Many adult health problems such as sexually transmitted diseases, drug and alcohol addiction, and family planning, have strong social stigmas attached to them. Even less contentious issues, such as heart disease and cancer, or the needs of the elderly, proved challenging because the health department had to interpret the latest research results, and assist citizens in integrating these insights into healthy behaviour patterns.

During the 1950s as well, curative medicine took centre stage. Antibiotics and improved surgical techniques led the public to think that a new era was dawning. Public health professionals were less sanguine, especially when they became regarded as second class and second rate, since their work lacked the glamour and immediacy of curative endeavours. By the early 1960s, health departments in Canada and the United States were rethinking their priorities, adopting new approaches for reaching the public and evaluating their role in the current health care system. In Canada, the situation was urgent because the federal government was preparing to introduce a national system of health insurance, which did not include a significant preventive component.

During the late 1960s and early 1970s, as curative health care costs started to rise, governments in developed nations began to re-examine the potential role of prevention. In 1974, Canada's Minister of National Health and Welfare, Marc Lalonde, released *A New Perspective on Health for Canadians: A Working Document.* This paper epitomized many of criticisms of the medical care system which had arisen during the 1960s, as a new generation of social activists became involved in both the health industry and municipal politics. With its emphasis on prevention, health promotion and environmental issues, the Lalonde report was very topical for Torontonians. The voters had elected a reform administration in 1972 and the Health Department quickly became one of the rallying points for change. As the agency closest to the public offering advice and guidance on health and disease prevention, Toronto's Department, according to the reformers, had become mired in the past and oblivious to citizens' concern about deteriorating environmental conditions. When a group of ratepayers appeared before the local board of health to ask for assistance in dealing with lead contamination problems, the reformers initiated a lengthy campaign to reorganize the

Department's structure and to reanimate the staff. Health promotion and health advocacy became the foundation for sophisticated programs directed at specific target groups rather than the citywide focus of their predecessors. Modern systems management techniques, teamwork and decentralization ended medical dominance and the hierarchical structure which had predominated since 1910. When decentralization was completed in 1982, Toronto's Health Department entered its second century with renewed vigour and a commitment to the fourth phase of the international public health movement: health promotion.

The history of the development of Toronto's Health Department illustrates the way in which one of Canada's leading cities responded to the health hazards of urban-industrial growth. It also demonstrates the evolution of an administrative structure and the traditions which develop within the public service. By adapting the changing focus of the international public health movement to Toronto's circumstances, the staff were translating public health theory into services and programs, while consistently seeking to remain at the forefront of the crusade for health. The work they did is the subject of this study.

Chapter One

Activists and Advocates: The Pioneers, 1883–1929

"Good health is the bedrock on which social progress is built."[1] For Toronto's first four health officers, Drs. William Canniff, Norman Allen, Charles Sheard and Charles Hastings, serving as the city's medical health officer during the first fifty years of the Department's existence provided the opportunity to combine social service with medical expertise. Together science and reform zeal were the foundation for the Department's efforts to ensure that Torontonians achieved the good health essential for social progress. As Victorian-trained social reformers, these doctors lobbied to obtain the medical health officership because they wanted to apply their expertise to Toronto's pressing health problems. But first, they had to define their role and introduce international public health concepts to their fellow citizens.

All four were well equipped to do so because they had undertaken postgraduate work in Britain and were linked to the American public health crusade as well. These external models were vital because as amateur administrators, these men were pioneering a new municipal office and building a modern bureaucracy. To do so successfully required a clearly articulated vision, strong leadership skills and a prosperous economy since local public health work was completely funded by local taxes during these decades.

Although Ontario's Public Health Acts of 1884 and 1912 made legal definitions of the role of local health officers, they did not describe how such officials were expected to persuade ratepayers and aldermen to support the extension of inspection activity or the expansion of the civic bureaucracy. Clearly the personality and political acumen of each health officer was a factor in his success in this area, but the city's economic circumstances were equally important. Between 1883 and 1921, Toronto's population expanded from over 86,000 to approximately 521,000, and the council was hard pressed to provide roads, schools and other essential services before the national economy improved at the beginning of the twentieth century. Until the 1912 Public Health Act made dismissal a provincial prerogative, Toronto's medical officers walked a fine line in their dealings with the council on issues of hiring additional staff and increasing their efforts to eliminate environmental abuses because the Health Department was not a revenue-generating operation. Indeed, many of its activities prompted opposition from the public and the business community.

To combat this, Canniff, Allen, Sheard and Hastings all participated fully in the reform movements of their era. They worked through lay and medical organizations to publicize the benefits of the reforms that they proposed and acquired a high public profile as a result of their activism. Such personal involvement in reform crusades demonstrated the extent of their commitment to social change and the very gradual evolution of the concept of the impartial bureaucrat.

By 1915, Toronto had an international reputation as an innovative leader in modern public health administration. Building on the work of his predecessors, Charles Hastings had expanded his staff, added health education to the sanitation and disease control efforts which were the foundation of municipal preventive efforts, and introduced modern management principles. But the forces of change were already at work. As the older generation of reform enthusiasts retired, they were replaced by professional administrators who preferred to work within the political system rather than to lead reform crusades. Public interest in and support for expanding municipal services also diminished during the 1920s. When Hastings retired in 1929, his successor inherited a Health Department whose credo of active community service was being modified by changing social and economic circumstances.

Laying the Foundation: The Canniff Years

"Indubitable integrity, strength and independence of judgment, suavity combined with firmness, a good knowledge of sanitary science and men, indefatigable energy, and... acquaintance with civic affairs" were the characteristics which the *Canadian Practitioner*, one of Toronto's leading medical journals, stated were necessary for the city's new medical officer.[2] But did the city's aldermen agree? In the previous decade, the city had grown from 56,000 to over 86,000 and inhabitants were questioning the politicians' reliance on ad hoc measures to deal with environmental problems and contagious disease. Why not imitate British and American cities and appoint a permanent medical health officer?

In 1883 the municipal politicians responded to the demand because of intervention from the senior levels of government. The Macdonald administration provided the proverbial carrot by offering a conditional grant for the collection of mortality statistics to all Canadian cities over 25,000 people who had permanent salaried medical health officers. A year earlier, the Mowat government had passed permissive legislation to create a Provincial Board of Health to supervise local health work and this body was actively encouraging the creation of a medical health officership in the provincial capital. Toronto's aldermen, however, were more interested in rationalizing the city's medical services than they were in implementing the British and American approaches to sanitation and disease control. As a result, by-law 1317 which defined the medical officer's duties limited his preventive role to offering advice to the mayor, the Markets and Health Committee and the city's General Inspector of Licenses. In addition, the new appointee was to provide expert assessment of people applying to the city for medical relief, to care for injured civic employees, and to conduct monthly vaccination clinics.[3]

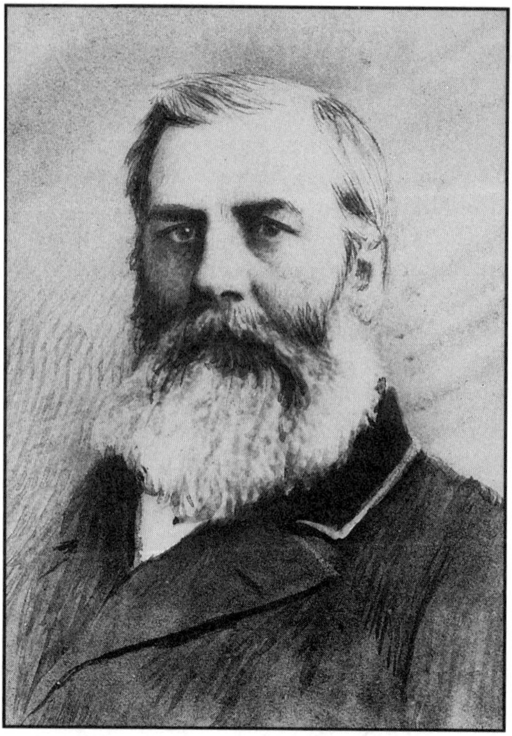

Dr. William Canniff, MHO, 1883-1890.

In spite of its stress on curative tasks and limited preventive responsibilities, the position interested several Toronto doctors, all of whom lobbied council members for their support. The front runners were Edward Playter, Parkdale's former medical officer, a noted public health activist and Liberal, and William Canniff, a former Dean of Victoria Medical School, well-known surgeon and amateur historian, and staunch Conservative. Canniff had the added distinction of being the chairman of the Canadian Medical Association Committee which had convinced the Macdonald government to pay for the collection of urban mortality statistics, and he informed council members of his desire to see the system implemented effectively. On March 12, 1883, the aldermen voted 18 to 9 in favour of his candidacy, not because he was well versed in sanitary science but because he was a Tory.[4] For some of the aldermen, the medical officership was another patronage plum. As they were to discover, the new medical officer viewed it as an opportunity to use his medical expertise to benefit all his fellow citizens.

In 1884, Canniff outlined the challenges which he had faced during his first year in office to the delegates at the Sanitary Convention sponsored by the Provincial Board of Health, held in Ottawa that year. According to the new official:

> The city of Toronto has, during the last few years, grown very rapidly and assumed the characteristics of a great metropolis. The result has been that the private premises of many citizens were in a condition far from satisfactory from a sanitary standpoint. As the summer advanced I became painfully aware of the fact that while, as nominally, the Medical Health Officer, I could not be absolved from responsibility, I was powerless to act. I had no assistance, no inspectors, no executive authority. When midsummer had arrived, I was, nevertheless receiving daily numerous complaints of sanitary evils from citizens.[5]

These complaints were the start of his campaign to build an effective Medical Health Department. Canniff justified expanding his activities beyond the limits imposed in by-law 1317 on the grounds that the public needed education in sanitary matters and by virtue of his medical training, he was the expert who could offer such advice.

To do so effectively, the medical officer had to have a better understanding of the city's sanitary condition, a legal definition of his preventive role, a corps of inspectors and financial and political support from Toronto's aldermen. In 1883 he was stymied in his attempts to evaluate the city's sanitation problems until Major Frank Draper, the city Police Chief, offered to assign policemen to serve as inspectors. As he told his audience, Canniff was "a novice...in inaugurating (such) a system" but he quickly devised an inspection questionnaire and met daily with the policemen to assess their reports and be brought up-to-date on "problem" cases. In this manner, he laid the ideological basis for the Department's work culture by insisting on "education rather than coercion."

Like many of his contemporaries, Canniff's commitment to preventive medicine and public health was rooted in his belief that "by the application of proper sanitary laws great saving might be effected in the public interest by preserving the health, giving comfort, and by keeping the breadwinner free from disease."[6] These views had been inculcated during his postgraduate study in Great Britain in 1855 and were common among Victorian social reformers on both sides of the Atlantic. Taking a broad view of their responsibilities, men like Canniff, Playter, Isaac Ryall, Hamilton's health officer from 1876–1900, and the medical members of the Provincial Board of Health used newspapers, voluntary groups and active lobbying to educate the public to support their demands for stronger legislation, increased funding and higher sanitation standards.

At the beginning of his years in office, Canniff quickly became aware of the political nature of his position. Recognizing the "indifference or aversion" to sanitary reform which dominated the growth-conscious aldermen, he set out to change their perceptions. In 1884, amendments to the Ontario Public Health Act strengthened his focus on prevention by making the annual appointment of a local board of health mandatory and requiring the board to provide a yearly report of the city's health status to its provincial counterpart. The legislation caused controversy in Toronto when a non-elected board was proposed. This attempt to add interested professionals, such as an architect, an engineer and a philanthropist, to what previously had been an aldermanic committee, foundered after a year's trial. Fortunately, the arrival of a reform contingent on council in 1886 and 1887 gave Canniff the political support he needed to respond to the city's increasing sanitation problems.

From 1886 to 1889, lawyer Phillip Drayton, whose father-in-law Dr. Charles Covernton was chairman of the Provincial Board of Health, served as the chairman of Toronto's local board of health. Through these years, the health officer was constantly under attack for failing to have "nuisances" removed promptly by citizens who passed their complaints on to Drayton and other aldermen. By 1888 and 1889, Canniff's patience was wearing thin and he pointed out to the mayor and the local board that it was "unjust to make his department a scapegoat" for long-standing environmental abuses because all these problems had been investigated continuously and he and his staff had made frequent recommendations for abatement. In his annual reports, his monthly summaries of the Department's activities and his public addresses, the medical officer ascribed the criticisms which his department received to lack of legal power to compel clean-ups "lest the interests of some alderman's particular friend be hurt thereby" and to lack of funding from cautious ratepayers for essential urban amenities.

Gradually Canniff also realized that his faith in "persuasion" was somewhat misplaced. As all his successors were to learn, not every citizen was willing to adapt to the Health Department's sanitation standards and communicable disease control procedures. This discovery prompted Canniff to redouble his publicity efforts through forging links with local, national and international public health groups. In Toronto interested architects like Henry Langley and S.G. Curry, engineers such as Charles Sproatt, Kivas Tully and Allan Macdougall, businessmen like Oliver Howland and W.B. Hamilton, politicians like George Ross, the provincial Minister of Education, and Mayor William H. Howland joined doctors like Charles Covernton, Peter Bryce and William Canniff in forming the Toronto Sanitary Association. At its monthly meetings, lay and professional members heard noted experts discuss the city's environmental flaws and potential technological solutions to them.

As Canniff and his supporters prepared to attack the city's sanitary deficiencies, they turned to the American Public Health Association for inspiration. Founded in 1872, the APHA moved from city to city for its annual meetings as a means of spreading the gospel of preventive medicine. With a mixed membership of experts and interested citizens, the organization had a broad appeal and a wide range of interests. Controlling the spread of communicable diseases was one central concern and in 1884 while the American government was hosting an international cholera conference, Canada and Mexico were invited to join the APHA. Canniff and the other Canadian delegates accepted the invitation and offered to host the 1886 meeting in Toronto.

During the meeting, Canadian and American health officers formed a joint association of State and Provincial Health Officers to share information about the outbreak of contagious diseases such as smallpox and cholera, and to inform each other about the control measures which central and local governments intended to use to stop these diseases from crossing state or provincial borders. Peter Bryce, the secretary of the Provincial Board of Health, also used the 1886 meeting to organize an Association of Executive Health Officers of Ontario, partly to standardize public health practice in the province and partly to foster a sense of professional identity among medical officers.[7] As one of the chief organizers and participants in the conference, Canniff had an opportunity to meet the leading figures of the American public health movement, gain their support for the type of work he was doing, and initiate close links between Toronto and its American counterparts.

Even this professional support failed to convince Toronto's taxpayers to approve Canniff's cherished trunk sewer proposal, its aldermen to pass a by-law to eliminate privies in the downtown core, or its doctors to report promptly any cases of infectious disease they were treating to the medical officer and his staff. The decline of the reformers, an economic downswing, a turf fight with the city engineer over control of plumbing inspection, opposition from vested interests like the ice dealers whose livelihood he had threatened, and a smear campaign alleging that he had been seen drunk in Parkdale, led a bitter and disillusioned medical health officer to resign on September 17, 1890.[8]

As Toronto's first permanent medical officer, Canniff had pioneered the position. Given his British training, he naturally focused attention on environmental pollution problems and the creation of a disease control apparatus. But was he an employee of the city council or the province? In February 1890, Toronto's council had passed a by-law rescinding the provisions of the model by-law attached to the 1884 provincial Public Health Act, in an effort to assert control over the medical officership. By making council the paramount authority, the by-law challenged the medical profession's belief in professional autonomy. Canniff's immediate successors learned, as he had, that the medical officership was a lightning rod which attracted more criticism than praise.

Frustration in Office: The Allen Regime

After Canniff resigned, a hundred-man delegation of Toronto doctors persuaded the local board to hold a competitive examination to choose his replacement.[9] This was a marked contrast to the British and American approaches to the appointment of medical officers. In Britain, qualified medical officers advanced slowly through the ranks of the public health bureaucracy, while in most American cities, the spoils system prevailed and the health officership alternated between Republicans and Democrats.[10] In Toronto, the examining committee deadlocked twice as staff from Toronto's competing medical schools were unable to agree on an acceptable candidate. Dr. A.R. Pyne, Canniff's temporary successor was the son of the Ontario Medical Council's registrar while his chief rival, Dr. T.S. Covernton, was the son of a member of the Provincial Board of Health and a lecturer in sanitary science at the Women's Medical College.

Without a clear cut victor, the council turned to a compromise candidate, Dr. Norman Allen, and appointed him in March 1891. At twenty-six, Allen was a graduate of Trinity Medical School who had just returned from post-graduate training in Great Britain. Inexperienced and impulsive, his quick condemnation of the city engineer, for causing a typhoid epidemic by dumping human waste into the harbour near the water intake pipe, revitalized the simmering feud between the two departments. Worse was to come. In his annual report for 1892, he criticized the patronage appointment

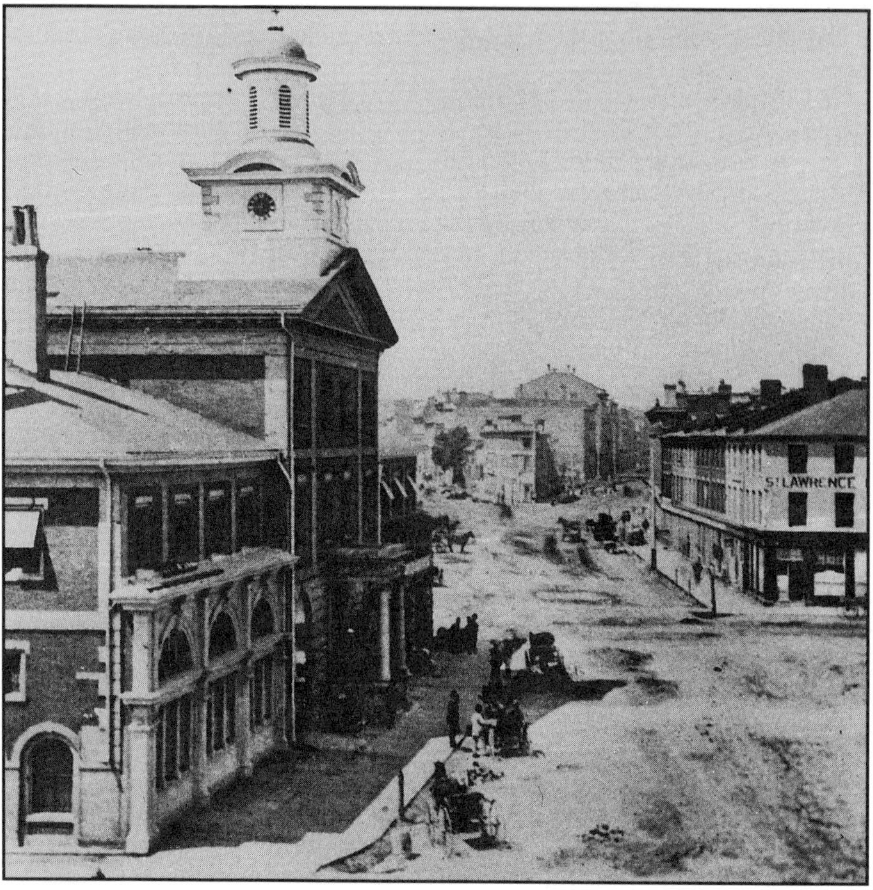

The Medical Health Department was located in Toronto's second city hall from 1883-1899.

system and announced that he had appointed trained sanitary inspectors. The young medical officer also consulted members of the Provincial Board of Health about Toronto's notorious "privy menace." Lacking the political acumen of his predecessor, Allen failed to realize that Toronto's Tory councils distrusted administrators who depended on the Grits at Queen's Park.

But the cause of his downfall was his inability to direct the department. In January 1893, the city council's executive committee reported that "the business of the Department has been carried on in a most unsatisfactory, extravagant and unbusiness-like manner." They were alluding to Allen's inability to produce accounts from the city's new Isolation Hospital and his bookkeeper's incomprehensible records of city spending on health activities. When the medical officer was unable to refute the charges, he was fired.[11]

Applying Science to Society: The Sheard Administration

Although the Toronto *Mail* was concerned that Allen's firing represented excessive interference by the mayor and other politicians, and the politicisation of the Health Department, the controversy did not deter able candidates from applying for the post. In March 1893, on the recommendation of the local board of health, the council appointed thirty-five year old Dr. Charles Sheard to the position. The son of a former mayor, Sheard had the contacts and maturity which Allen lacked. A noted teacher at Trinity Medical School, former editor and co-owner of the *Canada Lancet*, and a surgeon, he had been elected president of the Canadian Medical Association in 1892. As an independently wealthy real estate tycoon, Sheard combined the medical expertise and business ability which the aldermen were seeking.

He also represented the second phase of the public health movement because he had been trained to accept the germ theory and devoted much of his time to publicizing it among the public and his colleagues. As well, Sheard promoted the professionalization of public health practice. During his 1897 presidential address to the Executive Health Officers Association, he moved from commiserating with his colleagues about their "onerous, and sometimes exceedingly trying and irksome duties," to informing them that their work was just as much a specialty as any other form of medicine, and that they too must adopt the scientific method.[12] While noting the difficulty that many of his fellow officers had in collecting data, Sheard reminded them that "it is science which seams and scars the detested face of hypocrisy and lies...." Both his reverence for science and his stress on specialization suggested that Sheard, like other advocates of the germ theory, had narrowed the broad vision of the sanitary reformers to focus on individuals rather than the environment.

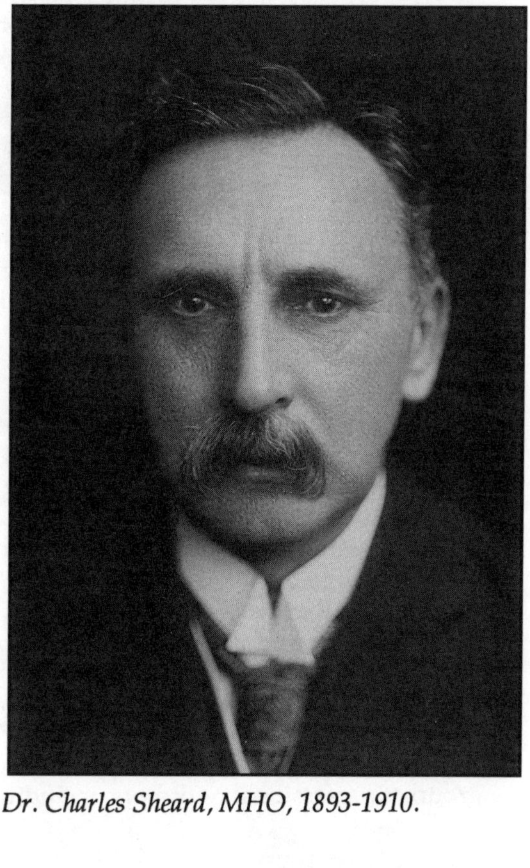

Dr. Charles Sheard, MHO, 1893-1910.

Decisive and sharp-tongued, Sheard served full-time for six months to reorganize the Department in 1893; he expanded its services to include those necessities of the bacteriological revolution — a laboratory and a well-run isolation hospital. After this task was completed, he returned to teaching on a part-time basis and divided his efforts between training the future generation and public service. When Trinity amalgamated with the University of Toronto Faculty of Medicine in 1903, Sheard was appointed Professor of Preventive Medicine. From this position, he and his supporters pushed for the creation of a diploma in public health, to ensure that future medical officers received post-graduate training like their British counterparts. In 1905, the election of a Conservative majority in Ontario paved the way for his appointment as the chairman of the Provincial Board of Health from 1906 until 1910. Using this vantage point, he and his colleagues were able to persuade the Whitney government to strengthen the position of local medical health officers by amending provincial health legislation in 1909 to put funding for preventive work on the same basis as taxation for school boards. All of these activities illustrated how closely knit the public health professionals were and how intent they were on upgrading their qualifications to enhance their status within municipal governments.

As an administrator, Sheard attracted attention in 1905 when the council shifted street cleaning from the city engineer's department to the Health Department. After firing virtually all the street cleaners, the medical officer received a visit from a former aldermen whose protest over the medical officer's attempts to improve efficiency prompted fisticuffs. One of the Toronto papers described the effect of "Sheardofritis" on the aldermen and sanitation staff:

> Each garbage worker hustles now
>   He's working you may bet
> He has no time to loaf in lanes
>   Or smoke a cigarette,
> He knows he must earn his pay
>   Without a single doubt
> For Dr. Sheard will get him IF
>   He Don't Watch Out.[13]

In fact, Sheard was attempting to apply contemporary business practices to the patronage-ridden sanitation department. Theoretically as impartial professionals, he and his contemporaries like Dr. Thomas Whitelaw, Edmonton's Medical Health Officer,[14] should not have had to resort to verbal or physical violence to assure public or political acceptance of their management decisions, but within the municipal sphere modern bureaucracy was just beginning to emerge.

For both these men, the prewar years brought conflict and co-operation with a variety of reform interests. In Toronto, prohibition, the social gospel, women's rights, juvenile delinquency, and crusades against contaminated milk and infant mortality were the focal point for social reformers' activities. Structural reformers preferred to alter urban government and discuss municipal ownership of utilities and transportation companies. And a new group of professional reformers, including doctors, sanitary engineers, and social workers, united to demand the introduction of modern management techniques. In 1904, Vancouver's city council voted to appoint a medical officer who would have complete charge of the Department and its staff because the "principle of professional management under responsible directorship, widely accepted in the world of business, was becoming acceptable in city government as well."[15] Professional management meant scientific analysis of activities, a hierarchical and centralized bureaucracy, and the creation of a divisional structure. By 1913, Vancouver had a staff of 35 in ten divisions for a population of over 100,000.[16]

Although Sheard was aware of these currents of change, he did not introduce such innovations. Instead, he directed seventy sanitary inspectors, one public health nurse, a part-time city analyst, and the staff of the Isolation Hospital, in a small health department with a tightly controlled budget. As a wealthy taxpayer himself, he was trying to protect the city's

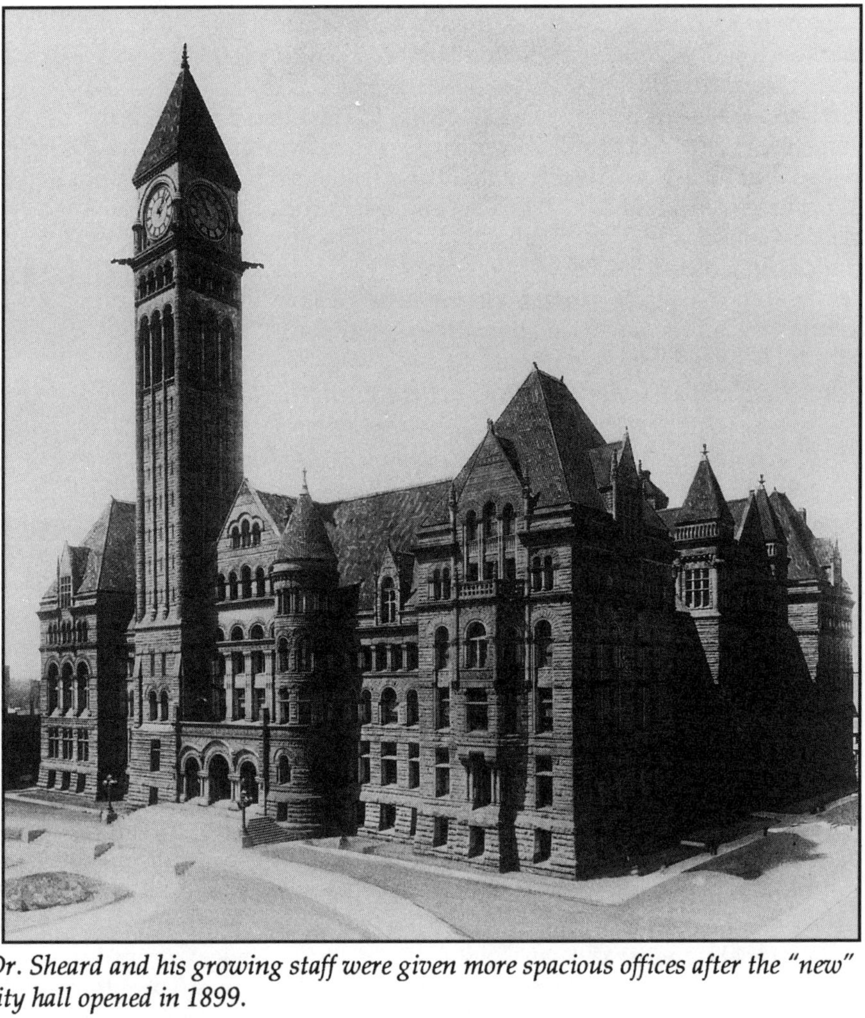

Dr. Sheard and his growing staff were given more spacious offices after the "new" city hall opened in 1899.

reputation for economy and efficiency. Although Toronto went into a recession in the winter of 1907-08, buoyant optimism characterized the city during the decade as the population expanded from 208,040 in 1901 to 376,538 in 1911. For many reformers, the medical officer's caution and limited spending were an affront in light of the problems which they saw in city streets.

By 1910, Sheard was tired of the constant criticism directed at his Department. The final straw was a typhoid epidemic which erupted in February. After introducing chlorination to stop the outbreak, Sheard resigned in March. As the outbreak continued, his departure was short-lived, but by September he had the epidemic under control and was able to retire again. In his letter of resignation, he noted that it was time for a "new broom" who "has the qualifications, mental and physical vigour, independence and universal knowledge, as will place him beyond all possible influences which constantly tend to effect their desires through a Municipal officer in Toronto."[17] This call for an independent expert administrator marked the transition from gifted amateur health activists to professional health bureaucrats.

During his seventeen years in office, Sheard had expanded the inspection staff, convinced ratepayers to support a referendum favouring a trunk sewer, and initiated ties with fellow professionals. He had not responded to reformers' demands that the Department introduce milk depots, school medical inspection, and other personal health services, such as well baby clinics. As a result, Toronto lagged behind cities like Vancouver and Providence, Rhode Island, which had restructured their systems in preparation for moving into a new field — health education.

The Modern Conception of Public Health: The Hastings Years

On October 1, 1910, the headline in the *Toronto World* read "Dr. Hastings The Man So Profession Declares." A fifty-two year old obstetrician, Charles Hastings was on the verge of retiring to British Columbia when the medical officership became available. His interest in community health was longstanding. In 1885, after he graduated from Victoria University, he assisted Canniff as a vaccinator during the smallpox epidemic that year. When he returned from post-graduate study in London, Dublin and Edinburgh and set up practice as an obstetrician, his clientele included citizens from all social ranks. Gordon Sinclair was one of the babies that he delivered in working class Cabbagetown.[18]

A staunch Presbyterian, Hastings was also a social activist. In 1908, he became deeply involved in the Canadian Medical Association's milk committee, and in 1910, he was a founding member of the Canadian Public Health Association, whose structure, rationale and membership were similar to its American counterpart. Through these activities, he developed a network of contacts with Canadian, British and American public health professionals and was keen to introduce their services or programs to Toronto. His success in developing public health work in Toronto resulted in his election as president of the American Public Health Association in 1918. In his presidential address, Hastings philosophized on the meaning of democracy and informed his listeners that:

> Every nation that permits people to remain under the fetters of preventable disease, and permits social conditions to exist that make it impossible for them to be properly fed, clothed and housed, so as to maintain a high degree of resistance and physical fitness, and that endorses a wage that does not afford sufficient revenue for the home, a revenue that will make possible the development of a sound mind and body, is trampling a primary principle of democracy under its feet.[19]

This statement of his deepest beliefs showed him to be a Victorian meliorist like his predecessors. His interest in personal health services, however, demonstrated his "modern conception of public health" and made him a suitable candidate in the eyes of Toronto's reform groups. Such views appealed to his medical colleagues and they also praised him for having "good sound judgment, an unusual amount of common sense and excellent executive ability." All of these factors convinced the council to appoint him.

Hastings' enthusiasm and the city's good economic position until the depression from 1913-15, transformed the Health Department into a modern bureaucracy. As soon as he took office, the "new broom" started to expand his staff and introduce scientific management practices. By 1915, he had established fifteen divisions, all of which reported to him. By subdividing inspection and nursing duties this way, each staff member had a specific task that could be monitored to ensure efficiency and cost effectiveness. A new division which collected vital statistics gave Hastings the factual foundation for his political lobbying. And to combat the poverty which he saw as a root cause of ill-health, the new medical officer created a Division of Public Service in 1914.

Shortly after he took office, Hastings gained two advantages which his predecessors lacked: legal backing for his position and permanent tenure during "good behaviour" and residency. In fact, the provincial Public Health Act of 1912 not only renamed him as the Medical Officer of Health, but more importantly, made him both the chief executive officer of the local board of health and the administrative head of his department. The structure of the local board of health was also altered, and its status was changed from being a council committee to being a corporation. Each of these changes reflected the Whitney government's recognition of the problems which previous boards and health officers had faced, and its commitment to modernizing public organizations.[20]

Like many progressive reformers, Hastings believed that experts should direct municipal services with little interference from local politicians, and the provincial legislation gave him more freedom than any of his predecessors. He was also fortunate that two reform mayors, Horatio Hocken and

Jimmy Simpson, shared his views and supported his efforts during the first decade of his administration. In contrast to the eight man board which had overseen his predecessors, Hastings's board was small, consisting of three resident ratepayers and the mayor *ex officio*. Consequently, he had to undertake more publicity of his Department's activities among both the council members and the public.

In 1915, the Bureau of Municipal Research assessed his efforts to verify Hastings' oft-repeated comment that "public health spending is an investment not an expenditure." The Bureau's researchers were impressed with the Department's performance during its initial expansion phase and stated that taxpayers were getting value for their dollars. In administrative terms, the survey team thought there was room for improvement. The Bureau recommended the appointment of an assistant for the medical officer, simplifying the number of divisions, improving accounting systems, and hiring clerical assistance to relieve the nurses and inspectors of some record-keeping duties.[21] This study epitomized modern evaluation techniques and was intended to forestall political criticism of further expansion.

By 1920, Toronto's Health Department was considered such a model administration that the Rockefeller Foundation sent international students to study at the University of Toronto so they would be eligible to do field work with the city department. Five years later Hastings was invited to join the American Public Health Association's Committee on Administrative Practice, a new group established to develop evaluation criteria for city health services.[22] Although Toronto was never formally evaluated by the APHA, the Local Appraisal form was used for self-evaluation by the

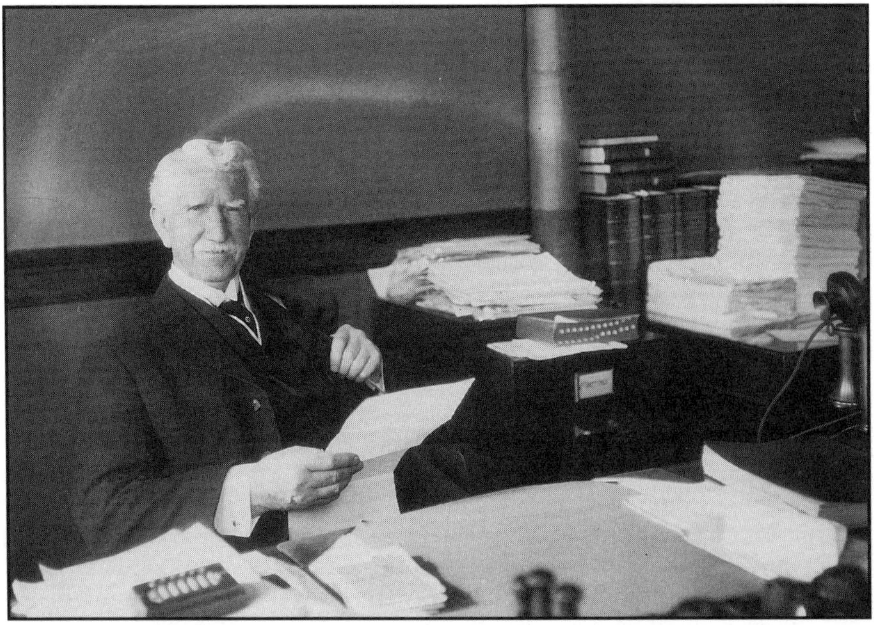

Dr. Charles Hastings, MOH, 1910-1929.

Department's divisions during the 1930s. Such efforts served a dual purpose: they measured the city's performance against impartial criteria and they reminded the aldermen and residents of the excellence of the services they received.

By the 1920s, the city's financial status had been eroded by wartime inflation and further undercut by the post-war depression. Retrenchment was the order of the day. In 1923 the Board of Control pointedly reminded the local board of health and the medical officer that it had the final say in authorizing spending for conference attendance. To Hastings, this was a threat to his staff's professional development, and he brusquely told the Board of Control that the provincial Public Health Act gave him the authority to fund his staff on these excursions. Three years later a more serious challenge came from Alderman John Winnett, who moved a motion in the local board of health to request the medical officer to present reports detailing proposed policy changes to the board, before they were published in the city's newspapers.[23] In the critical climate of the 1920s, the tactics which had fuelled the demand for the expansion of city health services prior to 1914, were evidently no longer acceptable.

In addition, as the largest health department in the country, employing 379 staff by 1920, Toronto was frequently raided by other municipalities, the federal and provincial governments, educational institutions, and voluntary groups looking for senior staff. Dr. Grant Fleming, Hastings' second deputy medical officer became the director of the Montreal Anti-Tuberculosis and General Health League in 1923, while his successor, Dr. H.C. Cruikshank left to join the Ontario Health Department in 1926. As early as 1919, Hastings reported to the board of health that twenty-eight of the Department's nurses had left to take administrative positions elsewhere in Canada and in 1923, two senior district supervisors, Mary Millman and Florence Emory, joined the new Department of Public Health Nursing at the University of Toronto. The turnover meant that younger district nurses and inspectors were able to see promotion possibilities if they fulfilled the necessary educational requirements and gained experience in their present positions.

Hastings' ability to replace large numbers of staff lost during the decade was hampered, however, by new employment criteria and salary schedules drawn up between 1924 and 1927. In 1926, the local board of health tried to clarify the Health Department's anomalous status within the city bureaucracy by asking the city solicitor if the board had the "absolute power" to appoint staff. The city's lawyer replied that the Public Health Act permitted the board to recommend further appointments but that the ultimate decision rested with the city council.[24] As a result, the Health Department had to conform to the city's requirement that anyone seeking employment be a veteran or a resident.

During the 1920s as well, the reform coalition that had originated with Canniff and supported many of Hastings' projects and services disintegrated. For the prohibitionists, the war had been disillusioning. For the social gospellers, concern about the effect of church union overrode interest in secular reform. But the most important change was the ideological shift from the worldview of the Victorian meliorists, who believed that people were perfectible, to the perspective of twentieth century behavioural scientists, who argued that "conversion" was not the goal of health education efforts.[25] The latter succeeded in excluding lay members from the American Public Health Association in 1922 and from the Canadian Public Health Association in 1928. Such changes signalled the increasing dominance of professionalism.

Within the Health Department, the conflict between these two perceptions was played out in the Social Welfare Division. Originally created in 1921 to provide assistance for the unemployed during the post-war recession, the new division quickly became a bridgehead for the introduction of American social work techniques and procedures. The concept of "distancing" or professional detachment did not encourage participation in community programs to address poverty and other systemic problems.[26] Instead, it stressed the importance of the individual. By 1929, Hastings was stating that public health workers found people in distress and referred them to social workers, whose professional training enabled them to make a "social diagnosis" and deal with the client's needs.[27] The complete split between health and welfare work occurred two years after Hastings' retirement when a separate municipal Department of Public Welfare was established.

The 1920s also witnessed a change in professional preparation for the medical officership. In contrast to Canniff, Allen, Sheard and Hastings, each of whom developed his administrative skills after being appointed, subsequent medical officers had an opportunity to take further training. The University of Toronto offered a diploma in public health beginning in 1904, but the first one was not started until 1912 because of lack of interest and lack of teaching staff.[28] The 1912 Public Health Act made a diploma in public health a prerequisite for employment, and since then, all of Toronto's medical officers have completed the qualification. Hastings's successor, Gordon Jackson, received his diploma in 1922 while Leon Pequegnat won his in 1926, A.R.J. Boyd took his in 1936, and G.W.O. Moss completed his in 1948.

This type of advanced training for professionals fulfilled Sheard's demand for specialization. In the 1920s, students taking the course studied bacteriology, general hygiene, immunology, sanitary engineering and chemistry, public health organization, legislation and vital statistics, and the history of preventive medicine and epidemiology. They also visited baby clinics, the Island Filtration Plant, venereal disease clinics, and other health care activities which the Department supervised.[29] For the graduates of this program, working in a health department was a career decision not the vocation that it had been for the early health officers. As impartial experts, the mid-twentieth century public health staff were professional administrators not fervent reformers.

Public attitudes also changed. During the 1910s, there was little opposition to home visits by the public health nurses or the inspectors. After the war such intervention and activities, like smallpox vaccination, were sometimes criticized as representing "Kaiserism." In 1919, conflict over the imposition of compulsory vaccination revealed the growing cleavage between the medical officer and the public. By 1927, Hastings was compelled to admit that:

> No health department can force the citizens to use this pure water or safe milk, nor, can they force them to subsist on a properly balanced diet, although every item of it be inspected before its sale. Only the individual can do this and the part of the Department of Health is to teach him what to drink, what to eat, how to arrange his life to secure the maximum of efficiency together with the maximum of health.[30]

Indeed, he and his growing staff of district medical officers, dentists, dental hygienists, and public health nurses had concluded that "they have not only to instruct the public but also to unteach many erroneous ideas that have been prevalent for many years."[31]

Between 1910 and his retirement in 1929, Hastings modernized Toronto's Health Department, persuaded politicians to increase its budget from approximately \$85,000 to nearly \$900,000 and to increase its staff from 70 to nearly 500. His publicity efforts in Canada and the United States brought visitors from around the world to see his system in operation. In 1924, an admiring Toronto alderman, Frank Denton, wrote an article entitled "Toronto Leads the World in Public Health Service." After explaining the services which the Department provided to the *Star Weekly*'s readers, Denton noted that Hastings did not think that his administration had reached "perfection" and that "he is constantly on the war-path, visiting his field forces, not merely sitting at his desk, seeking for improvement and enlargement of its scope."[32] Although he had modernized the Department's administrative structure and increased its staff, Hastings' system had flaws that would become apparent in the decades which followed. His genial personality and strong vision stimulated his young, energetic staff, and influenced politicians and the public. But how would the Department function without such a committed and dynamic leader at the helm during the Great Depression?

Conclusion

Between 1883 and 1929, Toronto's first four health officers laid the foundation for a modern health department. As gifted amateurs who learned to administer a growing staff while on the job, they were able to innovate by choosing to emulate the British or American model which seemed most appropriate to Toronto's needs. As Victorian social reformers, they believed strongly in the perfectibility of human beings, and in their duty as experts to contribute to social change. This active conception of their role led them to participate in the reform movements of their day, and to lobby politicians and citizens for support for their projects.

For the first forty years of the Department's existence, the vision which the health officers propounded was shared by supportive colleagues, other reformers, and certain mayors and councils. After 1920, however, new factors entered the equation. Economic restraint in the post-war world limited Hastings' ability to hire additional staff and to introduce new programs. The professionalization of public health training and the hierarchical nature of the divisional structure meant that the medical officer could no longer practice the type of personal management that Canniff and Sheard had offered. But the most significant change was the transition from social activism to professional detachment. Subordinating the reform ethos to bureaucratic imperatives signalled the end of the Department's dynamic growth phase, and marked the transition from the medical health officer's active leadership in the public health crusade to a focus on professional development and expert administration.

Chapter Two

Professionalizing Public Health: The Medical Bureaucrats

> With the discovery of the germ origin of disease came a change in the status of organized Public Health. The revelations of Pasteur and the many famous workers who have since followed, have raised Public Health administrators from the position of glorified broom squads to that of intensive scientific investigators.[1]

When Gordon Jackson made this comment to his colleagues at Toronto's Academy of Medicine, he was describing his generation's intellectual justification for the shift from the reform ethos of the pioneer medical officers to the professional orientation of their successors. The process of professionalization began while Jackson and his successors were studying medicine and continued during their preparation for the diploma in public health. In keeping with widely accepted views, the latter course inculcated the belief that civil servants should be impartial, neutral administrators not social activists. The bureaucratization of the medical officership had many expected and unexpected consequences for the development of public health services in Toronto as consensus-building among medical colleagues and politicians replaced active participation in reform crusades.

Factors beyond the jurisdiction of the city's medical officers also affected the public perception of their role. During the 1930s as medical science became the source of new knowledge and new treatment for many age-old scourges, medical officers in Britain, the United States and Canada had to redefine their role by proclaiming that preventive activity was an important link between medical researchers and the public. As one component in the health care spectrum, public health services competed with hospitals and practitioners for scarce financial resources. Since most preventive programs focused on long-term change, they lacked the immediacy of curative services and thus did not attract great public attention. As a result, senior administrators lost the public profile that their predecessors had used as an effective publicity tool.

The financial limitations of the Great Depression and World War II compounded the situation. During the 1930s, Toronto's mayors and councils balanced the city's budget by slashing annual appropriations and imposing pay cuts on civic employees. In spite of pressure from a variety of women's groups and charitable organizations, the Health Department was unable to introduce new services and was hard pressed to maintain existing ones. A decade of cutbacks led to a demand for evaluation of the Department's performance and in 1943, the Ontario Health Department's survey team reported that the city's Health Department was mired in the past.

The administrative changes which the Phair committee proposed did not lead to a significant renewal of the Department's activism because the city was more interested in creating a metropolitan government than in updating its Health Department. Indeed, a further study of the Department's work, conducted as part of the civic survey of 1957 by J.D. Woods and Gordon Limited, also suggested modernizing its administrative practices and decentralizing most of its staff. Although both these reports reflected contemporary views of administrative priorities, neither was fully implemented because each one threatened the Department's strongly-entrenched traditions and work culture, and prior to the late 1960s, there was little public demand for change.

During the 1950s, the public health movement itself was seeking a new focus. What issues should be the next field of activity? The elderly? Immigrants? Baby boom children? Adults? In addition to these questions, Canadian public health administrators also queried their place in a national health insurance plan. Was there a role for prevention or would curative medicine dominate federal-provincial cost-sharing? By the mid-1960s, a further factor was added to these concerns: the decline of public respect for "experts." Together all of these trends combined to challenge the traditional approach to public health policy and programs which Toronto's medical officers had been trained to implement. By the early 1970s, change was on the agenda as external forces united to redefine the role of the professional health administrator from medical bureaucrat to community advocate.

Facing Constraints: The Jackson Years, 1929-1951

When he assumed office in June 1929, Dr. Gordon Jackson had an experienced staff, a centralized bureaucracy and a formidable reputation to maintain. The new medical officer had not only completed a diploma in public health but had also worked as a district medical officer, director of communicable diseases and quarantine, and deputy medical officer. For Jackson and his successors, this type of career development differentiated them from their colleagues who practiced curative medicine. During the 1920s, the changes in Canadian medical education, which Abraham Flexner's 1910 report on medical schools in the United States and Canada had set in motion, were completed. Students now had five years of medical school followed by an internship. If the individual wanted to specialize, he or she had to complete further study before writing the Royal College of Physicians and Surgeons fellowship examinations. Although most medical schools offered courses in preventive medicine in the fifth year, few chose to make this field their life's work, and by 1946 the Canadian Public Health Association was searching for ways to recruit new blood into the field.

In the United States, public health practitioners had studied the educational options in their field during World War I. Charles Chapin, Providence's health officer from 1888 to 1932, conducted a study for the American Medical Association and recommended that public health institutes be set up to train expert administrators. In 1916, Johns Hopkins created the first Rockefeller Foundation funded school of hygiene on the continent.[2] The University of Toronto applied to the Foundation for support and in 1924 received a grant that enabled it to open its School of Hygiene three years later. Students from the School did field work with Toronto's Health Department, and its senior staff usually taught courses in health administration.[3] Since the Canadian Public Health Association also had its head office in the School of Hygiene until 1963, Toronto's Health Department staff served that organization as well. This mutually beneficial arrangement meant that the city was closely tied to the changing emphasis in public health work, and participated in a variety of research projects as the public health movement adopted the medical research model.

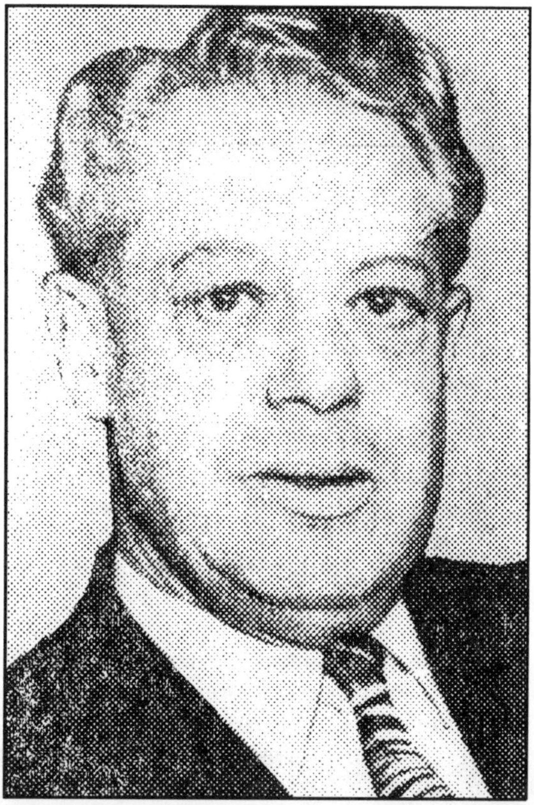

Dr. Gordon Park Jackson, MOH, 1929-51.

In both Canada and the United States, the 1920s were a decade in which many doctors began to challenge local health departments' maternal and child health services. Toronto's attempts to introduce diphtheria toxoid and pre-school medical inspection foundered, as local physicians objected to this infringement on their practices. When the Depression began in 1929, Jackson and his staff bore the brunt of such opposition. In 1930, the new medical officer addressed his colleagues at a symposium on State Medicine held by Toronto's Academy of Medicine. He reminded his audience of the services which his staff provided to them and to the public, and pointed out that his doctors and nurses shared the same professional culture and ethics as they did. Jackson called for more understanding between the two groups, and appeared to be urging his listeners to see preventive work as one part of the spectrum of health services, rather than as a competitor.[4] The medical officer's refusal to allow Toronto doctors to participate in a city-run diphtheria toxoid campaign in 1931 on legal grounds, however, jaundiced the physicians, and relations were cool except during polio epidemics when the emergency forced them to co-operate.

Throughout the 1930s, Jackson also faced opposition from the mayor, the Board of Control and some voluntary groups. In 1931, a Toronto woman died after her apartment was fumigated, and the mayor and Board of Control were perturbed when a coroner's inquest criticized the medical officer and his fumigation staff for dereliction of duty. In fact, the province had just introduced new regulations governing the procedure, and the city was trying to prepare a by-law to license fumigators when the tragedy occurred.

The following year, the *Toronto Star* unleashed a six month conflict within the Department by publicizing the death of Lillian and Matthew Kenny's baby. The Kennys charged that a public health nurse, Mary Bullick, had ignored their request for medical assistance for their dying child. When Jackson first investigated the controversy, he refused to believe that his staff were "heartless" and tried to convince the Board of Control that demoting Bullick was sufficient. The politicians, however, had been trying to bring the Health Department to heel since the 1920s, and this incident gave them their chance. In September Jackson fired Bullick, in spite of strong support for her from her colleagues in the Department, nursing groups in the province, and the Local Council of Women. When Bullick started a suit for wrongful dismissal, she was assisted by Eunice Dyke, the Director of Public Health Nursing since 1914. Dyke held a staff meeting to discuss the problem, collected donations for her nurse's legal fees, and went with Bullick to see the lawyer who was preparing her case. When she reported her action to the medical officer, he fired her.

As one of Hastings' original appointees and most innovative staff members, Dyke had an international reputation in her own right. Her expertise may well have posed a threat to Jackson's control of the staff, and he took the opportunity of her "disloyalty" to dismiss her. When the case reached the court, Bullick won. The Board of Control was inundated with petitions calling for the nurses' reinstatement and the council split on the issue. Neither the Controllers nor the medical officer were prepared to back down. Nevertheless, Mayor William Stewart was sufficiently upset by the incident, that when Jackson delivered a report on the matter to the Board of Control in December 1932, the mayor told him "Go back to your office, and step on it." As the *Canada Lancet* reported to its medical readers, the comment "was a piece of gratuitous impertinence."[5]

Within the Department the Dyke-Bullick fiasco strained the relationship between the nurses and district physicians to the point that Jackson had to order the nurses to speak to their medical colleagues. Over time the controversy died down, but one long-term consequence was further centralization of control in the medical officer. From 1932 onward, all correspondence had to be vetted by his office, and all requests for information by the press had to be relayed to his staff for a reply. By the 1960s, this administrative procedure was frustrating younger staff, but in the 1930s, a more deferential climate prevailed.

As a non-revenue producing department, the Health Department suffered cutbacks during the Depression. In 1933, Mayor Stewart suggested eliminating the city laboratory as a cost-cutting measure because he was sure that the provincial laboratories could provide the service. Although the transfer was not complete until 1967, appropriations for the Division of Laboratories were consistently cut. So was funding for new services such as high school medical inspection. The city's hiring policies also meant that there was little staff mobility during the decade, and that external candidates were automatically excluded unless they had been born in Toronto or could prove prior residency. And by 1938, the question of collecting fees from patients in the Riverdale Isolation Hospital had become significant. Jackson's careful response to each of these crises demonstrated his political astuteness rather than the reform zeal which had characterized his predecessors.

During World War II, the city began to plan for the future. In 1942, Mayor Frederick Conboy, the former director of Dental Services for the Ontario government, a lecturer in the Faculty of Dentistry, and a former member of the local board of health, proposed a survey of the Health Department and its activities. Arguing that the Department was recognized "all over the continent," Conboy justified his request to council for the funds for the investigation, by stating that the survey would ensure that the Health Department became "the best possible organization." He was supported by Aldermen Hiram McCallum and Robert Saunders, who pointed out that the Department had been underfinanced for years.[6] The council asked Dr. John Phair, Ontario's chief medical officer and the former director of medical services for the city health department, to appoint a survey team. For Phair, this was an opportunity to assess the province's most prestigious health department and to aid it in its postwar reconstruction, by applying the new criteria for municipal health services that the American Public Health Association had developed.[7]

The survey team reported on December 4, 1943. Much of its commentary was a critique of the influence of Charles Hastings. While expressing sympathy for Jackson's problems in exorcising his predecessor's ghost, the Phair Committee challenged the Department to adopt more recent management practices, and to reorganize its administrative structure. In particular, the committee recommended that the medical officer and his deputy realign their duties. They suggested that:

> The responsibility of the Medical Officer of Health should be largely concerned with over-all supervision, formation of policy in collaboration with the Local Board, co-ordination of effort on the part of the Department with other official and non-official agencies concerned with community health. The Deputy Medical Officer might concern himself with aiding the Medical Officer of Health in general departmental administration, with in-service education, health education generally, nutritional service, vital statistics as well as the control of venereal disease.[8]

To remain in the forefront according to the Phair committee, Toronto had to modify its administrative structure, appoint medical experts to head its divisions, and introduce modern planning procedures.

In response to the Phair Committee's *Report,* Jackson and his deputy, Leon Pequegnat, divided the administrative tasks between them. The medical officer had overall responsibility for the Department and took charge of the Sanitation, Food Control and Communicable Disease Control divisions, while the deputy was responsible for overseeing public health nursing, medical services including tuberculosis and venereal disease control, and specific services, like maternal and child health and school medical inspection.[9] This division of duties gave the deputy an chance to develop his administrative skills while his superior was readily available for consultation. Little wonder that administrative change appeared so slow to evolve, since each man continued to follow many of the precedents set by his predecessor. Moreover, the appointment of medically-trained division directors in response to the Phair Committee's recommendations entrenched the medical research model until the early 1970s, when these men retired or died in office.

Jackson's final years in office were marred by further controversy and ill-health. In 1947, he had to fight an attempt to combine the Health Department with the city's Welfare Department. Since he was the medical officer who had insisted on the separation of the health and welfare services in 1931, he was adamant in his opposition to re-unification. He also had to defend his staff during the city's salary reclassification survey. During the war, Toronto began to evaluate its employment practices, and in 1945, the city created a Personnel Department to develop criteria for hiring and promotion. The new department conducted a job classification survey and established salary levels for municipal employees. In 1947, the Department's nursing supervisors were upset to learn that they were not paid as much as the Welfare Department's supervisors, but the medical officer was unable to get their salaries raised. And a lengthy conflict over the appointment of a new director of mental health in 1950–51, led the *Toronto Star* to remark that Jackson was "one of the most discussed non-elected men at the city hall."[10]

When he died of a heart attack in August 1951, Jackson was president-elect of the Ontario Public Health Association, a group founded in 1949–50 in an effort to revitalize public health practice in the province. Membership was open to the public and strong efforts were made to recruit public health inspectors and nurses. Pressure for change was growing among public health workers in Britain and the United States too. The introduction of the National Health Service in 1948 altered the role of British health officers who became involved in home care, services for the elderly, and more general health education activities. In the United States, the American Public Health Association and the American Hospital Association issued a joint statement in 1948, which argued that: "Preventive and curative medicine have reached the stage where they are no longer separable, and it is necessary at the present time to bring them together physically and functionally."[11] For Canadians, the impact of the changing focus of the international

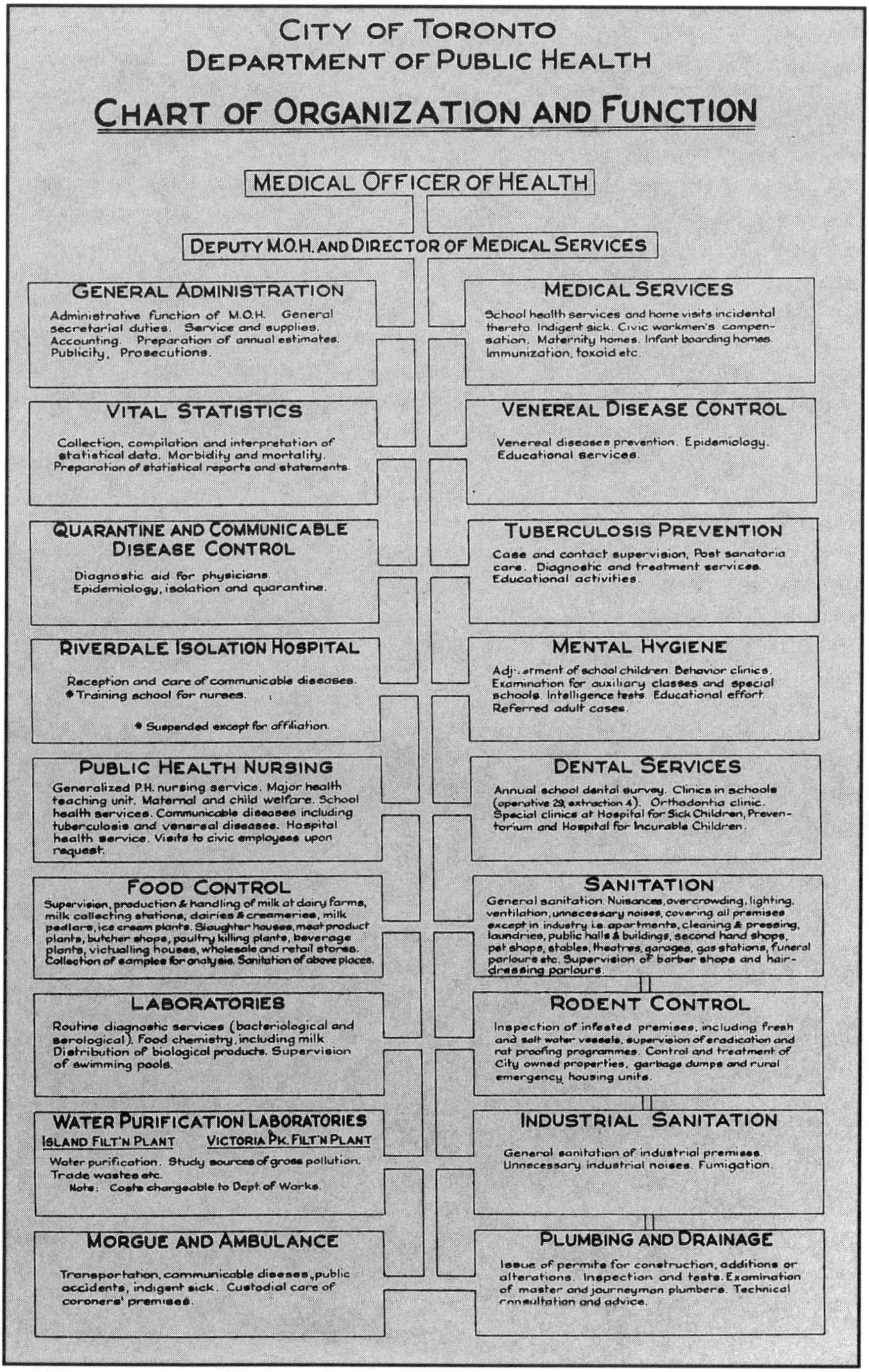

This chart illustrates the range of services which the Health Department offered in 1948.

public health movement was compounded by the slow development of this country's health insurance system. Jackson's successors then had to find a renewed sense of mission and identity.

Redefining the Department's Activities: The Pequegnat Era

Jackson's difficulties with the politicians led Alderman Nathan Phillips to question the automatic appointment of his deputy as the new health officer. A graduate in medicine and public health from the University of Toronto, Pequegnat served from 1924–5 as the eastern organizer for the Canadian Social Hygiene Council, a group dedicated to educating the public about the dangers of venereal disease. In 1926, he joined the Health Department as a district medical officer and was appointed the deputy in 1929. He served an exceptionally long apprenticeship and by the late 1940s, there were strong hints that he did not share Jackson's outlook on many issues. In fact, part of Mayor Saunders' motivation for the 1947 unification attempt may well have been conflict among the senior staff.[12] During the Board of Control's discussion of Pequegnat's appointment, testimonials from the Director of the School of Hygiene, the Registered Nurses' Association of Ontario, the provincial Health Department, the Health League of Canada

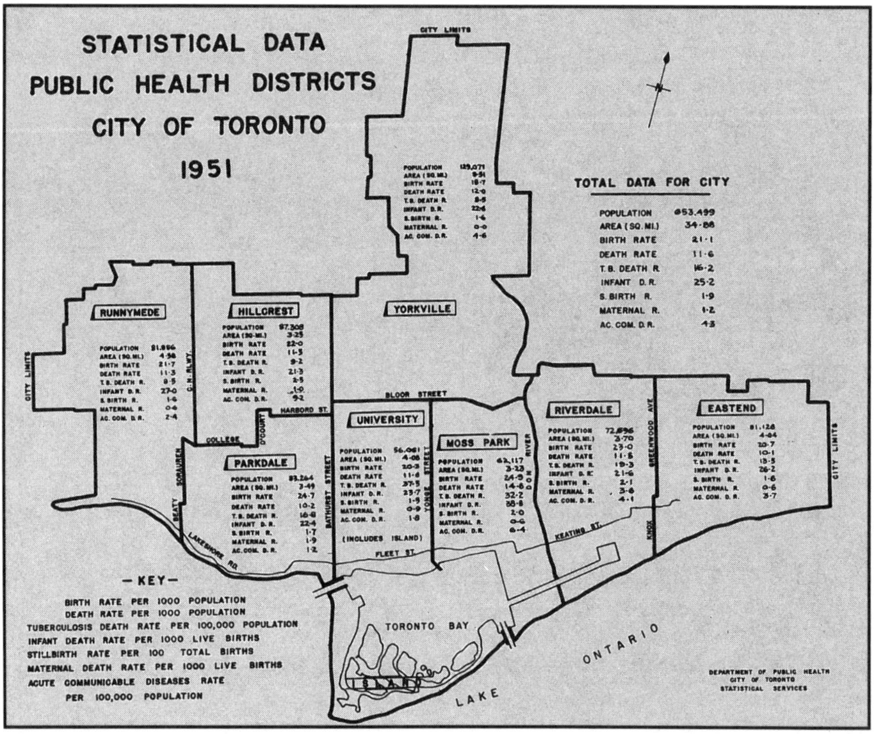

The Department's annual statistical compilation for 1951 reflected the city's health status, including the continuing high death rate from tuberculosis and the beginning of the baby boom.

and the Academy of Medicine were noted. The honours that he had received from the American Medical Association and the Royal College of Physicians and Surgeons of Canada were duly recognized, but the ultimate point in his favour was twenty-two years of dedicated service to the Department.[13] He was appointed by a vote of seventeen to one and served until 1958.

As Jackson's long-serving deputy, Pequegnat had experienced the conflict with the politicians and doctors, which had slowed the Department's adoption of new programs and services during the Depression and war years. When he became the city's medical officer, he expected to be able to expand the Department's services because the economic climate had improved and the federal government had introduced a system of national health grants to fund staff education, pilot projects, and surveys of health care personnel and facilities. In 1949, Toronto's Welfare Council, and the University of Toronto Schools of Hygiene and Nursing, petitioned the local board of health to consider setting up a demonstration area in one of the city's health districts. With the assistance of a national health grant, the Hillcrest District became the testing ground for innovative activities. By creating such a unit within the department, Pequegnat was acknowledging the growing stress on evaluation that was permeating Canadian and American public health practice. Through the 1950s, the Department's demonstration projects to evaluate the effectiveness of pre-school medical inspection, topical stannous fluoride applications for toddlers, skills training for developmentally delayed children, and home care for the elderly were carefully assessed before they were adopted throughout the city.

In his presidential address to the Canadian Public Health Association in 1957, Pequegnat discussed the "changing responsibilities in public health" that he had seen in his thirty years as a medical officer. From his perspective, the greatest change had been from dependence on police powers to control communicable diseases and remove environmental threats, to persuasion and health education. He predicted that his successors would have to deal with the information explosion and its exploitation by commercial interests. He noted the need to complete older services, "and to salvage precious time...for new ventures." To ensure that these were effective, he called for upgraded training for public health inspectors, better salaries and working conditions for staff nurses, and warned about offering new programs without first evaluating the necessity for them.[14] During his brief period in office, many of his efforts were affected by the city's changing ethnic composition and the council's concern with shifting some health duties to the new metropolitan government.

"Improving on Excellence": The Boyd Administration

Breaking with the past, Pequegnat had looked outside Toronto's Health Department for his deputy. In 1951, forty-six year old Dr. A.R.J. Boyd was appointed to the post. Boyd was raised in Saskatchewan, and educated at the University of Saskatchewan (1926), and McGill University Medical School (1931), prior to receiving his diploma in public health. After service in the

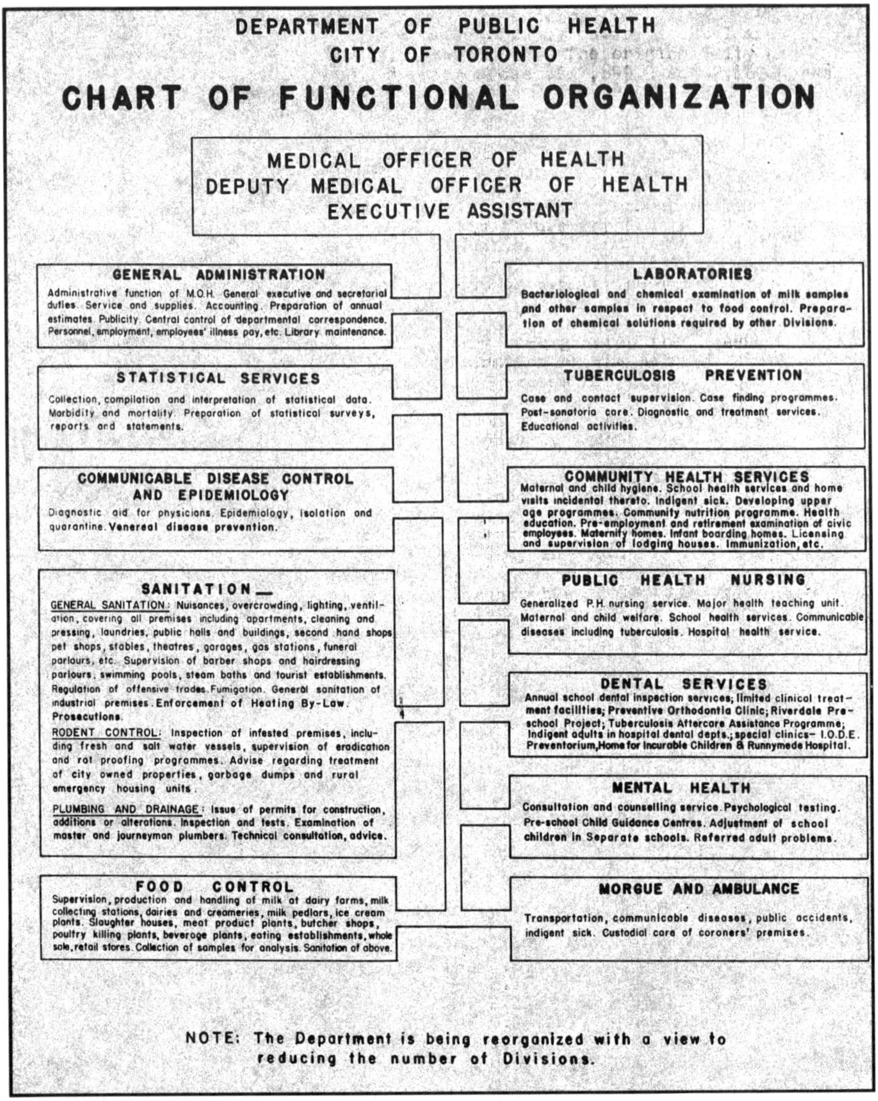

In 1958, the Health Department responded to the previous year's Civic Survey by starting to reorganize.

Royal Canadian Army Medical Corps during the Second World War, he became a medical officer in Vancouver and Kingston and taught public health at Queen's University before joining Toronto's Health Department. Both his military service and his civilian experience had accustomed him to expect deference to his expertise and respect for his position. During his years in office, he was a distant manager and depended on his senior staff to interact with middle management and field workers.

In 1957, he drafted the Department's response to the Civic Survey which

J.D. Woods and Gordon Limited carried out. The survey was undertaken after the formation of Metropolitan Toronto in 1953–4, because as Mayor Phillips noted: "We wanted them to tell us whether we were wasting time and money in duplication or archaic methods."[15] Woods and Gordon recommended that Toronto's Health Department decentralize into four districts with medical officers, inspectors, nurses and support staff, all sharing office space and focusing their work on responding to their area's specific needs. The report suggested that the medical officer and his deputy would remain at city hall and continue to carry out their legal duties, while also devoting more attention to planning for the future. Under this arrangement, all the current division directors would lose their administrative functions, and become expert consultants to the district offices.[16] Boyd's reaction to this proposal was that it did not take the discipline-based work relationships of the department into consideration, and that it was not feasible given Toronto's relatively small population.[17] Was the deputy defending the work culture that had evolved since the Hastings' regime? Did he distrust contemporary management practices? Or was he simply protecting the Department's independence within the municipal structure?

As a result of Boyd's arguments, decentralization was not attempted, but several divisions were amalgamated and the duties of the senior administrators were clarified. Tinkering with the administrative structure in this

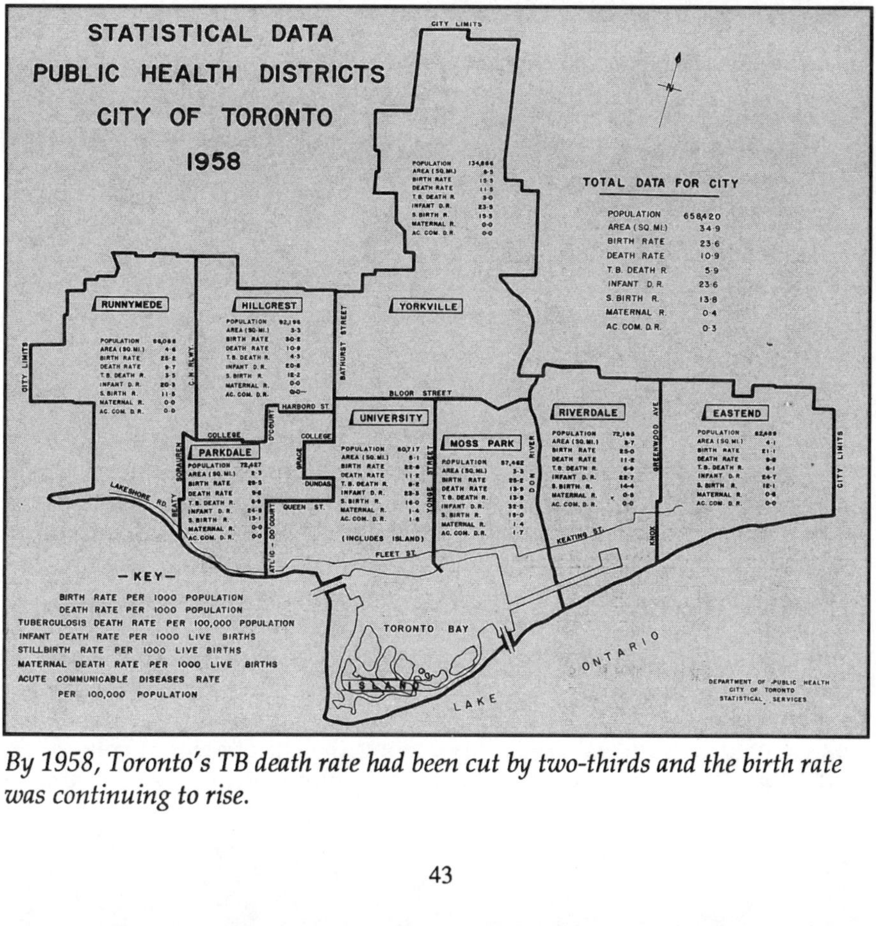

By 1958, Toronto's TB death rate had been cut by two-thirds and the birth rate was continuing to rise.

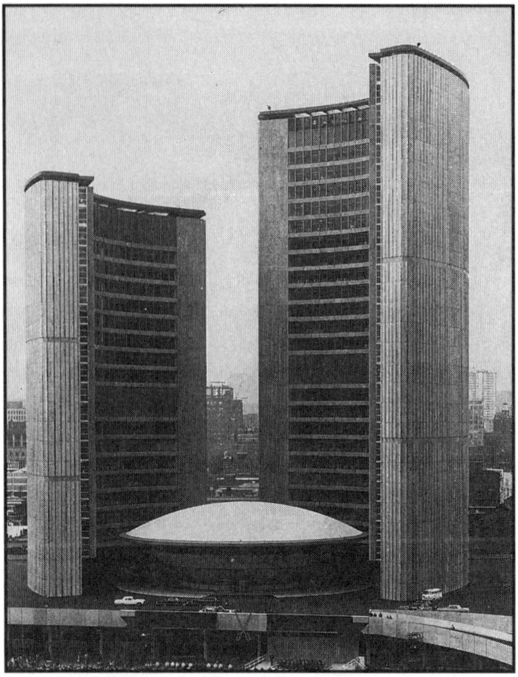

When Toronto's modern city hall opened in September 1965, Health Department staff were relieved to move out of their cramped offices in the "old" city hall and its annex.

fashion did not deal with the underlying problems inherent in such a large centralized bureaucracy. Beyond the Health Department, changes were brewing. By the 1960s, public health in Canada was in a state of crisis. When the Canadian Public Health Association prepared its brief for the Diefenbaker government's Royal Commission on Health Services in Canada, it opened by arguing for a new definition of health as a positive state of existence, "rather than accepting the negative concept that health is the absence of disease and that health services are synonymous with sickness and treatment services." The committee members who wrote the submission were reacting to thirty years of marginalization. Until the end of the 1920s, preventive medicine and public health had captured public attention, but since the late 1930s advances in surgery and drug treatment had undercut interest in prevention.[18] Public health personnel had suffered a corresponding loss of status, and the CPHA committee wanted the Hall Commission to recommend the creation of a career public service in the discipline. As the Association's own committee on recruitment argued, health departments would only be able to attract staff by "having the respect of other health services, providing interesting work and adequate remuneration."[19]

For Toronto, as for many other urban health departments, staffing remained a problem due to lack of funds and qualified personnel. In 1946, the Canadian Public Health Association had appointed its first committee on salaries and qualifications, to plan for the postwar era. The nation's rapid growth during the 1950s meant that the committee had to revise its standards constantly. By 1965, when Boyd was directing the committee, the criteria for the medical officership had been redefined to require either a diploma or degree in public health, certification from the Royal College of Physicians and Surgeons, and ten years of administrative experience prior to appointment.[20] In large measure, raising standards this way was intended to enhance medical officers' credibility among their professional colleagues. Their efforts were in vain because the Hall Commission did not recommend

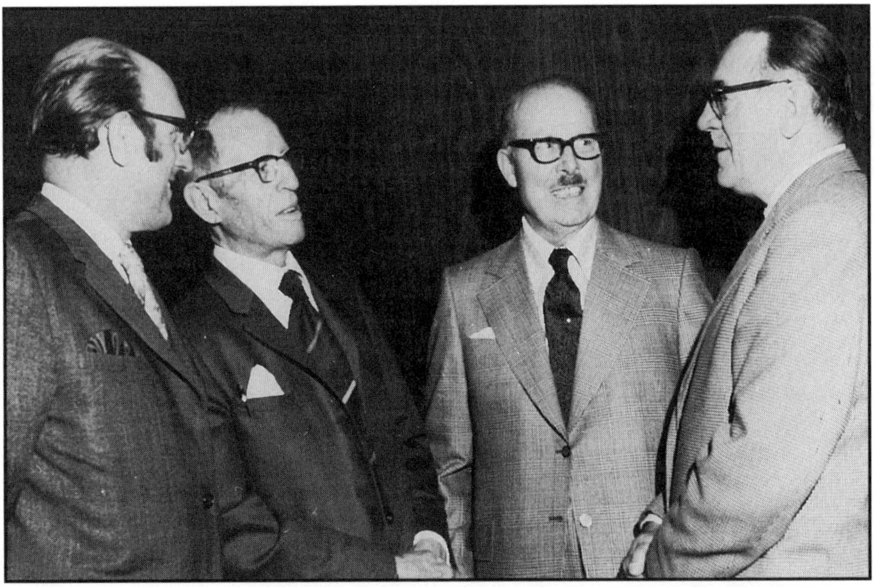

At Dr. A.R.J. Boyd's retirement dinner in 1972, both his predecessor and his successor joined Mayor William Dennison in honouring him. From left to right: Dr. George W.O. Moss, MOH, 1972-1981, Dr. Leon Pequegnat, MOH, 1951-58, the mayor, and Dr. Boyd, MOH, 1958-72.

a health insurance system which balanced curative and preventive activities and funding.

When he became the medical officer in 1958, Boyd faced a decade of strenuous public opposition to all forms of authority. Postwar affluence had produced a generation of youthful critics who attacked medical experts and all types of hierarchical organizations. For an individual of Boyd's background and temperament, the criticism that he received from all sides during the 1960s was galling. Beginning with conflict over the municipal abattoir in 1958, the quality of the Department's meat inspection staff in 1962, the slowness of its involvement in birth control clinics in 1965, and ending with the hepatitis controversy of 1968, Toronto's medical officer found himself under attack by politicians, women's groups and the press, for what they saw as his stodgy approach to current problems.

Early in the summer of 1968, the Department's inspectors discovered cases of hepatitis among the hippies living in Yorkville. With the approval of the medical officer, the district inspectors attempted to keep the situation calm by increasing their visits and using quiet diplomacy to ensure that potential disease victims were tested for the disease at nearby hospitals. In early August, Controller Margaret Campbell and several reporters broke the story, and a week later the provincial Health Department took over because of loud public criticism of Toronto's "lax" disease control efforts. The incident demonstrated the Department's vulnerability to publicity-seeking politicians and the differing perceptions of its statutory responsibilities.

In an interview with the *Toronto Star* in 1968, Boyd explained his reaction to the "epidemic" and stated: "When I came to Toronto, I knew I was joining a department with an excellent reputation. I'm proud of the department and its staff. I hope we have progressed, but it's very hard to improve on excellence."[21] What he failed to see was that the Department could no longer rely on its traditional approach to social and environmental health issues. Instead, both the medical officer and his older staff had to recognize the applicability to Toronto of the American Public Health Association's 1963 policy statement, that "the nature and scope of public health practice are not static, but must change with the needs and desires of the people and with progress in science and technology," because "public health planning is one phase of social planning."[22]

In 1971, the city council asked each department to "set out for public consideration a clear statement of [its] goals, objectives and priorities." Boyd defined the Department's mission as being "to promote and protect health and prevent or control disease."[23] This positive conception of health work was proposed by the World Health Organization and represented the next frontier in the public health crusade. Translating this rhetoric into policy and programs, however, challenged the status quo. When he retired in 1972, Boyd left his successor, Dr. George W.O. Moss, to cope with the changing political climate.

Challenge and Change: The Moss Years

Toronto born and educated, Moss had served with the Royal Canadian Army Medical Corps during the Second World War. After a brief period in private practice convinced him that he could do "more for more people" as a public health administrator, Moss accepted a provincial bursary to study for his diploma in public health at the School of Hygiene. Since the school had been accredited two years earlier by the American Public Health Association's committee on public health education, its training program was modelled on the APHA "Big Six" — control of communicable disease, epidemiology, maternal and child health, vital statistics, laboratories and health education. After a year of service in a rural health unit to fulfil the terms of his contract with the Ontario Health Department, Moss joined the Connaught Laboratories and was cross-appointed to the East York-Leaside Health Unit, where he supervised clinical trials of the polio vaccine. His interest in epidemiology and his initial professional experience conditioned him to believe that co-ordinating joint research projects with colleagues from the School of Hygiene and the University of Toronto Medical Faculty was a key aspect of his job.[24]

Through committee work for the Canadian Public Health Association, Moss was well acquainted with leading public health administrators, including Boyd, who asked him to join Toronto's Department in 1958.[25] As the Association's Honorary Secretary, he also participated in the early efforts to redefine the role of the Canadian Public Health Association. In 1967–68, the organization created a commission to review "the Association's present and future role and to...study its aims, objectives, structure, organization and operations." The following year, the commission suggested numerous changes, the most important of which was opening membership to the general public.[26]

Through the 1970s, the Canadian Public Health Association and its journal continued to question long-standing practices. Should the Associa-

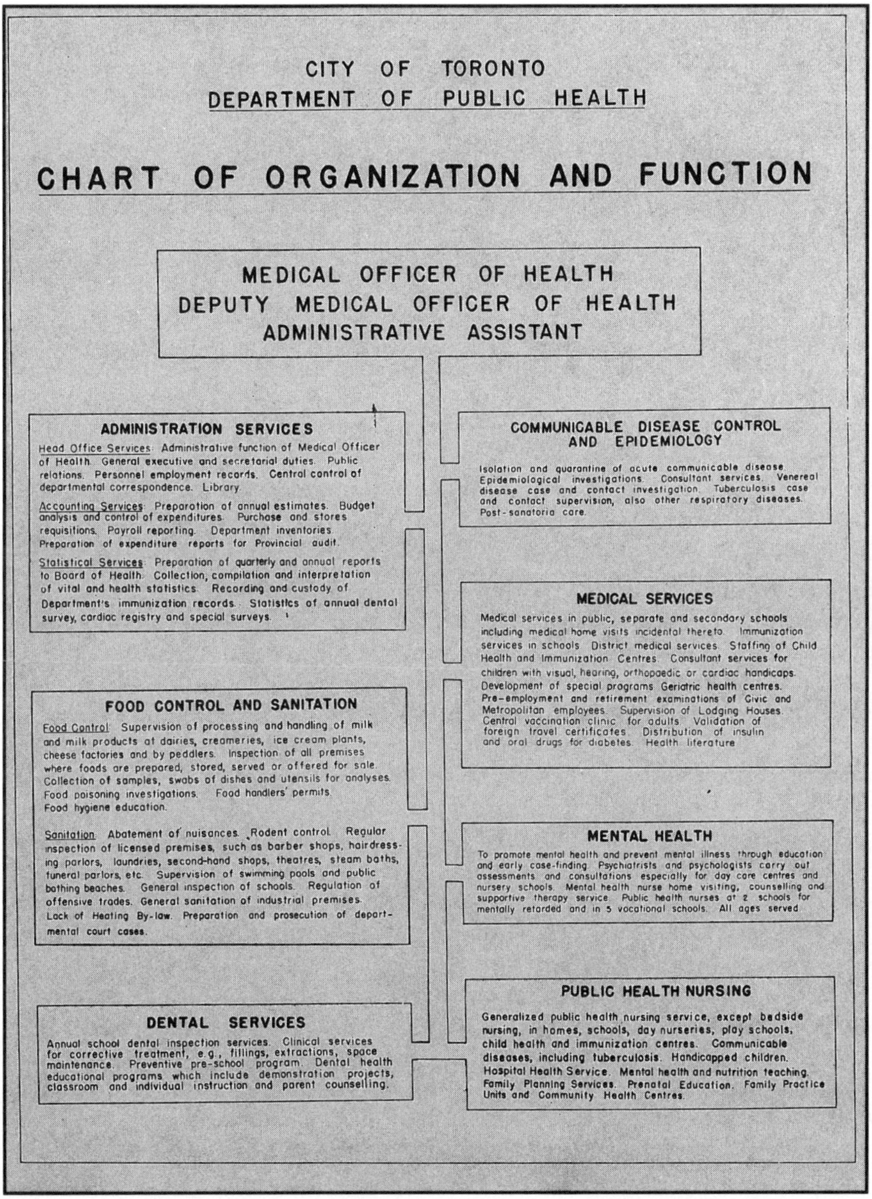

By 1972, the Department's administrative structure had been simplified.

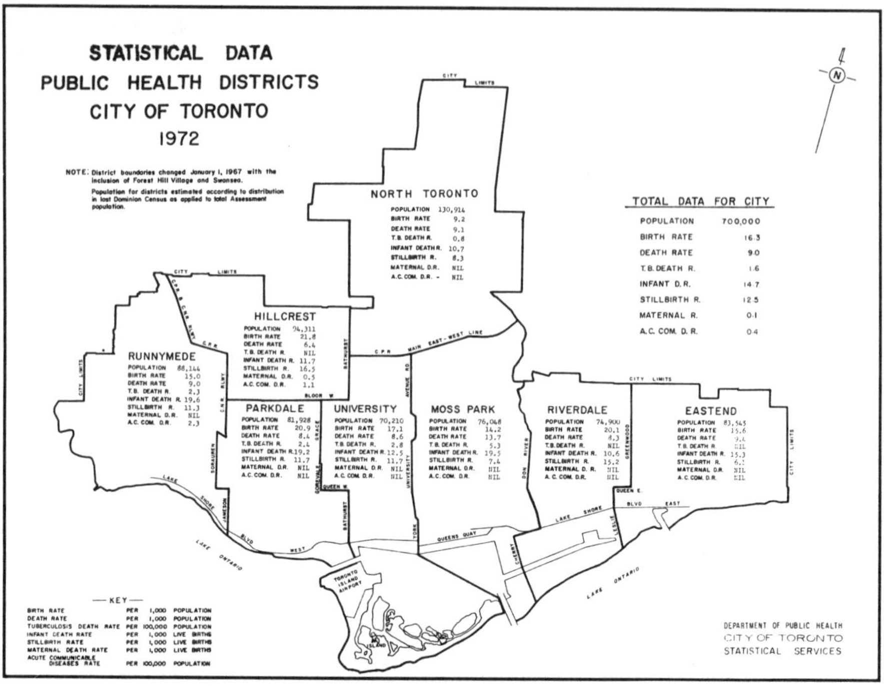

By 1972, Toronto's birth rate had fallen and its death rate from TB and other communicable diseases was negligible.

tion, for example, change its name to the Community Health Association in an effort to overcome the stigma attached to the term "public health"? Was there a role for local health officers, or should Canadian office holders be eliminated as British ones were in 1974? What type of education should be offered? Were the revisions to the School of Hygiene program which added courses in health administration to the curriculum in 1964, sufficient to prepare medical officers for the pressures they would face? Or should public health theory and practice be integrated into the medical curriculum? Between 1973 and 1975, the University of Toronto amalgamated the School of Hygiene with the Faculty of Medicine, and made community medicine part of every student's training. Would this solve the split between curative and preventive experts, or should Health Department employees be drawn from the growing ranks of health educators and community workers? All of these issues arose as a result of the turmoil of the 1960s, the continuing shortage of public health professionals and an attempt to reinvigorate the public health crusade.

In addition to these challenges, the very existence of Toronto's local board of health and its Health Department was threatened during the 1960s and 1970s. In 1967, the Robarts government recommended the amalgamation of all municipal health departments. To encourage the various municipalities to surrender their independence, provincial administrators offered to fund 75% of the costs of the new unit, just as they financed the operation of health units elsewhere in Ontario. When Toronto and the surrounding boroughs turned the offer down, they were restricted to 25% financing.

The introduction of the Ontario Health Insurance Plan in 1972, prompted the Minister of Health, Dr. R.P. Potter, to make another effort to end local autonomy. Potter proposed creating District Councils of Health to undertake long-range planning and co-ordination of services; eventually these groups would supersede local boards and their departments.[27] Once again this attempt at centralization and rationalization was rejected in favour of local direction of health programs. But the province's efforts to rationalize health care and its costs were not over, and in 1974, the Ontario Task Force on Health Services also suggested eliminating local health departments. Yet two years later, the Ministry of Health's own Health Promotion Branch prepared a report lauding the services and programs which municipal departments provided. The change reflected the impact of the federal government's working document, *A New Perspective on Health for Canadians,* with its stress on prevention and the role of environmental and behavioural factors in health problems, and the province's sense of crisis as curative costs spiralled.

With all these concerns as a backdrop, Moss assumed the health officership just as the forces which were to alter it became dominant. As the head of a Department, which members of the urban reform coalition perceived as hidebound and moribund, the new medical officer was put on the defensive when the lead issue erupted in January 1973. Within the Department, restive

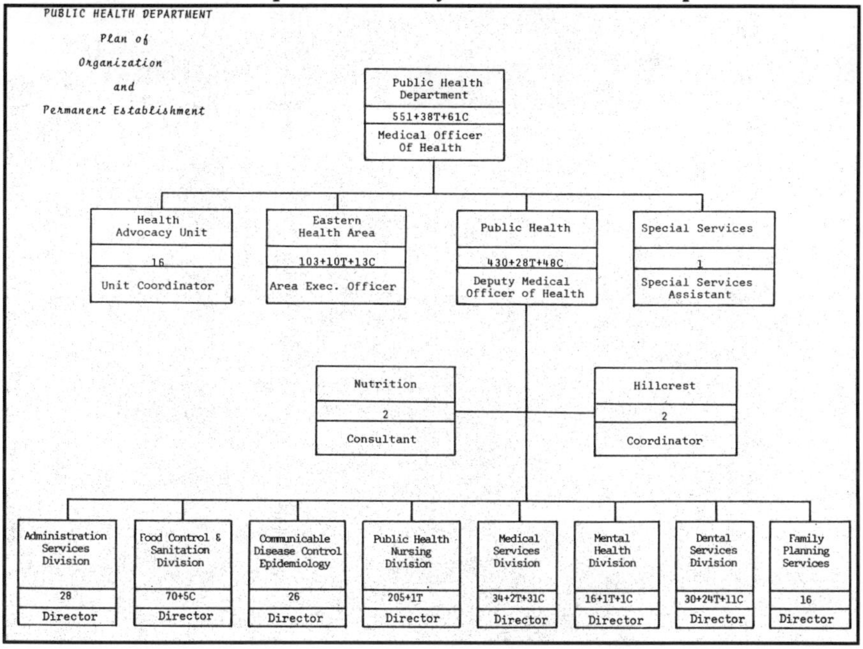

By 1980, the Department's administrative structure had been modified to include the Health Advocacy Unit and the Eastern Health Area.

younger staff criticized the layers of middle management, and the incremental model of change that slowed the Department's response to contemporary problems and limited its policy-making efforts. The political conflict that the lead controversy aroused, and staff discontent, resulted in the appointment of the Health Planning Steering Committee. This representative group prepared *Public Health in the 1980's*, a report which stressed the new orientation of the public health movement, and suggested a radical restructuring of the Department to achieve more extensive community involvement and to eliminate medical dominance. As these views gained support, the medical officer and other senior staff opted to take early retirement and to let their successors grapple with implementing decentralization, the team management system, and redefining the medical officership.

Conclusion

In 1980 when Toronto's local board of health was searching for a new medical officer, it announced that the candidate had to have experience in community organizing, excellent interpersonal skills, and a commitment to health advocacy. This description of the medical officership redefined the well-established pattern which Jackson, Pequegnat, Boyd and Moss's careers had followed. As professional administrators, these men had built on the legacy of their predecessors using an incremental model of change. The gradual modification of existing programs and the constant struggle for financing led some external observers to conclude that little was being accomplished. In fact, the Department's inspectors and nurses were involved in innovative activities in the various districts, but the pace of official change was slow. As the head of the Department, the medical officer was the target of criticism for the lack of dynamic development.

In some respects, such charges were unjust because through much of this period, public health experts in Britain, the United States and Canada, were attempting to redefine their goals and to offer an alternative to the curative system. In others, the opposition was valid because all organizations begin to decline after the initial creative period is over. Only charismatic and far-sighted leaders can overcome the stasis inherent in large bureaucracies, and such individuals are rare. By the early 1970s, the limitations of the traditional definition of the medical officer's role were evident to contemporary reformers, who wanted to restore Toronto's Health Department to its early twentieth century position of prominence, and they initiated the process of redefinition and renewal which has continued to the present.

Chapter Three

Forging A Professional Identity: Public Health Inspection and Public Health Nursing

According to late twentieth century management consultants, caring, committed staff are an essential component of successful organizations. This is particularly true in the public service, especially in the public health field where inspectors and nurses represent the human face of the Department's policies and programs to citizens. As the two largest occupational groups within the Department, the history of the inspectors and the nurses' efforts to forge a professional identity reveals the way in which the changing emphasis of the international public health movement and local developments united to shape the distinctive "work culture" which each group possesses. As current commentators have defined it:

> Work culture is a product of an occupation's history, shared experience, and social environment. It leads, over time, to a set of behavioural prescriptions and understandings that are taught to new members as normal, correct, and appropriate ways to act and think.[1]

In 1884, Ontario's Public Health Act permitted local boards of health to appoint sanitary inspectors to investigate environmental problems and to ensure that they were corrected. For many politicians, this provision added another patronage position to civic government. Public health reformers, however, started the long process of upgrading the inspectors' educational qualifications by rejecting patronage and encouraging potential staff to complete British-based certificates. Until 1935, however, no Canadian courses were available and most training occurred on the job. For Toronto's inspectors, close contact with their peers and supervisors contributed to the development of a shared outlook that stressed "persuasion not coercion."

When sanitary reform was superseded by interest in health education, the inspectors' public profile diminished and they were regarded primarily as technical advisors rather than full-fledged professionals. The introduction of the scientific management system contributed to this view because compartmentalizing the staff's activities limited opportunities for innovation and change. Of equal significance, the city's employment criteria, its limited recruitment efforts, low salaries, and lack of a pension plan until 1943, lessened staff turnover and entrenched traditional approaches. By the late 1960s, however, the appearance of new environmental problems had resulted in a demand for better trained inspectors. This provided the impetus for a reassessment of their status within the Department and resulted in the creation of an environmental services manager position, in the decentralized administrative structure that was introduced between 1979 and 1982.

Although the city's first public health nurse was not appointed until 1907, Charles Hastings' adoption of health education as the focus of the Department's activities produced a rapid increase in the number of nurses between 1910 and 1929. As nurses, these women shared their occupation's ideology of service, but unlike the majority of their colleagues, they chose to perform their duties in the preventive, not the curative field. In contrast to the inspectors, Toronto's nurses were required to have professional qualifications prior to appointment, and were encouraged to upgrade their educational training by pursuing postgraduate studies. Both the inspectors and the nurses were expected to join professional organizations and to participate in their meetings, in order to describe the "Toronto system" and to learn about innovations developed in other cities. By the 1970s, Toronto's nurses were aware of the fourth phase of the international public health movement — health promotion — and wanted to modify their activities to add this new dimension. Like the inspectors, they looked to decentralization with its stress on teamwork as the way to modernize their role.

From Policemen to Teachers: The Public Health Inspectors

"Officer, that's him! That's the man who was here yesterday." When he heard those words one autumn morning in 1888, rookie inspector Robert Wilson knew that the baker whose shop he inspected the day before had not understood the purpose of the visit. After the police sergeant who escorted him back to Police Station No. 3 learned from his colleagues that Wilson was indeed a Health Department inspector, he told the young man to ask the medical officer for more official proof of his appointment than a letter. As a result of this incident, Toronto's inspectors received metal badges to show to householders, shopkeepers, and factory owners, when they arrived to inspect either on a routine basis or in response to citizen complaints.[2]

In 1883, Toronto lagged behind Hamilton, New York City, Ottawa, Milwaukee, and most large British cities, because it did not have any permanent sanitary inspectors. When Canniff tried to persuade the local board of health to appoint inspectors in 1884, Alderman Moore "characterized the institution (the Health Department) as a gigantic fraud gotten up for the purpose of patronage."[3] In a society which lacked technical training and specific educational qualifications for such posts, these fears were well-founded. Nevertheless, the medical officer had decided that "Sanitary inspectors should be well informed on general sanitary matters. They should be instructors. They should have tact and judgment, and rarely resort to any authority which they possess."[4] With these criteria in mind, the local board appointed six temporary inspectors in 1885 to supplement the work of the police inspectors. With one exception, they were laid off at the end of October when house-to-house inspection stopped.

A year later, a reform-oriented board began to think in a more long-term fashion and passed a motion stating that "these men will have to satisfy the Medical Health Officer as to their fitness for sanitary work before being employed, and must be young and active men."[5] For Canniff, this was an opportunity to expand his staff and to create a probationary system to assess potential employees. But as letter writers Hygiene and Sanitas pointed out in the Toronto *News*, patronage remained the basis for appointment in spite of the medical officer's efforts to adopt British standards. By 1890, the Department's staff included one chief inspector, eight staff inspectors and two full-time clerks, serving a population of nearly 181,000. In comparison, Hamilton had four inspectors for roughly 49,000 people in 1891, while Montreal had a staff of twenty sanitary inspectors, four meat inspectors, and two milk inspectors in 1897, for nearly 300,000.[6]

Canniff's successors worked to increase the number of inspection staff and to define their qualifications. None of the provincial health statutes specified educational requirements for sanitary inspectors and no Canadian training programs existed. As a result, in 1906 Charles Sheard helped establish a Toronto branch of the Royal Sanitary Institute. The British-based institute had been created in 1876 by the father of the sanitary movement, Edwin Chadwick, and a group of his supporters. In 1877, the Sanitary Institute began to offer training courses for inspectors and to provide examinations leading to a certificate of competence. After receiving its royal charter at the end of the century, the organization expanded to the Dominions and opened branch offices in most provincial capitals.[7] Sheard and Hastings encouraged their inspectors to take the examinations and to supplement their on-the-job experience with in-service training.[8]

Like the medical officers, the sanitary inspectors were pioneering a new employment opportunity. To encourage a professional outlook among themselves, western Canadian inspectors formed a Sanitary Inspector's Association in 1913. By 1923, they had concluded that they should have a national organization, and that becoming a section of the Canadian Public Health Association would achieve this goal. The inspectors were reacting to the shift in public health practice from environmental activities to health education work. In the 1920s, leading Canadian and American health authorities such as H.W. Hill, of London, and Charles Chapin, Providence, Rhode Island's long-time medical officer, criticized local health departments for continuing to spend money on sanitation services. As the president of the Canadian Sanitary Inspectors' Association asked in 1924:

> Is it implied that no efforts are to be made to improve housing conditions, or conditions in industrial plants? Is there to be no City Department in our cities and towns charged with the duty of seeing that dwellings are kept in a habitable condition? Of what avail to spend large sums on child welfare work and the supervision of school children, if, after saving the infants' lives, they are to live in insanitary homes. The sick cannot all be hospitalized; surely their home should be made and kept fit for occupation.[9]

SANITATION

(*Thursday afternoon, September 12th*)
Time: 3 hours

---

1. John Smith, a contractor, proposes to erect a 6-room dwelling house on a lot sloping steeply toward Blank Street. He has sublet the contract for plumbing to James Brown, a master plumber who holds a licence from the municipality. The dwelling is to have the following fixtures: Three-piece bath on the second floor, sink in the kitchen and fixed laundry tubs in the basement.

(*b*) Illustrate by a sketch the essential parts of such an installation to the point where the connection is made to the sewer on Blank Street.

(*b*) Describe the procedure needed to obtain the approval of the municipal authorities for this installation.

(*c*) Describe the inspections that would be made by you, as an inspector of plumbing. When should such inspections be made? Include in your account any tests you might use.

2. (*a*) What diseases may be transmitted to humans by water?

(*b*) Describe the essential features of a properly located and constructed dug well.

(*c*) What are the purposes of water filtration? Name the types of water-filter plants used by municipalities and describe *one* type.

3. You have been appointed sanitary inspector of a town of 5,000 population. What information would you attempt to obtain by means of a sanitary survey and how would you proceed to conduct such a survey? Indicate the form of your report to the medical officer of health, giving suitable headings for the presentation of the findings.

4. (*a*) Describe the construction and principle of operation of a septic-tank installation for a rural home. Illustrate your answer by a sketch.

(*b*) Describe the construction and maintenance of one type of outdoor privy. What other types may be used?

5. Write short notes on the following:

(*a*) Methods of refuse disposal in an urban municipality.

(*b*) The control of flies.

(*c*) The chlorination of a municipal water supply.

He objected to foisting these responsibilities on police forces, and quite rightly argued that funds for sanitary work would not remain in health department budgets if the duties were transferred to other municipal bodies.

While the Sanitary Inspectors' Association was forming provincial branches, the Ontario organizer found a degree of suspicion about his organization's activities among Toronto's inspection staff. They were concerned about the benefits of membership since many appeared disillusioned by their previous links to the Royal Sanitary Institute. Like their colleagues in Ottawa and Hamilton, Toronto's inspectors wanted answers to questions such as "How can you get me an increase in salary?" "How can my status be increased?," and, "How can I get recognition as a man who has studied and understands certain phases of Public Health?."[10]

FOOD CONTROL AND LEGISLATION

(Friday morning, September 13th)
Time: 3 hours

1. (*a*) What diseases may be transmitted to man through milk?

(*b*) A farmer with a herd of twenty cows wishes to sell milk to a dairy in a nearby city. Enumerate the various points to be observed in making an inspection for the granting of a licence, indicating the requirements which would guide you in making your report.

2. A butcher in a town of 5,000 population wishes to erect a slaughter house on the bank of a small river on the outskirts of the municipality. What requirements should be made regarding the location, construction, equipment, and operation of such a slaughter house?

3. You are required to inspect a restaurant which seats 50 persons. The owner is very willing to co-operate but has limited finances since the restaurant is in a poor section of the town. Describe your visit to the restaurant, the points you would note, and the advice you would give the owner, with special emphasis on dish-washing methods.

4. Discuss the pasteurization of milk under the following headings: (i) definition (according to the regulations of your province), (ii) the essential equipment in a small pasteurizing plant, (iii) possible defects in equipment and operation.

5. (*a*) An outbreak of food poisoning has occurred in a city. All who suffered illness were customers of one bakeshop. Describe the investigation which you would make and the inspection of the shop. What products are most likely to be the cause of the illness?

(*b*) What are the purposes of meat inspection as conducted in abattoirs? Describe the method of inspection and enumerate the conditions which may be found requiring the condemnation of a carcass.

PREVENTION AND CONTROL OF COMMUNICABLE DISEASES AND RELATED SUBJECTS

(Friday afternoon, September 13th)
Time: 3 hours

1. (*a*) What are the characteristics of communicable diseases?

(*b*) Write a note on the modes of transmission of communicable diseases. Give examples of diseases spread by each mode of transmission.

2. A case of smallpox is reported in a lumber camp. Discuss fully the measures which should be taken for effective control of: (*a*) the case, (*b*) the contacts.

3. For what purposes is fumigation with hydrocyanic acid gas employed? Describe in detail the procedure of fumigating a dwelling house. What safeguards must be used?

4. In a retail fruit store having living quarters situated immediately behind the shop, a case of scarlet fever occurs in a child of 7 years. The family consists of three other children of school age and two adults. What steps would you take as quarantine inspector on being notified of the case of scarlet fever? What are the regulations relating to the occurrence of scarlet fever under these circumstances?

5. (*a*) State quarantine and isolation periods as required in your province for measles, diphtheria, and poliomyelitis.

(*b*) Name three diseases for which there are vaccines or serums for use in their prevention. Indicate in each instance how the preventive treatment is employed.

The Central Board on Examination and Registration was gratified with the results of the examination, which gave evidence that candidates are meeting the higher standards set by the Committee. Since the introduction of the examinations in 1935 two hundred and two inspectors have obtained the Canadian certificate.

May 31, 1941. J. G. CUNNINGHAM, *Chairman.*

This sample examination (above and left) illustrates the types of questions which the Department's sanitary inspectors had to answer to earn their certificates.

As a result of these queries, improving their training became a priority, and they lobbied medical and nursing professionals in the Canadian Public Health Association to support their objective. In the 1920s, the American Public Health Association's Committee on Professional Education did not pay much attention to the inspectors' educational needs, because they did not share the same professional model of university-based training as the doctors and nurses. The British offered a contrast, as the Ministry of Health and the Sanitary Institute created a joint Board of Examiners in 1925, and required candidates to possess the equivalent of university entrance qualifications before they attempted to complete the examination.[11]

In typically Canadian fashion, a compromise was worked out between the conflicting British and American approaches to educating inspectors. Interested Canadians were still eligible to take the Royal Sanitary Institute certificate examinations but the pressure for a Canadian course and examination was building. In 1934, the Sanitary Inspector's Association was incorporated as the Canadian Institute of Sanitary Inspection by the federal Secretary of State. The Canadian Public Health Association assisted in the birth of the new group, and arranged with the deputy ministers of all the provincial health departments for the creation of a course in sanitary inspection, and the introduction of joint ministry and Canadian Institute examinations. The course began in 1935, and many of Toronto's inspectors completed its requirements and took the exam to acquire the Institute's certificate. The city's Health Department also provided examiners for the new program. Deputy medical officer Pequegnat, Dr. A.R.B. Richmond, the Director of the Food Control Division, and various staff inspectors, joined Ontario's deputy health minister and a representative from the Canadian Sanitary Institute in preparing questions and administering the three day examination, which followed completion of the course. The exam consisted of three sections: sanitation, food control and legislation, and prevention and control of communicable diseases. Students had to pass each section to earn their certificates.[12] As one of the largest employers in the country, Toronto's Health Department had a vested interest in raising the educational standards for sanitary inspectorships.

This effort to forge a professional identity intensified over the next decades. In 1942, a correspondence course was introduced, but by the mid–1950s, Ontario and Quebec's health authorities were convinced that it did not provide sufficient field work and that inspectors needed classroom training.[13] During 1946, in an effort to ease the predicted shortage of inspectors, the CPHA arranged a special "fast" course and conducted three examinations for recently demobilized members of field hygiene units. In 1947, the city of Toronto made the Canadian Institute of Sanitary Inspection's certificate an employment requirement, because it guaranteed that the applicant had completed his or her junior matriculation and had acquired an appropriate educational background for the position.

At no time prior to 1950 were rank and file inspectors encouraged to pursue university training. In 1944, John Phair informed the Ontario branch of the Canadian Institute of Health Inspectors that degree studies were not necessary for their work as technicians. To maintain staff competence, however, Ontario's Chief Medical Officer stressed the importance of in-house training and focusing on educational rather than regulatory activities.[14]

During the 1950s, the Ontario government and the Canadian Public Health Association jointly sponsored the sanitary inspection training available at the School of Hygiene. When the provincial health department transferred its sanitary engineers and inspectors to the Ontario Water Resources Commission in 1957, it lost interest in this form of training. In 1960, Ryerson Institute of Technology started to administer the course, and by the end of that decade it had become a two year program. Both the provincial and municipal health departments paid the fees of interested staff who wanted to upgrade their qualifications, as long as they promised to serve the community for a set period. With the resurgence of environmental pollution problems in the 1960s and 1970s, the inspector's task became so complex that a four year training period was established. Today, some Health Department staff are pursuing master's degrees in environmental studies to keep abreast of trends in this critical area.[15]

Developing Esprit de Corps

Education, however, was only one factor in creating an effective inspector. Team spirit developed through shared experiences. From 1883 to 1890, the small but growing corps of inspectors shared the medical officer's office in St. Lawrence Hall. The smell from the Market was so strong that visitors complained to the medical officer about the health hazard and Canniff reported their concerns to the local board. Since the inspectors spent their working days walking around the city carrying out their duties, only the medical officer and the lone clerk had to deal with the odour. Much to everyone's relief the new city hall at the top of Bay Street was a considerable improvement, although the Health Department had cramped office space. Common problems and congested working conditions helped to create a strong sense of group cohesion.

With the formal creation of Divisions of Sanitation, Meat Inspection, Plumbing and Drainage, Housing and Industrial Hygiene, Food Inspection and Laboratories in 1911, Toronto's Health Department became a bureaucracy. Now the inspectors functioned in a centralized hierarchy. Veteran inspectors from the Canniff years like Robert Shutt, Robert Wilson, and W.H. Meadows were appointed to senior supervisory positions. Younger experts like veterinarian A.R.B. Richmond, and chemists Dr. Fred Adams, Norman J. Howard and Dr. Ambrose Moffatt, were made division directors. Hastings was ensuring that his staff received professional direction, and he encouraged his division directors to maintain their memberships in the Canadian and American Public Health Associations, as well as organizations such as the American Waterworks Association, and the International Food Sanitarians Association. By presenting papers which described Toronto's inspection programs and research activities, these men added to the stock of knowledge and contributed to the development of a professional identity.

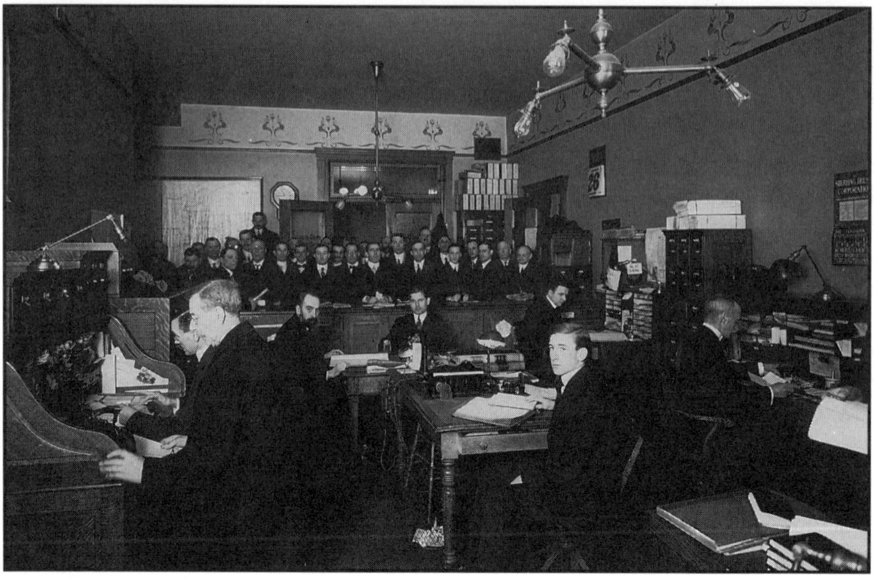

Morning roll call January 27, 1915 for the Department's sanitation, communicable disease control, housing and industrial hygiene inspectors.

In 1915, a city photographer captured the early morning roll call in the Sanitation and Food Control divisions. The staff inspectors crowded against the office counter while their directors sat at their desks. The Bureau of Municipal Research argued that such organized confusion created a poor impression on the public. It also noted that the Division of Meat Inspection's office was a board on top of a radiator in front of a window which the lone inspector shared with the members of three other divisions. The Bureau's investigators argued that "it is doubted if there is a more congested corner anywhere in the British Empire."[16] Such close contact in a centralized setting enabled the senior staff to foster the talents of ambitious junior inspectors. In Toronto, as elsewhere, experience was the primary criterion for promotion, and specialization in a variety of activities was encouraged through frequent transfers among the various units.[17]

In 1927, the city standardized wages and salaries and introduced employment criteria. Although the Bureau of Municipal Research had recommended competitive examinations for Health Department positions in 1915, the city merely required staff to be residents of Toronto or veterans of the Great War. According to the Phair Committee, these restrictions and the small annuity which the city paid to former employees, encouraged inspection staff to continue working long after their duties had become redundant. In its harsh criticism of the inspectors and their entrenched approach to their responsibilities, the investigators ignored the loss of younger staff to the war effort. Underlying their comments was the anti-inspection bias which Chapin had so carefully fostered two decades earlier.[18]

For the inspectors, the long years of the Depression and the dominance of people like Robert Wilson, who served for more than forty-seven years, meant that efforts to update their image were vital. In 1942, Melville Matthews, one of the city's senior inspectors, presented a paper to his colleagues at the Canadian Institute of Sanitary Inspectors' annual meeting. His theme was the transformation of inspectors from policemen to teachers, because "nothing is more undesirable than a domineering, officious approach" when trying to solve sanitation or disease control problems.[19] He urged his colleagues to stress the educational elements of their role as a means of developing "a public health consciousness" in citizens. His views were echoed through the 1950s as sanitary inspectors began to redefine their work after the creation of Metro and the transfer of the city laboratory to the province ended their responsibility for water quality and microbiological analysis.

Other changes had also affected them. In 1943, the long-awaited city pension plan was introduced and older staff members could retire with dignity. Female inspectors were pleased that they would receive more than the $9.00 a week pension that had been offered in 1939 to two women staff, who had served the Department for twenty-five and twenty-eight years by that date.[20] The creation of a city Personnel Department in 1945 and the unionization of inspection staff and other municipal employees, introduced complex bargaining procedures and external elements to the hiring process. According to the Ontario Health Survey Committee, Toronto had 74 full-time food control and sanitation division staff in 1948. In the rest of the province, 61 inspectors served municipal boards and 45 worked in health units.[21]

Through the 1950s, continuing staff shortages plagued the Department. Did sanitary inspectors have an image problem? In Britain, sanitary inspectors agreed to rename themselves as public health inspectors in 1956, and eight years later, the Canadians followed their example in an attempt to make this job sound more attractive.[22] But during the 1960s and 1970s, staff shortages occurred as a result of non-competitive salaries and the frustrations which many inspectors experienced in the specialized system, which had been implemented in 1911. Promotions were slow, and the inspector's position at the bottom of the administrative structure frustrated attempts to expand the Department's services to examine new environmental problems. Just as efforts to correct these problems were being made, the lead issue emerged. The increased workload and the switch from enforcing regulations to advocacy, challenged staff and contributed to a rising resignation rate.[23]

To overcome this and to respond to contemporary needs, the Divisions of Food Control and Sanitation were united in 1974, under the direction of a public health inspector rather than a veterinarian. When the University of Toronto's Community Health Department assessed the Health Department's activities in 1977, they found that the inspectors were far happier under the new system than they had been, because the generalized system eliminated boredom and lessened the inspector's "fear of mistakes syndrome."[24] The introduction of modern management techniques, including setting goals and objectives and creating evaluation procedures, also marked a significant change from the past with its emphasis on tallying the number of inspections and prosecutions that the staff had carried out. On the eve of decentralization, the public health inspectors were moving back into a position of prominence.

Health Guardians and Guides: Public Health Nursing

"Hats off to the District Nurse!" was the opening line in the Toronto *Sunday World*'s description of the many daily activities of Toronto's public health nurses. Written in 1924, this story illustrated how public health nursing had evolved since Toronto's lone tuberculosis nurse, Janet Neilson, had joined the Health Department in 1907. Neilson's appointment was part of a slowly growing movement in Canadian, British, and American reform circles. To break the cycle of poverty and ill-health, social activists funded demonstration projects such as the nursing service provided by the Henry Street Settlement in New York City at the turn of the century; these activities illustrated the effectiveness of professional advice and supervision.[25] By 1905, the success of these American ventures encouraged a Canadian philanthropist, Marjory Larkin, to pay the salary of a nurse appointed to do follow-up work for the Toronto General Hospital's Tuberculosis Clinic. In 1907, Dr. Harold Parsons, the clinic's director, asked Dr. Charles Sheard, who was deeply involved in the anti-tuberculosis crusade, to persuade the local board of health to support this work by taking over its nursing component. In contrast to his reaction to many of the other social reformers' proposals, the medical officer approved of tuberculosis nursing because it dealt with a significant cause of city mortality, so he willingly added the nurse to his staff. This episode illustrated the way in which lay groups introduced new activities, proved their worth, and then lobbied to have the municipal department make this type of work a permanent component of its services.

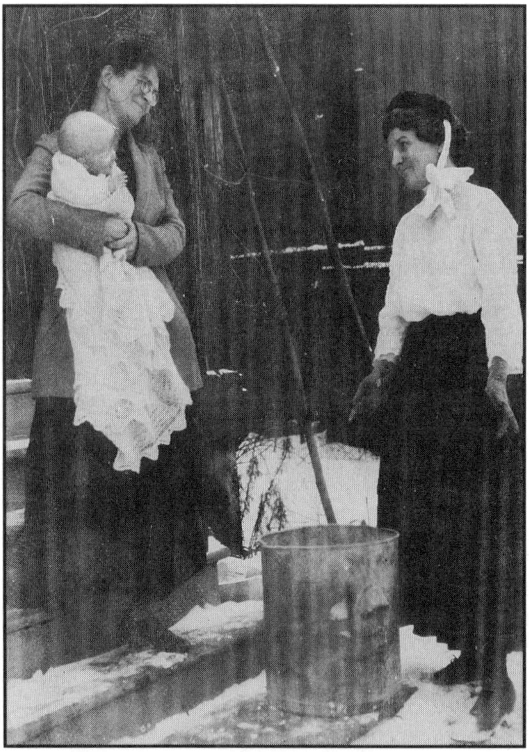

The Department's first public health nurse, Janet Neilson, giving a mother advice on waste disposal.

When Hastings took over the medical officership, he made the development of a public health nursing system a priority because "the entrance of the public health nurse into the field of preventive medicine has opened a new era in public health inasmuch as most of the real, lifesaving...public health activities today have been made possible by the public health nurse."[26] In 1911, he appointed Eunice Dyke as the city's second tuberculosis nurse. Toronto-born, Dyke had trained at Johns Hopkins' School of Nursing, one of the most prestigious and progressive institutions in North America. Her course work included a short stint of district nursing in Baltimore, but after she contracted tuberculosis, Dyke had to spend a year in the Muskoka Sanatorium to recover.[27] Both her background and her training fitted her well for creating the "Toronto system" of district nursing in 1914, when she became the Director of Public Health Nurses.

When she started her work, there were several other groups providing nursing service and health education. The Victorian Order of Nurses and the St. Elizabeth Visiting Nurses Association did bedside nursing, while settlement house nurses offered guidance in the milk depots and baby clinics which sprang up at this time. In 1910, the Board of Education had established its nursing system as part of school medical inspection. Since these groups concentrated on helping less affluent Torontonians, duplication occurred as nurses from different public and voluntary agencies visited the same home.

To complicate matters, the Health Department initially divided its nursing staff into tuberculosis, measles, and child welfare nurses. As Dyke and

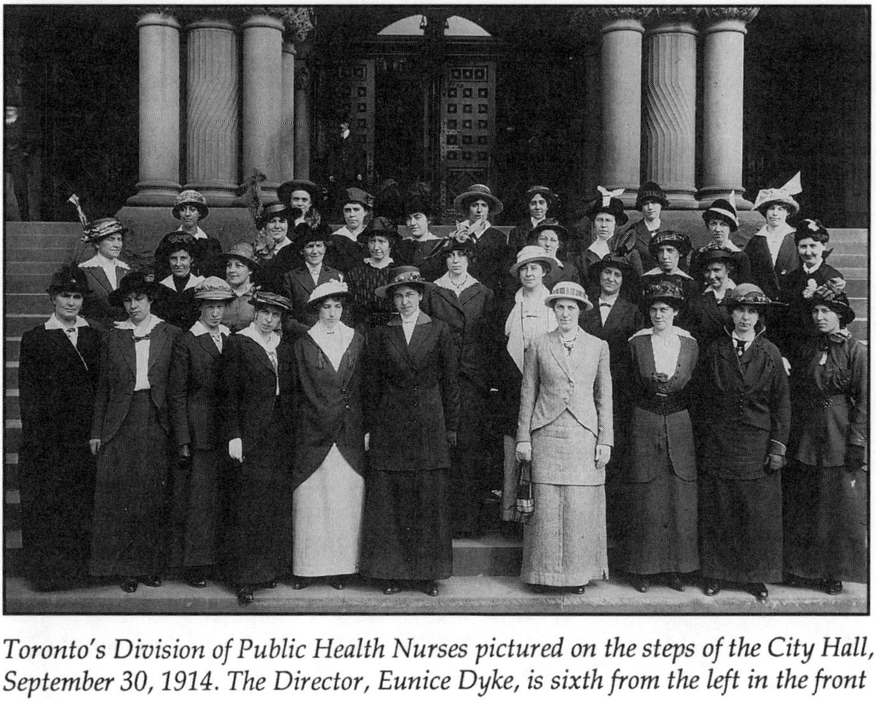

Toronto's Division of Public Health Nurses pictured on the steps of the City Hall, September 30, 1914. The Director, Eunice Dyke, is sixth from the left in the front row.

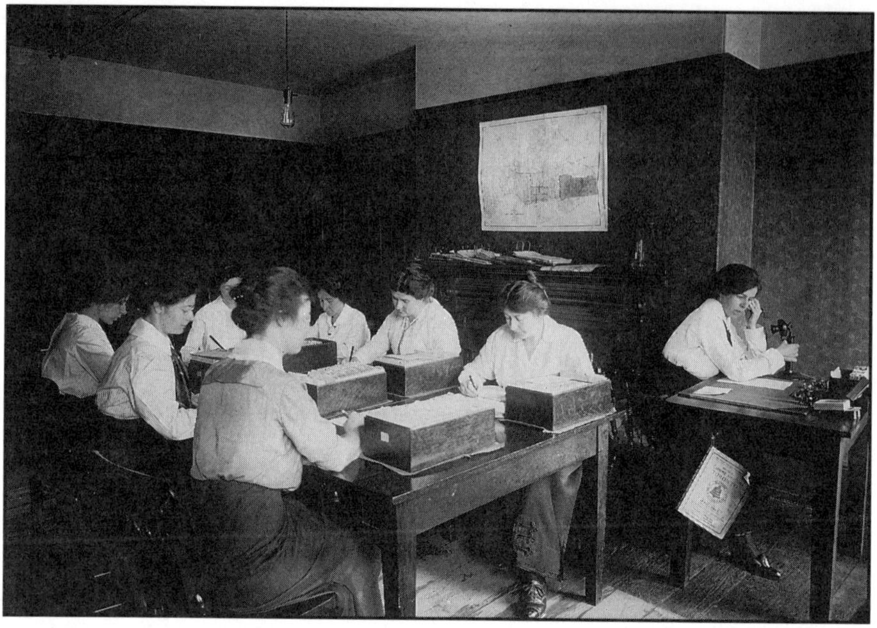

The University District nursing staff completing their daily reports in June 1915 while the district superintendent contacts local doctors and charitable groups by phone.

the other staff quickly realized, their work too overlapped. The "Toronto system" of generalized district nursing emerged from this chaotic situation in February 1914, when the Department united its nursing staff in a single division, took over nursing staff from several of the milk depots and baby clinics, and set up three district offices. Although the VON and the St. Elizabeth Visiting Nurses remained separate organizations, they co-ordinated their efforts with those of the Health Department. In 1917, Dyke and Hastings rounded out their nursing system when the Board of Education's staff was added to the Health Department.[28]

In contrast to the specialized systems which operated in Detroit and other American centres, Toronto chose to experiment with generalized nursing. Both Hastings and Dyke believed that the family, rather than the individual, was the target of the advice which the nurses were expected to offer. As a result, the Division of Public Health Nurses had a small central office executive consisting of the director, the assistant director, five special supervisors of maternal and child health, venereal disease control, school services, mental hygiene, tuberculosis and hospital social service, and essential support staff. In each district, a superintendent supervised eight to ten nurses, a clerk, students visiting for field experience, and neighbourhood volunteers. The district superintendent was also expected to make links with local charitable groups, and after 1918, to participate in the Neighbourhood Workers' Association, an umbrella group for Toronto's social welfare work. This duty reflected the reform impulse which led Dyke to remark: "It is hoped that the permanent results will prove to be co-operation between civic and private agencies and the establishment of a body of public health nurses capable of sympathetic services and wise initiatives."[29]

When the system was introduced in 1914, Toronto was divided into three districts and each nurse was assigned a segment of the city in which she was responsible for pregnant women, babies, and people suffering from tuberculosis and other communicable diseases. As the staff expanded, the number of districts increased to eight by 1923 and nine by 1927. The district offices, like Toronto's city hall, were usually cramped. In the early years, the nurses were based in local police stations, but by the 1920s, they were sharing accommodation with local welfare groups. One former nurse who joined the Department in the 1940s, recalled that when she became the senior nurse in the Riverdale district, she and another staff nurse shared the superintendent's office, while the district medical officer had a table and chair under the stairwell. In 1955, nurses in the eastern districts were pleased when the new Health and Welfare centre opened at 430 Broadview Avenue because they now had adequate office space for consultations and administrative tasks.

Like the inspectors, the nurses spent relatively little time in the office. After 1917, they devoted mornings to their districts' public or separate schools. At noon, they returned to the district offices for lunch and administrative activities. Most afternoons, armed with lists from the central office of births, recently released hospital patients, diabetes sufferers, sick school

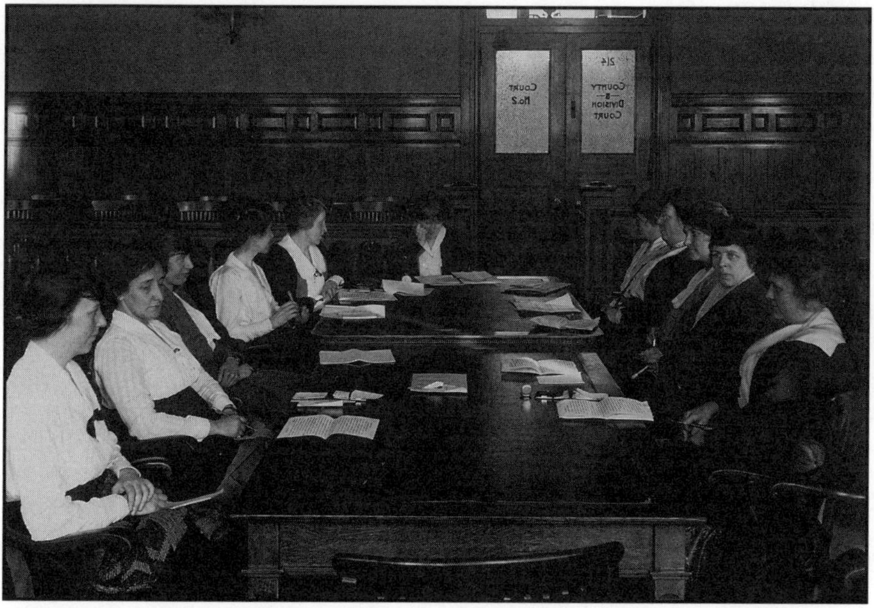

The district nursing superintendents met weekly with central staff to discuss current matters, share innovative approaches and plan for future nursing activities.

children, municipal compensation cases, and TB or venereal disease contacts, the nurses made home visits. During these calls, the nurses quickly assessed the family's economic status and made referrals to appropriate social services for financial or other types of assistance. Home visits also allowed the nurses to educate women and disease victims. In the 1910s and 1920s, the nurses occasionally did the dishes or prepared meals for harried homemakers because Dyke had trained them to think that "one who serves...therefore may teach."[30] Public health nursing thus required women with tolerance, a sense of humour and independent judgment.

Educating Public Health Nurses

When the Department initiated its nursing system, no training courses existed in Canada. Since Dyke and Hastings believed in the importance of professional training, only registered nurses were hired. Even this qualification did not satisfy the senior administrators, because the majority of the staff had been trained in hospital-based nursing schools and were not fully prepared for the demands of district nursing. To help nurses adjust to their new positions, Dyke introduced a probationary period in 1913 and set up a two week preliminary field course in 1915. The acid test was still how well the nurse worked at the district level and whether she remained with the Department. During the early years, there was a rapid staff turnover because women retired when they married, left to join the armed forces, departed to work for other agencies, or, as one nurse put it, resigned because she felt that the Department's policies were "too aggressive."[31]

In 1917, Dyke and Hastings joined the Graduate Nurses' Association of Ontario in demanding university-level nursing education from the Hodgins Commission on Medical Education. Although Justice Hodgins was sympathetic to the idea, it took the influenza epidemic of 1918-19 to demonstrate the need for better trained public health nurses in Toronto and elsewhere. When the 'flu epidemic broke out in October 1918, the Health Department swung into action, making 17,108 visits to stricken homes, and supervising the activities of the volunteer groups which sprang up to aid the 150,000 victims and their families. At the end of the outbreak 1,750 Torontonians had died and the need for an expanded staff was evident.

The Canadian Red Cross decided to continue its service activities in the postwar years, and the impact of the influenza epidemic led it to fund the creation of university-based courses in public health nursing as a three year demonstration project in Ontario, Quebec, Nova Scotia, Manitoba, Alberta and British Columbia. Just before the war began in 1914, the University of Toronto had created a Department of Social Service, which had provided social workers and public health nurses with courses that were pertinent to their disciplines. During the war years, Toronto's nurses had been required to take them, but the staff were not convinced of the relevance of some of the material to their work and agitated for more appropriate studies. In 1920, Red Cross funding was used to create a one year certificate programme in public health nursing based in the Social Service Department. The director of the University's Department of Public Health Nursing, E. Kathleen Russell, had spent a year with Toronto's Health Department, and intended to create a course that mixed classroom studies and field work effectively by drawing on the city Health Department's nursing staff.

Using instructors from the university's Faculty of Medicine and School of Household Science, Russell designed a curriculum that was similar to those offered at the Universities of British Columbia, McGill and Western Ontario. Students, who were required to be nursing graduates, had to take courses in preventive medicine and hygiene, psychology, methods in health teaching, principles and practice of social work, nutrition and dietetics, infant hygiene and child hygiene. Their elective options included courses in medical problems such as venereal diseases, tuberculosis and communicable disease, oral hygiene, mental hygiene, and social economics. Each of the instructors in medicine, oral, and mental hygiene was also a division consultant for the Health Department, and Dyke's special supervisors in maternal and child health, and social services, taught for Russell too.

In 1926, the University's Department of Public Health Nursing introduced a four year degree that included two years of university work and two years of clinical training at Toronto General Hospital. Clearly, the nurses were attempting to upgrade the educational qualifications essential for public health practice. As Dr. George M. Weir's survey of nursing education, conducted between 1928 and 1930, demonstrated, Canadian public health nurses were already better educated than their hospital-based colleagues, and in general, more satisfied with their careers. Yet his report noted that only 1,500 of Canada's 15,000 nurses specialized in public health work.

Why weren't more women attracted to the occupation? In an address to the Conference of Illinois Health Officers delivered in 1928, Dyke tried to answer this question. She argued that in some cities lack of interest or re-election concerns prevented the appointment of qualified nurses, while in others a "futile medical officer" was to blame. Of equal importance were the low salaries which senior staff received in comparison to colleagues working for private agencies. But the crux of the matter involved two related difficulties: first, the wide range of the problems facing public health staff meant that nurses "may not have the joy of maximum results in a selected field" and second,

> She may encounter contempt among her own profession for all services directed by public departments or an exasperating tradition that she should deal only with families too ignorant and difficult for private philanthropy to squander its energies upon.[32]

During the 1930s, public health nursing redefined its rationale and approach. Weir's survey identified a trend toward specialization and he argued that public health nurses now needed a stronger foundation in sociology and mental health than in the past, when service rather than education was the norm. To prepare effective public health nursing administrators, he recommended creating a textbook which used Canadian examples to illustrate supervisors' duties. The British Columbian concluded his analysis of Canadian public health nursing by urging nursing schools to accept Chinese, Japanese, Hindu, and native Canadian students.[33]

Weir's farsighted proposals sparked a response from Canadian nurses. In 1932, Esther Beith, the director of Montreal's Child Welfare Association and a former member of Toronto's Health Department, pointed out to her colleagues in the Canadian Nursing Association, that public health nursing had changed from its original focus on alleviating physical disease and health problems to an emphasis on education. Beith stated that previously the nurse's "success...was due rather to her personality, her prestige as a nurse, plus factual material. She superimposed her ideas on individuals and persuaded or dragooned them into certain health measures, but this was not health education."[34] Such comments typified the reaction of the second generation of public health nurses to the reform impulses of their predecessors. As social work concepts were integrated into public health practice, the service component diminished, and nurses devoted more attention to their educational work. Like Weir, Beith and her supporters wanted university degrees to become the basis for employment. When the University of Toronto's School of Nursing opened in 1933, it provided aspiring nurses with the chance to earn a baccalaureate degree, and by the end of the 1940s, Toronto was requiring its supervisory staff to have this qualification.[35]

In spite of the evolution of nurses' approach to health education in the city's homes and schools, the Phair Committee condemned it as ineffective. The committee also objected to the use of nursing staff as *de facto* heads of the maternal and child health and VD divisions. In his response to these negative comments, medical officer Jackson reminded the committee members of Toronto's international reputation as a pioneer in public health nursing, and of the toll which the Depression had exacted by preventing hiring. As he had pointed out to his colleagues at the Academy of Medicine in 1930, Jackson viewed the nurse as someone who "lives in a continued atmosphere of health and health education. Her one thought is health — her chief ambition, health promotion."[36] In holding these views, Toronto's medical officer was opposing the opinion of many doctors.

During the 1920s and 1930s, practitioners objected to public health nurses because they believed that these women were offering medical advice without a license and undermining the faith of the patient or his family in their doctor. To Jackson, such statements were surprising because in 1915, Hastings, Dyke, and the assistant director of Public Health Nursing, Nora Moore, had drawn up Standing Orders and Regulations to govern the nurses' conduct. The staff were told repeatedly that they could not recommend practitioners and that they must never dispute a doctor's orders. As Jackson informed his colleagues, practitioners were expected to report complaints about the nurses' behaviour to him in writing and in only two instances had these been justified. But Dr. A.M. Jeffrey, a general practitioner who had worked for Toronto's Health Department for a year, explained

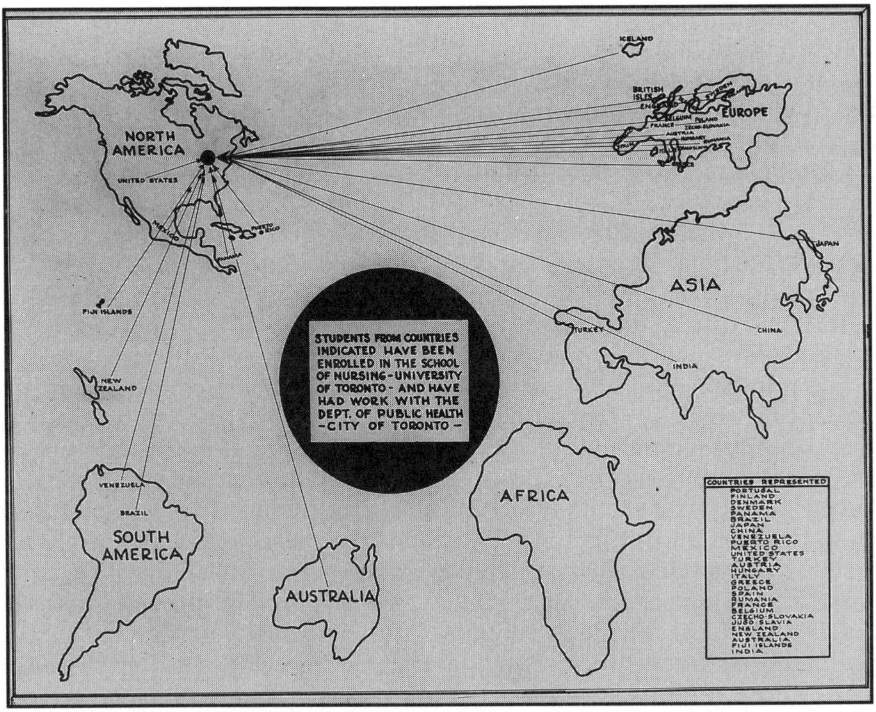

Toronto's international reputation as a pioneer in public health nursing had attracted Rockefeller-funded visitors from around the world by the early 1940s when this map was produced.

the fundamental conflict between the two groups when he argued that the nurses worked in a group setting and thought in terms of family and community problems, while medical practitioners had to struggle alone to build up their practices.[37] The potential for conflict continued until the 1950s when private prepaid medical insurance plans became widespread, guaranteeing most general practitioners economic security. During succeeding decades as doctors ceased making house calls and set up family practice units and health centres, a new, more positive relationship developed.

Within the public health bureaucracy, the nurses remained subordinate until the 1970s. Tradition, social convention, and nursing training conditioned public health nurses to defer to medical authority in most instances. Their work, however, demanded good judgment and independent action. Dyke and her senior staff fostered the nurses' sense of professional autonomy by encouraging them to organize in-service education, and to join and participate in the Canadian and American Public Health Associations, and the public health nursing section of the Canadian Nursing Association. During the 1920s, promising young staff were sent to American centres for field work, and in the 1940s, the Rockefeller Foundation awarded travelling fellowships to senior nurses. In 1941, Elsie Hickey, the city's third Director of Public Health Nursing, served as the chairman of the Canadian Public

Health Association's committee on nursing qualifications and her group recommended graduate training for nursing supervisors. By the 1960s, the assistant directors were studying for masters degrees in American universities in conformity with CPHA qualification standards, and the following decade the University of Toronto started its own graduate program.

Unity was also created through frequent social gatherings — a staff picnic in June, and a bowling league. From the 1910s to the 1940s, the daily lunch at the district office was the strongest integrating factor because new staff were able to share their concerns with experienced ones. Both groups benefited from the lunchtime visits of local social workers, central administrators, and district medical officers.[38]

Like the public health inspectors, the nurses were short-staffed most of the time. In 1946, the Canadian Public Health Association set up a committee to study the shortage of public health personnel. Five years later, the Ontario Health Survey reiterated the CPHA committee's findings that salary considerations determined career choice, and pointed out that the low birth rate during the 1930s meant fewer recruits for nursing. In many respects, Toronto was more fortunate than other Canadian cities because it was the site for field work by students in the University of Toronto nursing program and the hospital nursing schools. By the 1950s, the Department provided several hundred student placements annually. The experience was mutually beneficial because students received hands-on training while the Department's

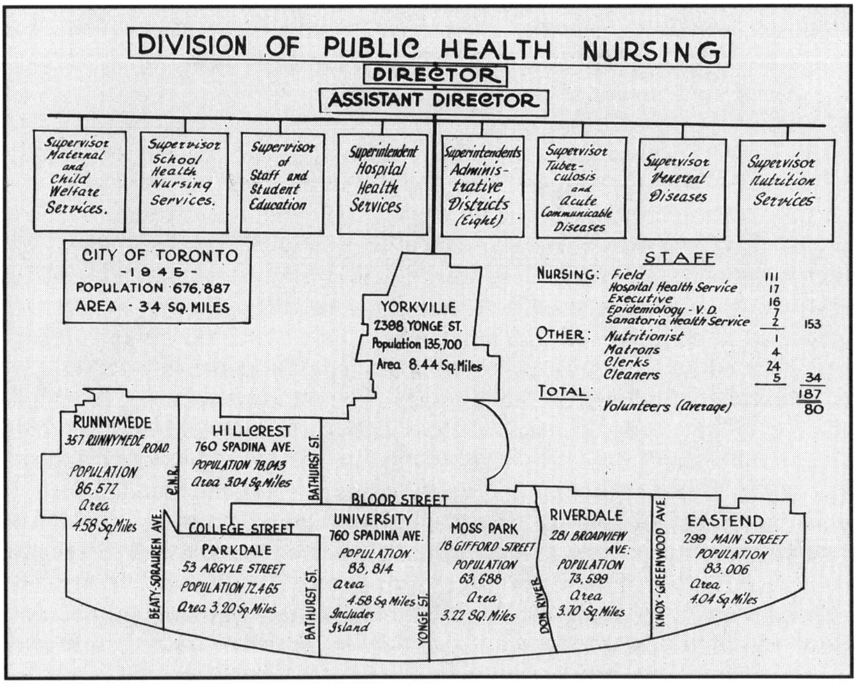

By 1945, Toronto had eight district health offices and a nursing staff of 153 serving a population of 676,887.

nurses were kept up-to-date with changes in nursing theory. As well, particularly promising students were offered jobs provided they completed their courses. Although a decade of staff shortages was alleviated by mass hiring of University of Toronto nurses in 1942 and 1943, the division remained under strength by the American Public Health Association's standards until the end of the 1950s.[39] At that point, the Department removed its restrictions on employing married women and continued its new policy of training and hiring nursing assistants.[40]

During the 1960s and 1970s, nurses began to question their place in the public health hierarchy. As the largest division within the Health Department, the public health nurses were also its most visible representatives. Through their district work, they uncovered new clients, such as the elderly, immigrants, and people with mental problems. Deference to medical authority gradually declined in importance as the nurses sought to deal promptly and effectively with these new needs. As a result, their training courses were modified to include social science methodology, and to emphasize "primary health care through quality nursing assessments via systems theory and community model."[41] When the University of Toronto conducted its study of the Department in 1976–7, the interviewers quickly discovered that public health nurses had more advanced views on the importance of primary prevention and health promotion than their medical colleagues. This produced friction within the Department and led senior nurses to lament inter-divisional gamesmanship and the loss of a unifying vision of the Department's mandate.[42] For many of the nurses, decentralization represented a chance to make what Eunice Dyke had described as the essence of public health nursing — "team play for health" — the core of future endeavours.

Conclusion

Ideology, professional training and shared experience all combined to shape the attitudes and behaviour of the Department's two largest groups — the public health inspectors and nurses. During the early decades, the staff drew their inspiration from the reform ethos which the health officers promoted. After 1930, however, the discipline-based divisional structure and the distant management style of the senior medical administrators diminished the sense of a common goal. Staff shortages, lack of funds for innovative programs, and external criticism from the Phair Committee in 1943 set the stage for change.

Through the 1950s and 1960s, both groups enhanced their educational requirements in conformity with the standards recommended by the Canadian Public Health Association. They were also affected by the influx of non-English-speaking immigrants, the appearance of new health concerns, such as air pollution and services for the elderly, and by challenges to their authority from the younger generation. This combination of factors led to internal pressure for modification of the existing administrative structure and for a new vision of public health.

Chapter Four

Improving the Quality of City Life: The Sanitation Division

"Do let the health inspector in" was the advice that Frank Drea of the *Toronto Telegram* gave to an angry reader who complained in 1971 that she was being harassed by "snoopers" from the board of health about a long-standing cockroach problem. When Drea investigated, he discovered that in response to neighbours' complaints, the health inspectors had called on the woman eighteen times, summonsed her twice, and were in the process of getting a court order granting them admission. As the columnist pointed out, "all they want to do is to show you how to get rid of the bugs. They say that you can't step fast enough to kill them."[1]

In spite of its tragi-comic overtones, this episode represented a classic illustration of the inspectors' work experience. From 1883 to the present, they have relied on the public to notify the Department about nuisances and other health hazards. Then they proceed to investigate, while using the visit as an opportunity to inform the owner or occupant of the relevant sections of the provincial Public Health Act or city by-laws. This educational function was backed by the legal power to issue abatement orders although medical officers and their staffs preferred to persuade, rather than coerce, citizens into action. Public health inspection, then, consists of routine duties and demand investigations. Both activities raise the vexed issue of compliance and have done so since the establishment of systematic work by the Department more than a century ago.

During these formative decades, the inspectors' work provided the ammunition for a variety of reform campaigns by the medical officers. Most of this activity occurred between 1883 and 1910 when the medical and engineering professions were in the process of defining their respective responsibilities in the fields of sanitation and water purification. After 1910, as noted American experts like Charles Chapin derided the sanitarians' focus on environmental issues, inspection became an expected, but not noteworthy, feature of Health Department work. Technological changes in house construction, refrigeration, and food control production ensured that the inspectors would continue to have work to do, but with the growing stress on health education, they lost their prominence. They were also affected by the loss of prestige which local health departments suffered after 1945 as the senior levels of government became active in housing and environmental issues. And in the 1960s, they faced a new challenge from the anti-establishment hippies who opposed the sanitation standards which had become a community norm. Public recognition of new environmental hazards in the 1970s brought the inspectors' role back to centre stage, as once again their efforts provided the information base for Health Department campaigns against new enemies.

"Persuasion not Coercion": Toronto's Sanitation Division

Toronto's twentieth century reputation as one of the cleanest cities in the world would have surprised many of its inhabitants in the 1880s. As a critical letter to the *Globe* pointed out in November 1884, the city's streets were a quagmire of slime, and its lanes and alleyways a disgrace with "unsightly heaps of rubbish and filth lying everywhere." Even worse, in the writer's opinion, were the "effluvia" rising from the privies and cesspools which were the major receptacles for human waste. Irate as the reader was, he failed to comment on the manure, produced by the horses that provided the major means of transportation and haulage for Torontonians. Similarly, he did not note the presence of cow byres, chicken coops and pig sties within the city limits. Nor did he mention the pall of smoke that hung over Toronto as a result of the coal-burning stoves and furnaces used in homes and factories.[2]

Smelly, dirty, and crowded, the city was a menace to the health of its inhabitants, according to the medical theory of the day. Although the germ theory was being adopted in progressive scientific and medical circles by the 1880s, its application was not yet clear. In contrast, the miasmatic theory, which the sanitary reformers in British and American cities used to justify their demands for pure water, effective sewage and garbage disposal, and household sanitation standards, did provide a scientific and intellectual justification for inspecting homes and businesses to make sure that they conformed to minimum requirements. As a committed sanitarian, William Canniff was determined to apply this theory to the city.

In 1883, he began his efforts by preparing a list of questions which the policemen assigned to him were to ask householders. Modelling his questionnaire on Chicago's, the health officer requested information about the owner, the occupants and their health, the number of rooms and persons per room, the inhabitants' water source, drainage arrangements and waste disposal practices, and the number of animals and the state of the stables. The British had used this type of sanitary survey since the 1840s as a means of "educating" citizens in their responsibilities.[3] Canniff's motives were similar. Of the 5,181 premises inspected in 1884, the sanitary police found 1,207 lacked any drainage, 3,374 had privies, 145 had "no water in use," 655 depended on wells, and 842 used cisterns.[4] These revelations led the medical officer to revise his list of questions in 1885, and to give his inspectors a set of educational guidelines on sanitation matters to discuss with householders. They also enabled him to start his campaign to persuade members of the local board of health and his fellow citizens to support improvements in Toronto's water supply and sewer system.

In spite of pressure from his police inspectors to apply the full strength of the law against the few citizens who refused to admit them or to clean up their premises, the medical health officer declined to do so because such

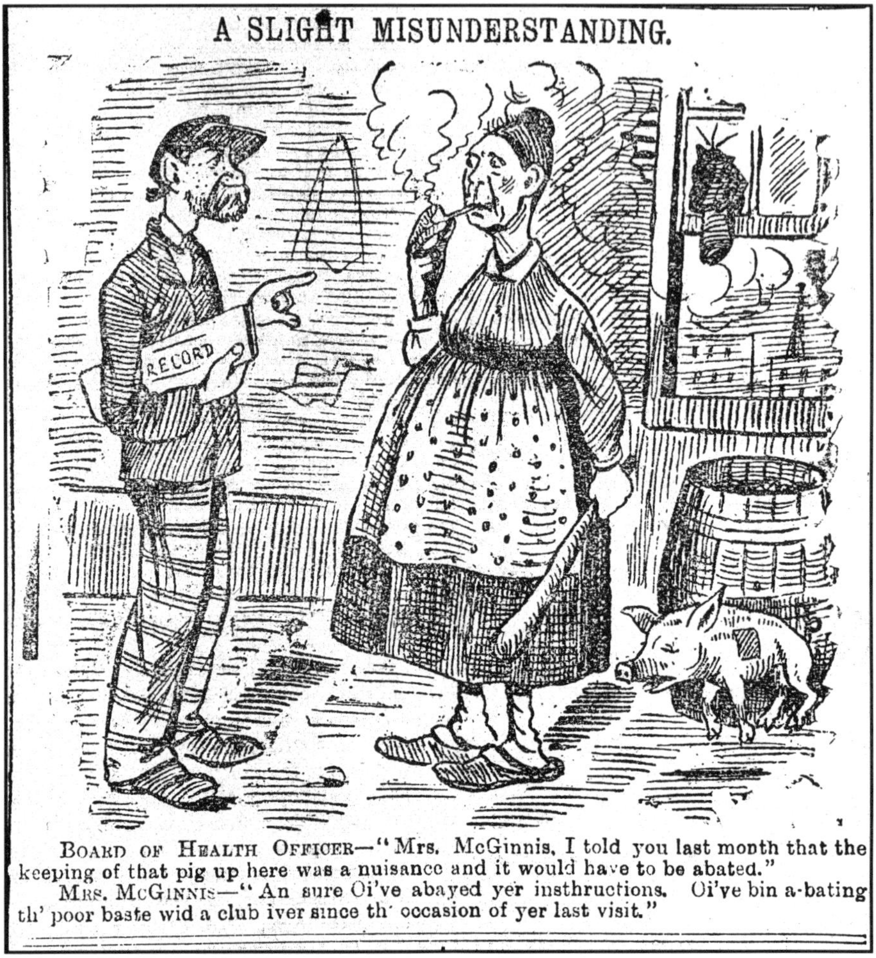

This cartoon illustrates some of the difficulties in educating the public to adopt improved sanitation standards.

action would "have tended to turn the public against me" and because "as the season advanced, many of the hostile or unwilling parties became ashamed of themselves and began to abate evils."[5] As all the Department's inspectors discovered, educating Torontonians in their sanitary duty was a time consuming process that often required numerous visits to convince the homeowners to hook up to the city's water or sewer systems. Cost constraints, and lack of sewer connections and water lines in the 1880s, were two factors in the continued use of privies, cesspools, and well water. Civic politicians' refusal to pass by-laws making conversion mandatory was another. Still, the inspection staff was slowly expanded and annual house-to-house inspections were conducted as part of the ongoing educational process until the 1930s. Toronto was by no means unique in providing this service. Ottawa appointed two inspectors in the 1870s, and Isaac Ryall, Hamilton's health officer, began house-to-house inspection in 1884.[6]

Much of the Department's activity stemmed from citizen complaints. As early as 1884, the city solicitor was warning the politicians that "a great many persons were trying to make use of the Local Board of Health to get a drive at their neighbours."[7] In spite of this, like their counterparts in British and American cities, Toronto's inspectors responded promptly to complaints and conducted thorough investigations. Injured parties, however, often took their complaints to the mayor and the aldermen if they felt that the Health Department was not responding quickly. Canniff's annual reports for the final three years of his health officership present a revealing picture of the slow pace of sanitary reform. In spite of his impassioned pleas for action by local politicians, long-standing environmental abuses were allowed to continue, and he had to write frequently to disgruntled citizens and local board members to remind them that he and his staff were doing their best.

During his tenure, the Department's standard procedures for dealing with complaints were established. After the Department was notified, the complainant was sent a postcard indicating that an investigation was being launched and asking the individual to contact the Department again if improvement did not occur. If the problem was not resolved after a verbal order was given during the initial inspection, a notice requiring the abatement of the problem was prepared. In 1888-89, the Department's inspectors responded to 6,000 citizen complaints; 1,422 of these received abatement notices and 5,743 follow-up visits to ensure compliance.[8] In Ottawa, the Health Department inspectors issued 30 abatement notices a day in the 1880s, while Hamilton's inspectors made 5,320 inspections in 1900. The growth of the latter city from 57,000 to over 100,000 between 1905 and 1908 nearly quadrupled the inspector's work load, and by 1912 they were making 19,223 inspections and 6,166 re-inspections.[9] Toronto experienced a similar population surge, and its staff carried out 17,849 inspections and responded to 3,980 citizen complaints in 1904.[10]

By the 1930s, the Sanitation Division's work load had increased to the point that it was sending out 13-14,000 typed notices of by-law infractions annually after carrying out more than 63,000 inspections. Was such activity really cost-efficient? Did it contribute to public health? The APHA Committee on Administrative Practice queried spending on inspection duties in its *Community Health Organization*, published in 1939.[11] Four years later the Phair Committee identified the main weakness of the Sanitation Division as "lack of adequate professional leadership and a shortage of personnel." The survey team wanted the staff to develop a "more positive type of approach" by eliminating irrelevant activities and providing "sustained supervision of potential sources of health hazards" instead of waiting for complaints.[12] But as the CPHA Study Committee on Public Health Practice recognized, the public was accustomed to reporting any type of sanitation problem to health departments and changing its expectations would be a long-term project.[13]

Staff shortages through the 1950s also limited the modernization of inspector's work. Three decades later, the public health inspectors made 23,987 inspections and gave over 23,000 verbal notices for abatement of various sanitation problems.[14] In the 1880s, Canniff estimated that his men needed three visits to eliminate a problem. Today, fewer visits are required because the standards, which were such a novelty a hundred years ago, are widely accepted.

Canniff's successors continued his emphasis on persuasion rather than prosecution, but when all else failed the Department went to court. During the 1880s, Police Magistrate George Denison often refused to convict and fine people charged under the 1884 model by-law, but his successors generally supported the Health Department's efforts to raise sanitation standards. With adequate proof, the inspector in charge of prosecutions usually won a conviction but legal action was clearly the last resort. The defendant was given every opportunity to complete the necessary repairs and improvements, and as the following statistics demonstrate, many of the cases were withdrawn. During 1888-89, the Department launched 234 prosecutions, had 581 cases remanded, 170 withdrawn because the work was completed, and collected $54.00 in fines from 12 successful prosecutions.[15] In 1924, a similar pattern was evident. The sanitation and food control inspectors prosecuted 245 cases, but 208 were withdrawn after the work was done. Only 23 cases were fined, and as Hastings observed: "We might state here that police court action is only resorted to when other means have failed, and we figure that the fewer the number of prosecutions, the greater the credit to the inspectors."[16]

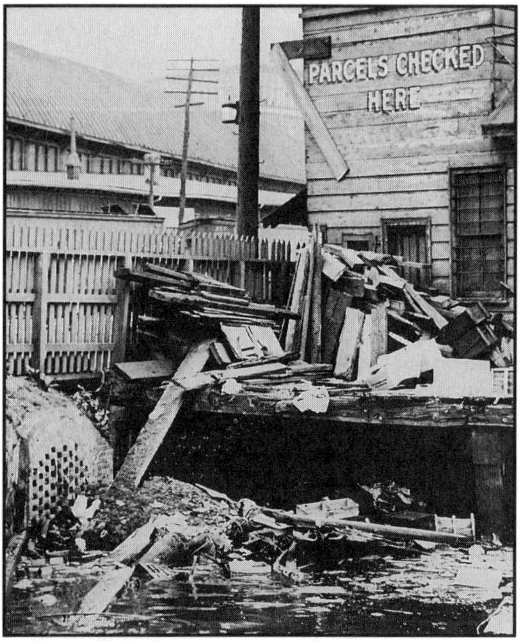

Health Department sanitation inspectors regularly inspected unsanitary businesses such as this one at the foot of Yonge Street in 1911.

As traditional sanitation problems such as foul privies and unsanitary stables declined in importance, the staff attacked other issues. During the 1920s and the 1930s, the sanitation inspectors began to perform routine and demand inspections of beauty parlours and barbershops, second hand stores, laundries, department and retail stores, and institutions like hotels and hospitals. When apartment buildings began to appear in the 1920s, the Department's role was expanded to include assessment of heating and sanitation. In 1954, Montreal's inspectors carried out similar duties; according to that city's medical officer, the members of his five unit sanitation division were responsible for "le contrôle de la salubrité des milieux, bâtiments, logements, etc."[17] In both cities, the inspectors' efforts were usually accepted without opposition.

By the early 1960s, however, the situation began to change. Inspectors working in Toronto's downtown core faced obstruction from non-compliant individuals, many of whom were described as hippies. A decade later, the problem of recluses and the Department's responsibility for them received great publicity after several elderly citizens died. How were the staff to deal with people who either did not, or could not, conform to the community's sanitation standards and by-laws? In keeping with its existing policy, the inspectors modified their approach to these people and tried to "cajole" them into compliance.[18] Only if they failed to achieve action did they turn to the courts. In 1967, six obstruction cases were prosecuted. This increased to nine in 1970, but declined to five by 1980.[19] Implementing the team approach to problem solving during the 1980s made dealing with recluses easier, while amendments to the inspectors' right of entry and the prosecution procedures under the 1983 Health Protection and Promotion Act, altered the staff's overall approach to non-compliant or obstructionist individuals.[20]

Health and Housing

"Be it ever so humble, it can be made a home." With these words, Leon Pequegnat informed the members of the Academy of Medicine that Toronto's Health Department still considered household sanitation to be an important aspect of its work. Although the city's major growth spurts lay in the past by 1935, they had long-term effects on the amount and quality of housing. Industrial development and commercial growth prior to 1913 enlarged Toronto from roughly 90,000 in 1883, to 376,538 by 1911. The prosperity of the 1920s provided a further impetus to rapid expansion and by 1931 the city's population had reached 631,207.[21] In addition, the city expanded territorially from 17 to 39 square miles through a series of annexations of nearby villages and towns in

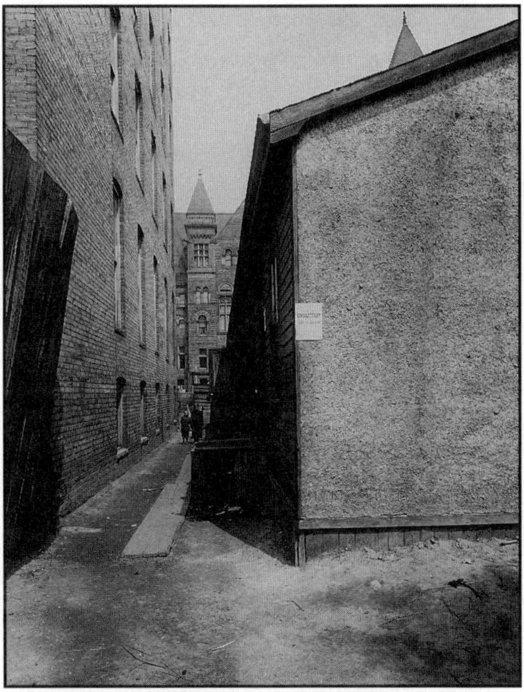

In May 1913, these houses were labelled "Unsanitary — Unfit for Habitation" by city inspectors. Ironically, the 1899 city hall overlooked this slum area.

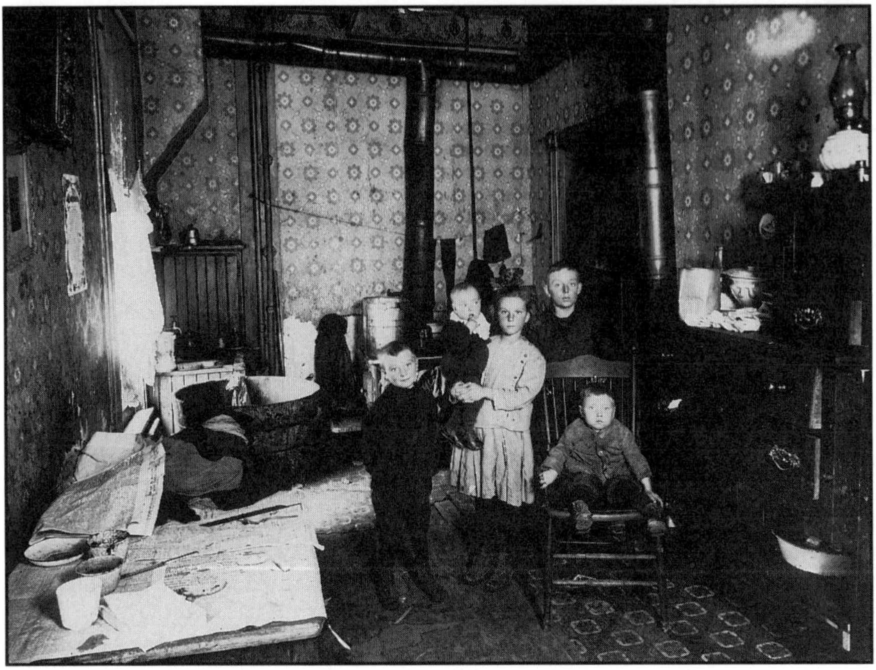

Housing reformers such as Charles Hastings used photographs like this one to justify their demands for municipal action prior to 1914.

the 1880s and the first two decades of the twentieth century. This rapid population and geographical development strained Toronto's housing resources and raised questions about the role of the Health Department in inspection and enforcement of minimum standards. In 1911, Hastings responded to these changes by creating two new divisions, Housing, and Industrial Hygiene, and dividing other sanitation activities between the Sanitation, and Plumbing and Drainage divisions.

Like most other North American cities including Montreal, Hamilton, Edmonton, New York City, Newark, and Milwaukee, Toronto's council relied on private builders to construct new homes. These men built in outlying suburbs for a middle class clientele who expected houses with the latest in heating and sanitation equipment.[22] Even when the city and the province gingerly moved into housing construction by supporting non-profit groups immediately before and after World War I, they targeted well-to-do workers rather than the urban poor and immigrants.[23] In Toronto and Hamilton, private enterprise remained dominant, and the two Health Departments were assigned the unenviable task of persuading homeowners and landlords to upgrade older housing.

As the first step in the battle to improve existing housing, Canniff, Allen, Sheard, and Hastings used their inspectors' reports to lobby the local board of health and council for a by-law that prohibited the use or construction of privies in any city building. Although the stench from uncleaned privies was unbearable on hot summer evenings, the major health reason for banning them in built-up areas was the well-founded fear that their presence contaminated water through subsoil seepage, and possibly food supplies (through fly-borne pollution). From an administrative standpoint, the amount of time which the Department's inspectors devoted to complaints concerning noxious privies was excessive. During his brief period in office, Norman Allen launched a campaign to eradicate privies and hence the "nuisance" complaints which he estimated consumed 60% of the inspectors' time.[24] His colleagues in Montreal and Hamilton made similar criticisms, but found few listeners during the recession of the 1890s and the frantic expansion after 1900.

When engineering technology was sufficiently advanced to enable builders to construct inexpensive bathrooms in homes, Allen's successors joined city engineers and other sanitarians in pressing city council for legislation that would eliminate these "relics of barbarism" from the downtown core.[25] In October 1913, the council finally passed a by-law that enabled Torontonians to have the city install indoor plumbing and add the cost to the individual's taxes. This represented the culmination of efforts that had begun in 1886 when Canniff had advocated that Toronto issue Sanitary Improvement Debentures, similar to those that Newark had introduced four years earlier to eliminate the "privy menace." By 1924, only 335 of the 18,000 privies which the Department's inspectors had discovered in 1912, still existed.[26]

Toronto's experience in convincing the council to support the abolition of privies through municipal construction of sanitary facilities in private

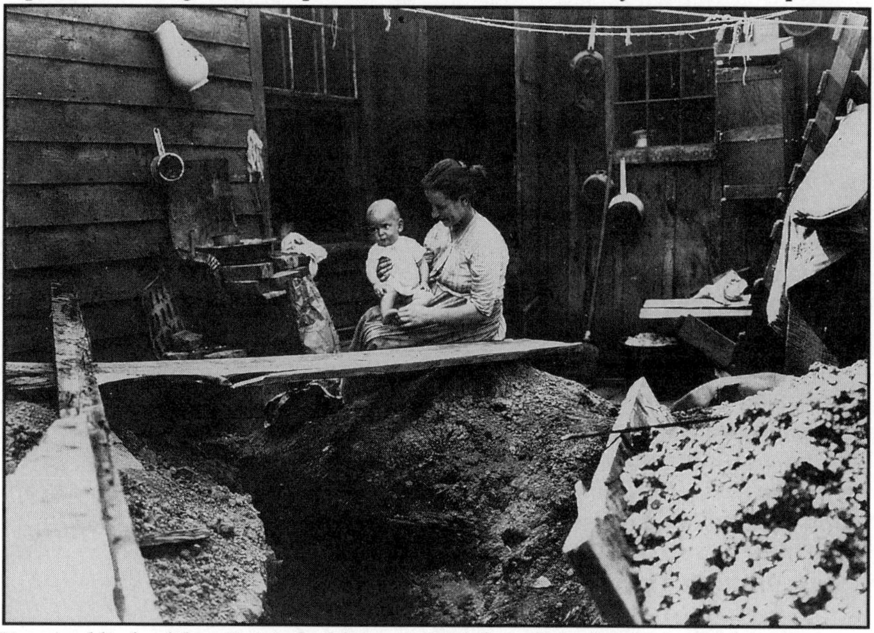

Since public health activists had long argued that removing household wastes was vital to protect children's health, connecting all the city's homes to its sewer system was essential.

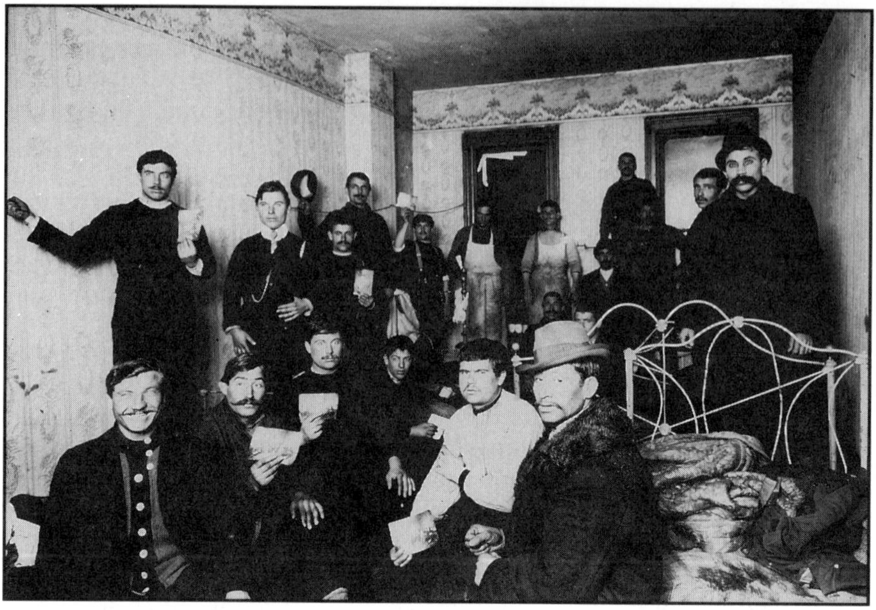

Overcrowding, particularly among immigrant workers, was a source of concern for health authorities.

homes was not paralleled in Edmonton. In the prairie city, the postwar economic recession from 1919–1923 prevented the Edmonton city council from passing a by-law similar to Toronto's and making "sanitary conveniences" a charge on the citizen's tax bill. By 1927, conditions had improved sufficiently that Edmonton was able to introduce the legislation, but the Depression quickly slowed down its implementation.[27]

The adoption of indoor plumbing solved only one aspect of Toronto's housing crisis. From 1896 to 1913, Toronto experienced an influx of immigrants, with the result that many families were forced to share sub-standard rental accommodation because of the housing shortage. Overcrowded conditions among the city's non-English-speaking immigrants had been noted in 1888, but by 1911, many citizens feared that Ontario's capital was in danger of repeating New York and Winnipeg's experiences with unsanitary immigrant ghettos. In 1911, Charles Hastings produced a *Report on Slum Conditions* which shocked middle class Torontonians into the realization that progress had produced poverty and urban blight. J.S. Schoales, one of the Department's inspectors, further highlighted the horrifying discoveries of the Sanitation Division staff:

> In 1912, we found 8,000 insanitary houses, alleys and rear dwellings; 1,500 houses practically unfit for habitation; 4,500 houses overcrowded as tenements, with from three to ten families in each; six, eight and ten of a family living in single rooms; 600 cellar dwellings,

damp, dark and overcrowded; over 500 filthy hovels in a most ruinous condition, surrounded by dirty foul-smelling undrained stables...; manure heaps, cesspools of slops, filth and garbage; evil-smelling privies, in some cases one for two or more families.[28]

Such appalling conditions had prompted Hastings to hire new inspection staff. Starting with four women appointed as "municipal housekeepers" in 1911, the staff of the Housing Division expanded to eleven, five of whom were women, by 1925. With their work focusing on immigrant and slum areas such as the Ward, the Housing Division staff gave advice on "cleanliness, sanitation and Canadian methods of housekeeping."[29] Such efforts represented both a humanitarian desire to help these people improve their living standards and a conscious attempt at assimilation to middle class values. Ironically, immigration declined during the 1920s as a result of exclusionary policies and was further limited by the Great Depression. Equally significant, the success of social work in professionalizing its case work method meant that the moralism implicit in the Health Department's home visits became passé in progressive circles.

Neither inspection nor education were expected to solve Toronto's housing crisis. Like many of his reform-minded Canadian and American contemporaries, Hastings became an outspoken champion of municipally-funded housing such as the British had undertaken. He used presentations to the Canadian Public Health Association, local women's groups, and the pages of the Department's *Health Bulletin* to alert citizens to the challenges

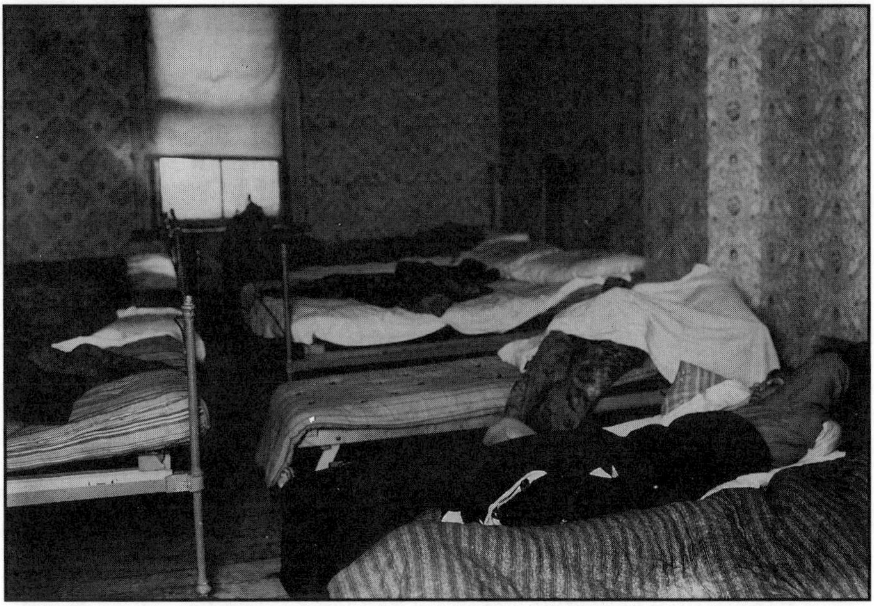

The Department's inspectors worked to eliminate congested boarding houses.

ahead. During the war years, his arguments, like those of colleagues in Hamilton, Edmonton, and Winnipeg, were in vain. In the climate of retrenchment that dominated the 1920s, few supporters could be found for such proposals, proving that the reform impulse of the previous decades had died out in the rush to return to normalcy.

The Great Depression reopened the housing question. In 1934, a survey conducted for Toronto's city council by the Lieutenant-Governor of Ontario, Dr. Herbert Bruce, and his committee, revealed that many of the slum conditions which Hastings had so graphically described in 1911, were still evident in the Ward and Moss Park areas. How had this happened given the continuous work of the Department's inspectors? Several factors contributed to the problem. First, as the Bruce committee bluntly observed: "People live in slums because they have to; because they cannot afford to live in better surroundings." Other than arguing as Hastings had, for a fair wage for workers, this aspect of the problem was beyond the Department's jurisdiction. Second, the Health Department was hamstrung by the legal requirement to prove that an individual's health had been "definitely impaired" by living in a house (valued at over $2,000), which it wished to condemn.[30] Statistics which the Department provided to the Bruce Committee indicated that tuberculosis morbidity and infant mortality rates in Toronto's slum areas were double the city average, but that between 1929 and 1933, only 67 houses had been condemned. Jackson justified his staff's restraint by noting the hardship which evictions would cause at this time.[31] For the Bruce committee, the solution was publicly funded urban renewal and increased powers for the Health Department's inspectors. Although plans for inexpensive workers' housing were included in the *Bruce Report*, the Depression and World War II prevented their immediate implementation, and in the interim, the provincial government did little to amend the Public Health Act's sanitation regulations.

Most other Canadian cities faced worsening housing problems in the 1930s. Montreal, Vancouver, and Winnipeg suffered from extensive overcrowding as unemployed people from rural areas flooded into the cities looking for accommodation and relief. As Mayor Ralph Day reported to the local board of health, Montreal's city engineer told the 1934 Canadian Public Health Association annual meeting that overcrowding had increased greatly since 1932, and that many "dwellings...owing to their age and condition, are neither advantageous to their occupants nor profitable to their owners, and for this reason could be repaired and remodelled." He also noted that Montreal did not have any slums as defined by its Health Department, which considered them to be dwellings "that it is unhealthy to live in."[32] In Edmonton, the city's health inspectors demolished a shack town which the unemployed had created, and then discovered that there was little they could do to provide alternative accommodation.[33] And like other Ontario cities, Hamilton's inspectors noted a decline in sanitation standards and supported the appointment of a special committee to investigate the problem. In 1937, the federal government finally moved to establish a housing program, but it supported the construction of new homes and contained only limited loan provisions for renovating existing ones.

During the 1930s and 1940s then, Toronto's inspectors, like their counterparts in Edmonton, devoted their attention to maintaining housing standards and preventing deterioration. A typical day's work for the sanitation inspectors during these decades was summarized like this:

> Report & sign in at City Hall at 7:50 a.m.
> Turn in previous days[sic] work & get work for day.
> Leave City Hall at 8:30 & go out to district.
> Investigate complaints sent in, re-inspect previous complaints, report on progress of work done. Complaints consist of general inspection of dwelling houses, plumbing & drainage, roofs and eavestroughs, wet cellars, garbage disposal, heating of premises, condition of furnaces, temperature of rooms in cold weather.[34]

Such a narrow focus on specific housing deficiencies demonstrated the increasingly legalistic posture which Jackson instructed his staff to adopt.

In 1943, Toronto's city council created a Reconstruction Committee, one of whose tasks was to investigate urban redevelopment. For the next two years, Toronto's Planning Board and the Citizen's Housing Association pondered the location of the first project, its design criteria and funding arrangements. Neither group sought input from the Health Department, although improving the residents' health was one of the project's goals. Why wasn't the Health Department an active participant? For an underfunded administrator like Jackson, public housing was the responsibility of city planners and architects, not health officers or inspectors. The medical officer's limited perspective on this matter was surprising, since the American Public Health Association had produced a series of studies in 1938 to demonstrate the health hazards of substandard housing.[35]

In spite of this evidence of a return to the crusading enthusiasm of prewar reformers in the United States, Toronto's Regent Park public housing project was begun with federal funding in 1947 under the direction of a group that did not include health workers. Presumably, the Department's senior staff did not want to be involved in the "petty political interference" which the CPHA Study Committee on Public Health Practice believed characterized this type of municipal activity.[36] No clearer illustration of the contrast between the social activism of the Victorian public health activists and the professional reticence of their successors could be found. Still, a survey conducted in 1953 indicated that the public health nurses had noticed a definite improvement in the sanitation of the new homes and in the inhabitants' hygiene practices.[37]

Prosperity in the 1950s slowed the demand for further public housing in spite of additional revelations of the abysmal conditions in the Ward.[38] And at the beginning of the 1960s, interest in rebuilding the downtown core and constructing a new city hall took precedence over public housing because Mayor Nathan Phillips and Metro Chairman, Frederick Gardiner, both

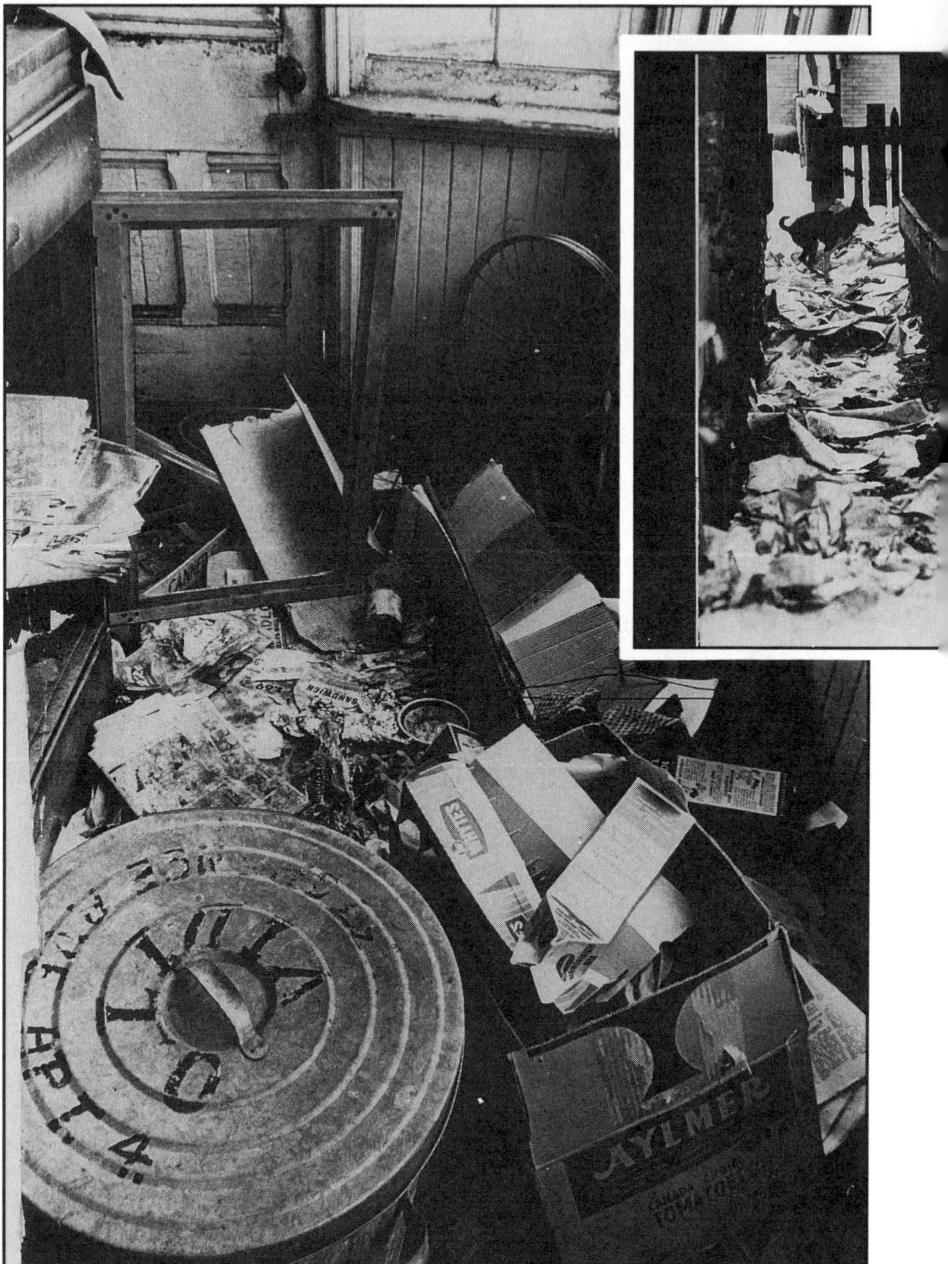

By 1965, living conditions in the houses slated for demolition (above and right) for the St. James Town project were abysmal. The Department's inspectors condemned this housing and prosecuted the landlords who owned it.

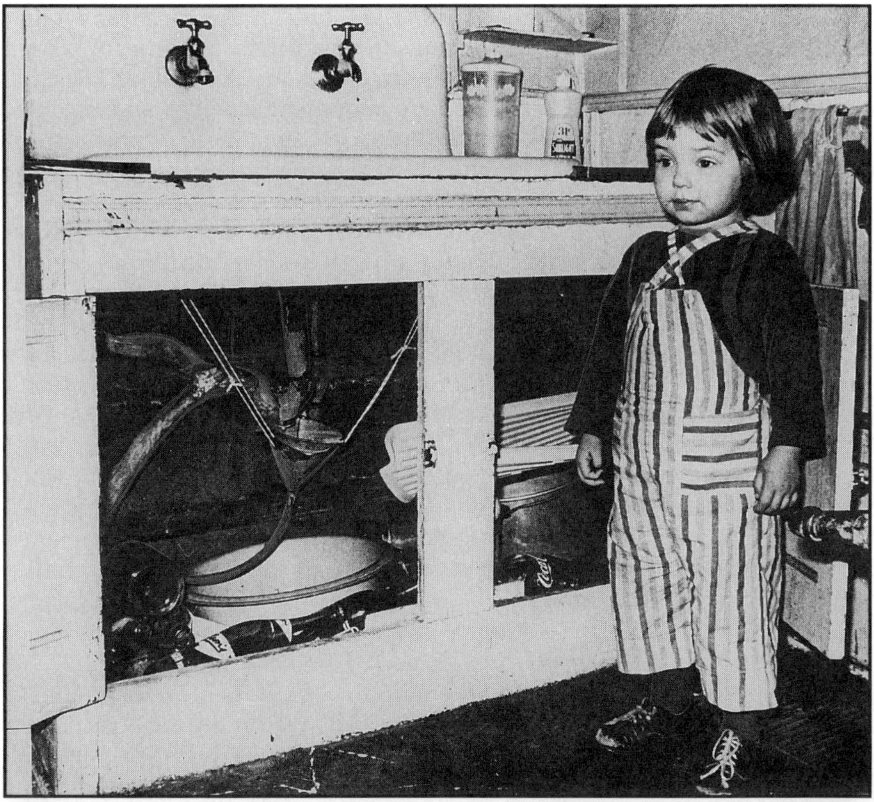

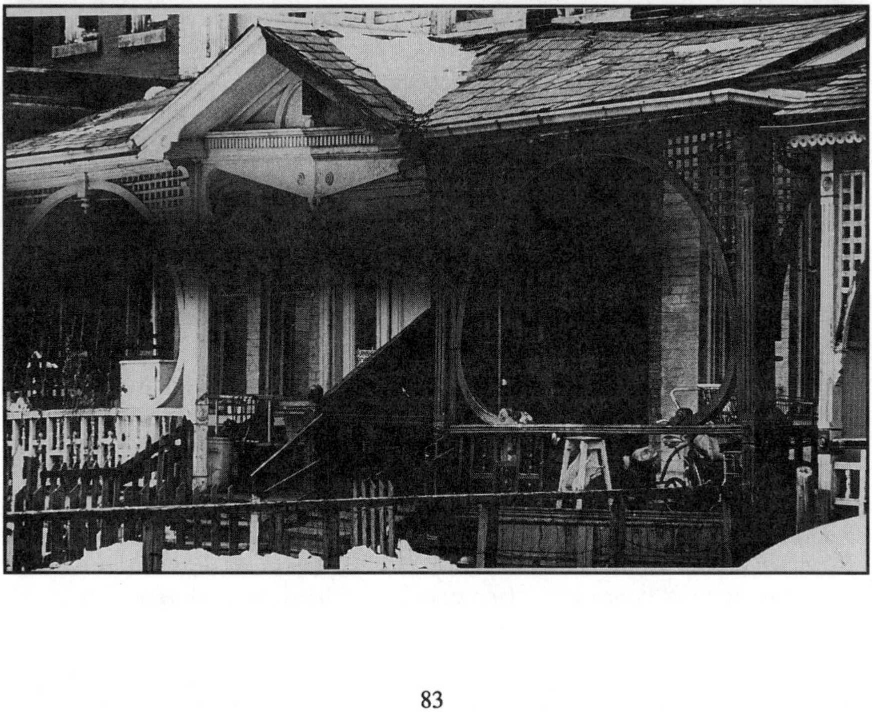

believed in the benefits of unrestricted development. The plight of welfare families, however, moved the politicians to seek public funding for several new housing projects including Alexandra Park and Don Mount. The city's executives also encouraged private redevelopment schemes and accepted Belmont-Meridien's proposal to raze slum housing along Parliament south of Bloor and replace it with a planned high rise community called St. James Town.

Prior to the construction of St. James Town's fifteen buildings, welfare and low income families rented the run-down houses scheduled for demolition. Conditions were so dreadful that the *Toronto Telegram* ran an exposé called "Ghetto of Poverty" to shock its readers into demanding action. In fact, the sanitation division inspectors were doing their utmost to locate the "adroit dodgers" who were renting out these houses, but found that little could be done to convince these speculators to fix glaring problems. Bedbugs, cockroaches, broken plumbing and lack of running water were health threats which the sanitation inspectors saw daily.[39] Although Toronto's inspectors had traditionally avoided condemning unfit housing unless alternatives were available, conditions had deteriorated so badly in the St. James Town area that many houses were closed through court action because they were "unfit for habitation."[40]

From 1965 to 1967, the sanitation inspectors also participated in the St. James Town Neighbourhood Unit project. This community-oriented and community-directed project was intended to assist low income families to relocate, with a minimum of disruption and maximum assistance from social service groups including public health nurses. The inspector's role was to inform the group's agencies of families in need whose rental accommodation was being condemned.[41] This project demonstrated the potential for fruitful interaction between two key components of the Health Department staff, many of whom had already established an informal network of information-sharing about clients.

In the late 1960s, the annual influx of flower children produced an accommodation crisis. The hippies took over abandoned buildings or camped out on vacant lots, in spite of opposition from neighbouring homeowners and businessmen. After extensive negotiations, health inspectors organized hostels or youth tent cities to ensure that their "realistic but improvised" sanitation standards were observed by "one of the most difficult segments of society."[42] The opening of the Rochdale co-operative apartment in 1968, created even more headaches for the sanitary inspectors because the people who lived there consistently violated the city's sanitary code.[43] Plugged toilets, overflowing garbage cans, cockroaches, mice, vermin, and an illegal pizza-making operation challenged the sanitation inspectors' tact and ingenuity, because in contrast to the working poor who tended to accept the inspectors' recommendations, the middle class hippies opposed any threat to their civil liberties.[44] By 1972, Rochdale had become a focal point for public opposition to the drug culture and the threat which the alternate lifestyle posed to Toronto's sense of order. Canada Mortgage and Housing foreclosed on it that year, and after complete cleaning and renovation, the building reopened as the Senator David Croll apartments for seniors and the disabled. From 1883 to the present, protecting the quality of Toronto's housing supply has been a central feature of the inspector's duties. Their efforts have been frustrated by the intractability of the problem.

Inseparable Issues: Sewage and Water Quality

The waste that people produced inside their homes generated great concern in the nineteenth century. For Canniff, removing human excrement as quickly as possible was essential to prevent typhoid, diphtheria, and cholera — all of which he considered "filth diseases." In the 1880s, water closets and sanitary sewers were sanitarians' solutions to this problem. Toronto's health officer publicized this option through the Toronto Sanitary Association, a voluntary group made up of architects, engineers, doctors, politicians, builders and philanthropists. With the support of a reform-oriented board of health and Mayor Howland, two referenda on constructing a trunk sewer were held in 1886 and 1888. In the first campaign, Howland publicized the medical officer's typhoid mortality statistics at a public meeting organized by the scheme's west end opponents. During the mayor's speech, a member of the audience interjected to support his claims about the health benefits of waste removal with "God Bless you. It's me that's suffered from it."[45] In spite of such evidence of the need for modern sewage facilities, both referenda were defeated because ratepayers feared higher taxes and the type of administrative incompetence that had led to corruption in the waterworks department, and shoddy workmanship on public works projects, such as the Garrison Creek sewer and dredging Ashbridge's Bay.

Toronto's rapid expansion and the endemic presence of typhoid led several councils to hire noted British and American civil engineers to investigate the problem and make recommendations. None of these plans was implemented because of lack of capital and public demand. Such reasons were not acceptable to the Provincial Board of Health which had been trying to persuade the aldermen to support modern methods of sewage disposal since 1884. When Charles Sheard joined the Provincial Board in 1906, he acquired a strong base of professional support for his attempts to end the problem. But why was the health officer intervening in a technological matter?

Both the "sanitary idea" and the science of bacteriology posited a close relationship between human waste and disease. As the leaders of the medical profession and responsible public servants, Canniff and Sheard would have been remiss had they not adopted the reform rhetoric and campaign strategies of their British and American counterparts. Their efforts also reflected a refusal to see the problem solely as the city engineer's responsibility, despite engineering's emergence as a separate profession. In 1907, Sheard addressed Toronto's business élite at the Empire Club to build support for sewer and waterworks construction. Warming to his theme, he informed his audience that their hopes for the city's future depended on their willingness to pay $3.5 million for an intercepting sewer system to deliver Torontonians' waste to a sewage treatment and filtration plant. The sophisticated technological approach that he recommended had been developed in the United States, after research teams at the Massachusetts Institute of Technology proved that sewage was not purified by lake or river currents. As the provincial capital, Sheard wanted Toronto to set an example of enlightened management for the cities around Lake Ontario by filtering its effluent and thus not contributing to further pollution.[46] In 1908, the medical officer's rhetoric and the civic boosterism of his business and professional supporters carried the day. As a result, by 1913 Toronto had an effective system in operation, and Charles Hastings was able to divert staff inspection efforts from this activity, and instead, to assign responsibility for monitoring the extent of sewage contamination to the Island Filtration Laboratory.

With improvements in water filtration and the construction of additional settling tanks for the city's effluent, the trunk sewer functioned effectively until the end of the 1930s. During the 1920s, Toronto's growth strained its ability to treat the waste water because the sewage plant had been built to treat 33 million gallons of waste a day and the city was producing 66 million by 1938. Starting that year, the medical officer warned the board of health that a new plant was essential. On May 1, 1939, the council appointed an Engineering Review Board consisting of two American experts and three Canadians, including Dr. A.E. Berry, the Director of the Ontario Health Department's Division of Sanitary Engineering, to look into the matter. The majority report recommended constructing an activated sludge plant in Ashbridge's Bay at an estimated cost of $9.5 million. Although they were loath to saddle taxpayers with the expense, the council held a referendum on the matter in 1940.[47] Strong voter support for the project failed to initiate construction and by 1941, the fecal coliform count was increasing according to the Department's hourly water tests. In spite of pressure from the board of health and the medical officer, little was done because during the war steel was unavailable for civilian projects.[48] The new sewage treatment plant was finally opened on Ashbridge's Bay in 1951.

Although the city's sewage was now 95% treated, the new facility could not purify the harbour waters because suburban development polluted the Don and Humber Rivers north of Toronto and washed up on the city's beaches. Since the health inspectors had been appointed to monitor the quality of water at Toronto's beaches in 1928, they remained involved even after Metropolitan Toronto was created in 1953 and jurisdiction over water and sewage was transferred to the Metropolitan Works Department. As part of its efforts to regionalize services and modernize management through long-range planning, the Ontario government established the Ontario Water Resources Commission in 1956 and the Metropolitan Toronto and Regional Conservation Authority in 1957. Controlling upriver pollution was assigned to these bodies, but by 1959, Boyd was closing Toronto's beaches, and in 1961, the *Globe & Mail* was printing editorials demanding additional treatment plants for the suburbs.[49]

Gross sewage contamination was only one part of the problem. Studies conducted during the 1970s revealed more than 400 different chemical contaminants in the waters of Lake Ontario and the Niagara River.[50] As European and American researchers demonstrated the carcinogenic properties of these products, reform groups arose to criticize the chemical industry and to lobby the federal and provincial governments. In contrast to the nineteenth century, when reformers naturally turned to local governments and Toronto's health officers had spearheaded the crusade for sewers and sewage treatment, twentieth century environmental advocates were slow to contact either the local board of health or the Health Department, because they did not believe that local authorities had the power, will, influence or funds, to deal with regional or international water pollution.

During the 1970s, health inspectors conducted weekly tests on the city waterfront. A slight improvement in water quality kept the beaches open until 1983, when severe thunderstorms and high temperatures pushed the coliform count above acceptable limits. Through the decade, senior staff argued that the beaches should be a recreational area not a wasteland, and in 1974, the federal Health Department also indicated interest in air and water pollution as environmental factors which required long-term commitments from all levels of government. The growing consensus among those favouring health promotion led the members of the Health Planning Steering Committee to include recommendations for Health Department advocacy activities in opposition to chemical contamination of air, water and food supplies.[51] And monitoring such concerns was included in the core programs which the health inspectors now carry out in their health areas.

Water Quality: A Perennial Problem

The purity of Toronto's water supply has always been inseparable from its waste disposal practices. Before the age of refrigeration, water was important not just for drinking, but also for producing ice to preserve food supplies. Although the city had purchased the waterworks in 1872, complaints that it produced "drinkable sewage" dominated discussion in the 1880s because Toronto took its water directly from the heavily polluted harbour. In 1884, Canniff started to publicize the water quality problem by asking visiting British experts to test its purity. Not surprisingly, they found it contaminated. After storms, citizens like insurance executive W.H. Orr, discovered mud and "a sort of sea-horse...with antlers and numerous legs" in their drinking glasses.[52] Legally there was little that the medical officer could do to combat such visible contamination because he did not control the scandal-plagued Waterworks Department.

During the 1890s two significant developments occurred. In 1893 the wooden water intake pipe on the floor of Toronto Harbour broke and floated to the surface. The influx of polluted harbour water caused a typhoid epidemic, which led to renewed public interest in water purification. The same year Charles Sheard appointed noted chemist E.B. Shuttleworth as the city's part-time laboratory head. Shuttleworth's systematic analyses of the water demonstrated the impact of storms, changing water levels and seasonal variations on the number of fecal coliform bacteria present in the city's supply. His test results enabled the Health Department to warn citizens through "orchestrated shrieks from the press" when it was necessary to boil their water to prevent typhoid.[53]

Sheard, however, wanted a long-term solution to the problem, and agitated for the construction of a new waterworks system based on the best British and American technology. Construction began in 1908, but the outbreak of typhoid in 1910 enabled him to experiment with a new approach to

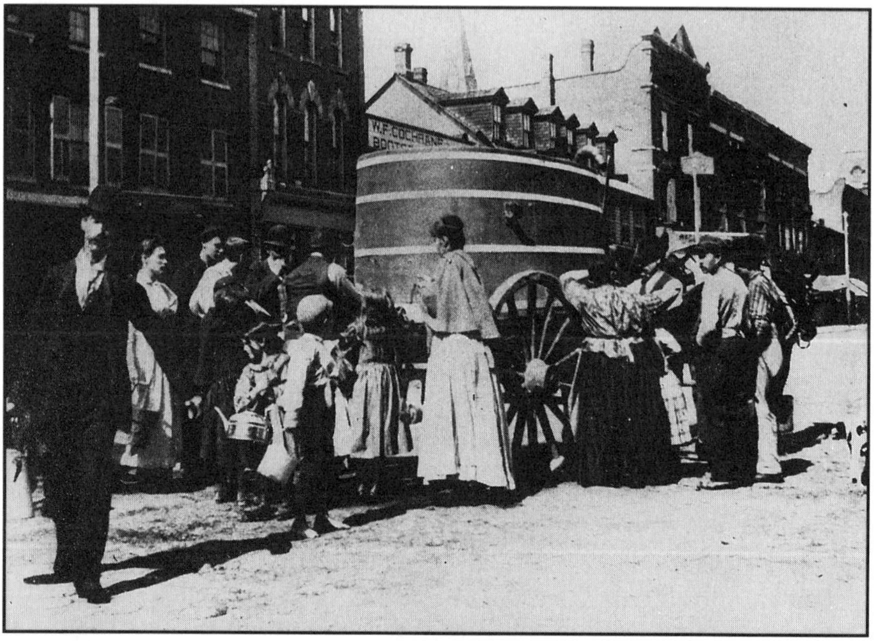

In September 1893, when the city's water intake pipe broke and a typhoid epidemic occurred, Torontonians had to turn to water carts for household supplies.

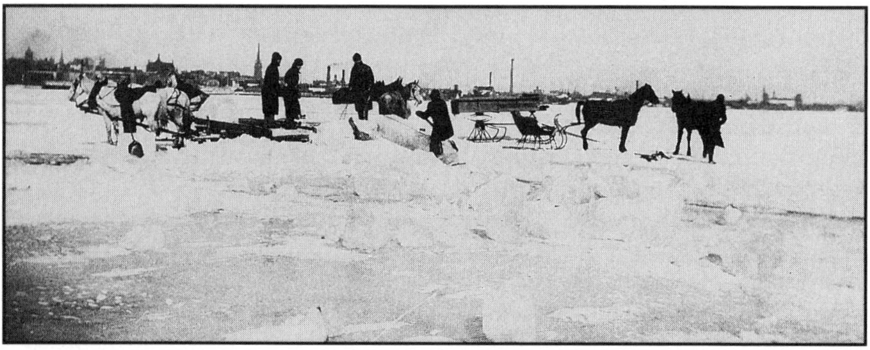

In the 1880s and 1890s, the Health Department organized a permit system for ice cutting. By 1900, Toronto harbour waters were too polluted to allow ice cutting for refrigeration to continue and many ice companies moved to Lake Simcoe.

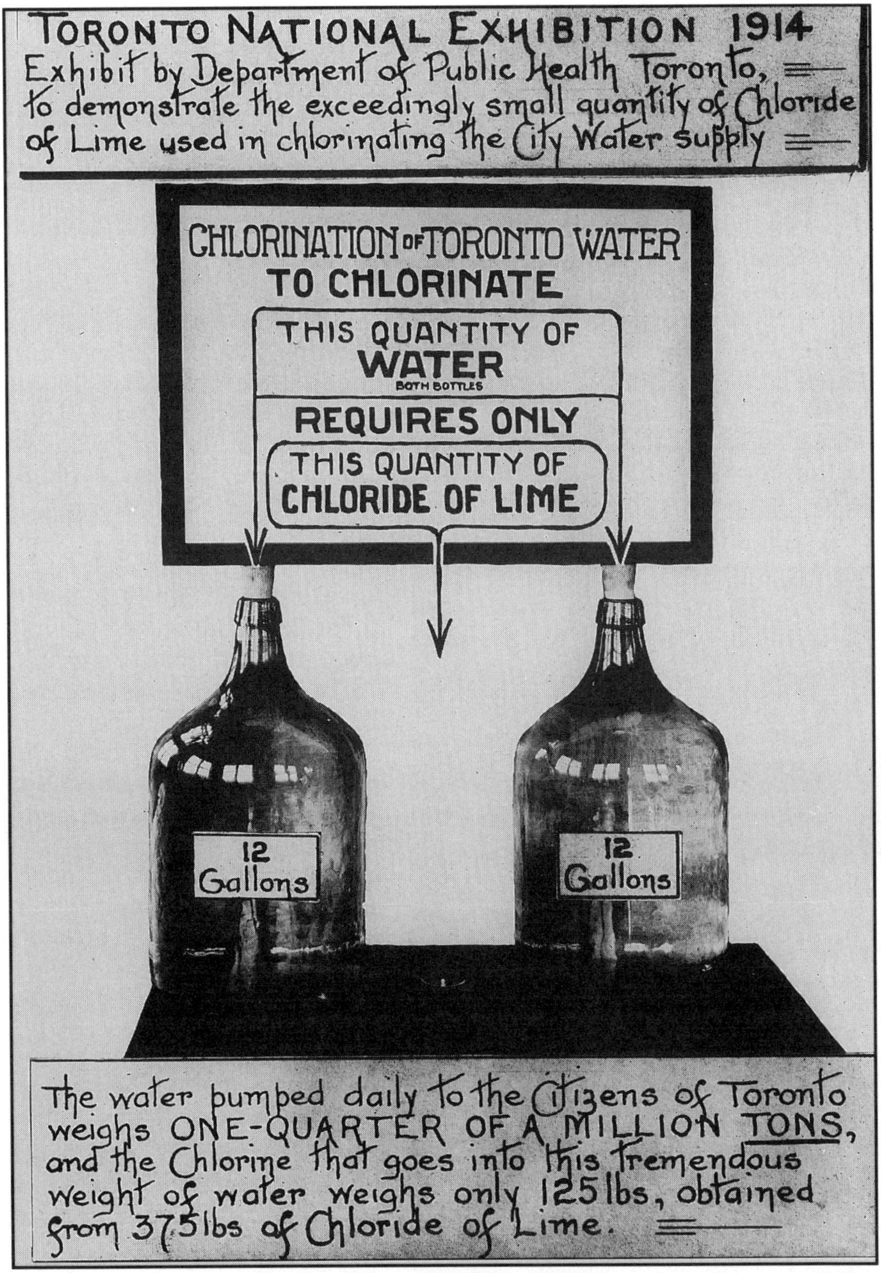

In response to public complaints about the excessive amount of chlorine used to purify Toronto's water, the Health Department prepared this display for visitors to the Exhibition in 1914.

water purification: chlorination. Toronto was among the first North American cities to use this method to control an epidemic and then to continue to use it for everyday purposes. By 1911 cities like Albany, New York, Philadelphia, Hartford, Nashville, Kansas City, Montreal, and Ottawa, had joined Toronto and Chicago in chlorinating drinking water.[54]

The impact of chlorination was evident in the declining death rate from typhoid. In 1910 typhoid claimed 40.8 victims per 100,000 cases; in 1914 only 7.7 per 100,000 died, and by 1915 this had diminished to 1.9 per 100,000.[55] Such a sharp drop in the number of cases and deaths signified the effectiveness of Sheard's use of the most recent American innovation and enabled Charles Hastings to declare the water purification campaign at an end.

But was it? By 1915, Hastings was contending with complaints from citizens concerning the water's taste. He assured these critics that the Department did not use any more chlorine than was necessary to kill the comma bacilli and that the"fishy, weedy, or chemical" taste was a result of chlorine "hooking up" with other chemical compounds, particularly trade wastes like coal tar. This explanation, and displays at the Canadian National Exhibition of the small amount of chlorine used on a daily basis, eased criticism until 1927. At that point, in response to a request from the local board of health, the city laboratory implemented taste prevention treatment after conducting hourly taste and odour tests. On the basis of their results, the staff chlorine operators adjusted the amount of the chemical that they used, to maintain water quality while avoiding any mustiness. Toronto's approach to this aspect of chlorination was so effective, that by 1937, Norman J. Howard, the Director of Water Purification, had become a well-known expert in the field and Toronto's work was copied by British and American cities.[56]

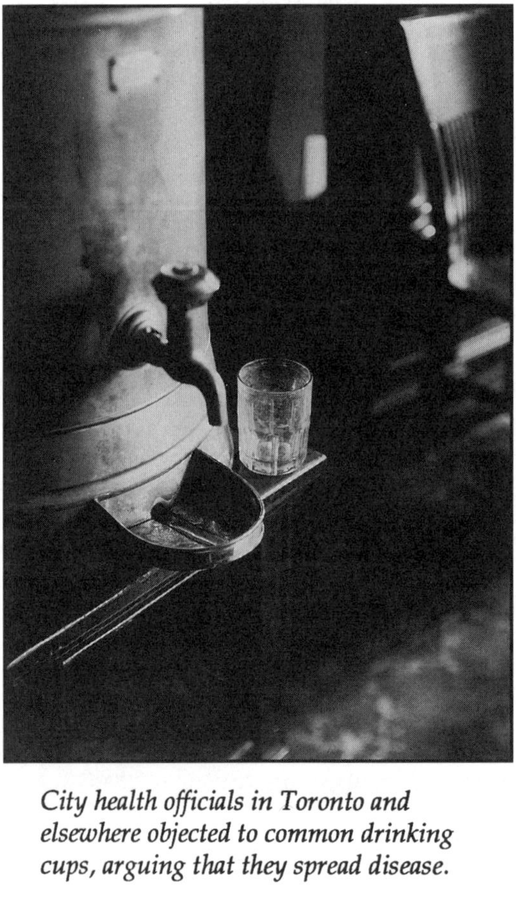

City health officials in Toronto and elsewhere objected to common drinking cups, arguing that they spread disease.

In 1934, Howard reported that the Filtration Plant Laboratory had carried out 9,690 chemical and 12,568 bacteriological tests of city water, and 4,478 tests of raw water because of growing concern about pollution. The daily bacteriological tests of tap

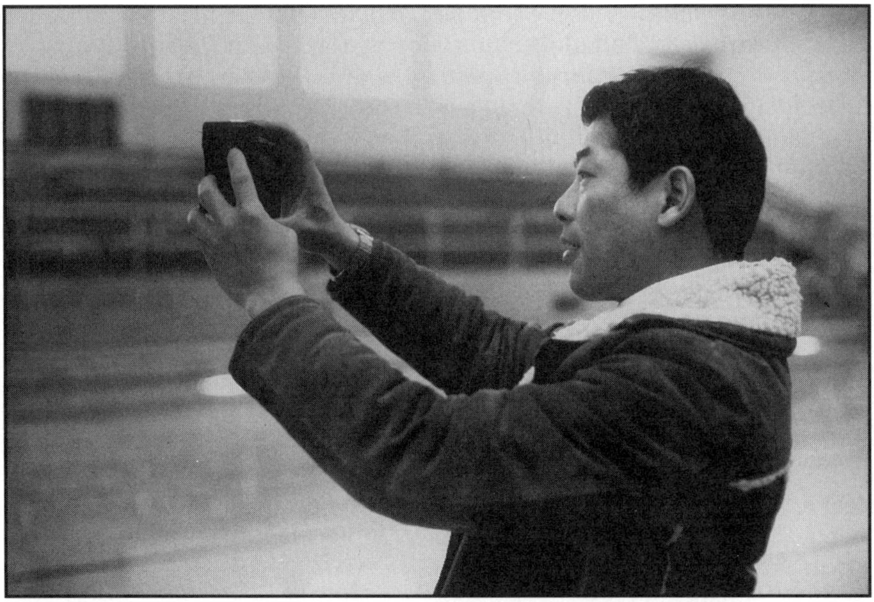

Swimming pool inspection has been one of the inspectors' duties since the late 1920s.

water were graded on a scale that was more demanding than the standards set by the American Public Health Association, in order to protect the quality.[57] Howard continued his contributions to the field by participating in the Canadian Public Health Association's Committee on the Bacterial Examination of Water and Sewage in 1942.[58]

Although its responsibility for ensuring water quality ceased with the creation of Metro, the Health Department continued to receive citizen complaints and to monitor the city supply. Both the Department and the board of health were approached for advice and support by individuals and groups concerned about water pollution. In 1963, the local board of health received a request from the Wentworth County Council asking it to assist the Hamilton-based group's effort to obtain provincial legislation banning mineral-based detergents. Recognizing the limits of its jurisdiction, the board did not act on the matter because the Metropolitan Works Committee was assessing it. Even more important, the medical officer, Dr. Boyd, did not have any evidence to indicate that detergents posed a health threat.[59] At this time, the board was not prepared to assume an advocacy position without valid scientific proof.

That proof emerged in the following two decades. In the 1970s, banner headlines warning the public about the latest chemical hazard found in the water created a climate of unease. Toronto's best known environmental group, Pollution Probe, was formed in 1969 to research this and other contentious environmental issues. It produced two highly critical reports, *Toxics on Tap* (1981) and *Drinking Water: Make It Safe!* (1983). The educational aspect of these studies was overshadowed by their political intent which was to serve as an external goad to action by the Health Department.

In 1983, the Department appointed a three woman research team to investigate the quality of Toronto's water in comparison with that of other Canadian cities and bottled sources. The researchers were also asked to assess the existing methods of water filtration and purification. Like their bacteriologically-oriented predecessors, these members of the Health Department were using the most up-to-date scientific methods to respond to public demands for information. In their report *Toronto's Drinking Water: A Chemical Assessment* (April, 1984), the researchers stressed the international dimensions of the pollution problem in Lake Ontario, and pinpointed chlorination as one significant factor in the mutation of the various chemicals found in the water. By conventional standards, Toronto provided its citizens with acceptable water, but the research team argued in favour of stricter standards and more comprehensive monitoring by the Metro Works Department and the provincial Ministry of the Environment. They urged the Health Department to advocate further research into the impact of various chemical combinations and to encourage public participation in the resolution of this problem.[60]

Conclusion

From 1883 to 1910, Toronto's sanitary inspectors laid the foundation for the modern city. By educating their fellow citizens to adopt basic levels of urban sanitation and reasonable water quality standards, these men and women were preparing the way for the application of the germ theory to Toronto's water through laboratory analysis, and enabling the public health nurses to educate their clients about tuberculosis, rather than typhoid and other water-borne diseases. But some problems were beyond their jurisdiction.

Housing was the prime example because the Department's inspectors were powerless to deal with the root cause: poverty. The quality of the city's water supply was another intractable issue since the water was polluted beyond the city's boundaries, and international co-operation was needed to clean up Lake Ontario. But most importantly, the decline of public and professional interest in sanitation and environmental problems after 1920 marginalized the inspectors and their contribution. Not until chemical contaminants proliferated after 1950 would the public again recognize the importance of establishing standards and monitoring health hazards. Then they turned once more to public health inspectors, whose expertise had been finely honed after a century of health education through "persuasion not coercion."

Chapter Five

From Producer to Consumer: Protecting Toronto's Food Supply

"You are what you eat" is a contemporary slogan which reminds consumers of the importance of assessing the nutritional value of the foods that they purchase. Today few shoppers pause to wonder whether the meat, milk and other products which they are buying have been processed under sanitary conditions and inspected by qualified representatives of municipal or federal departments. A century ago, citizens were not so sanguine about the quality and healthfulness of the foods that they bought, because Toronto only had a single food inspector, Robert Awde, who was hard pressed to carry out his duties.

When the Health Department was established in 1883, Awde assumed that some of his tasks would be transferred to the new organization, and in fact, Dr. William Canniff took on the responsibility of inspecting meat and milk supplies for visible signs of contamination and putrefaction. His inspector also visited dairies, cow byres and slaughter-houses to examine their sanitation standards. Such activities were derived from inspection practices in American and British cities and represented the sanitary reform phase of the international public health movement. As an understanding of the germ theory of infection spread among the public and the medical profession, pressure grew for federal and provincial authorities to establish scientific standards for food supplies. Municipal health departments were charged with carrying out inspection and analysis duties, and this brought them into conflict with citizens and businessmen. Like their colleagues in the Sanitation Division, the Food Control inspection staff quickly developed effective negotiating skills, and worked to persuade food producers and restaurant owners to conform to city by-laws.

By the 1960s, the staff of this division were also involved in health education activities. This work had grown out of the food handler education classes which Toronto's Health Department and the Health League of Canada introduced in 1944. In the post-war period, the arrival of large numbers of non-English-speaking immigrants added to the inspectors' workloads, as they had to translate their educational material into many languages and modify the Department's regulations to respond to different food production methods. Technological improvements in food processing since 1945 have also modified the inspectors' tasks and enabled them to devote more time to health education. Their activities have provided a secure foundation for the nutrition advice which the public health nurses and the Department's nutrition consultants offer.

The City's Food Control Division

When the Markets and Health committee was deliberating about the duties that should be assigned to the new medical health officer in 1883, the workingman's paper, the *News*, added its contribution to the proceedings by observing that:

> In his investigations of food, he will be expected to visit the boarding houses, and to experiment with every known variety of hash. The dwellers in these caravansaries will look to him to restrain the cook from mixing more than a legal amount of old boots, and the late lamented cats with the stews, and to insist that mules' ears be not fried in sand and played off for veal cutlets.[1]

In fact, the new Department's early food inspection activities were much more mundane, and restaurant inspection did not become important until the early twentieth century. In the 1880s and 1890s, meat and milk were the centre of attention because of the concern about the sanitation of the premises in which these commodities were produced. Neighbours' complaints about the stench and flies around slaughter-houses led Canniff to recommend the construction of a municipal abattoir, after his inspectors discovered that slaughter-house operators were dumping blood and offal into city sewers. The emphasis on environmental concerns reflected the contemporary belief that putrefying waste caused disease, and this prompted the Provincial Board of Health to set building standards for slaughter-houses within city limits. Since Canniff's call for an abattoir and the provincial

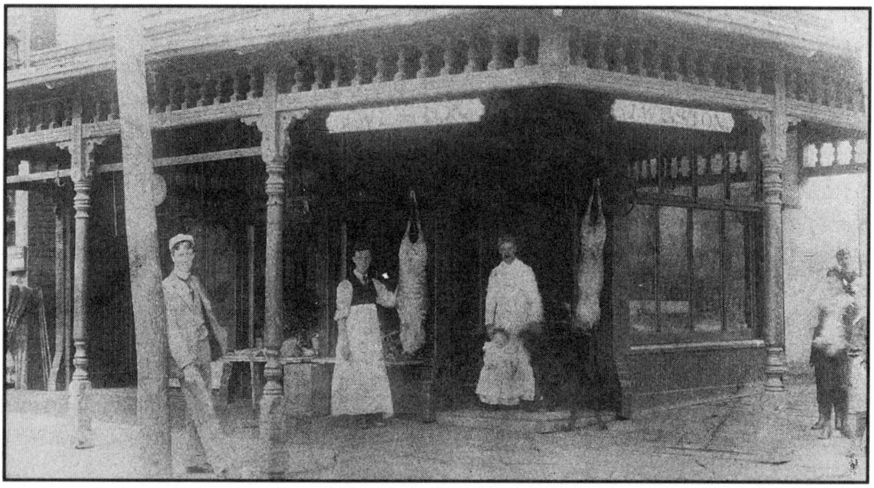

In 1896, Joseph Weston's butcher shop was one of the many commercial operations that the Department's food inspectors visited.

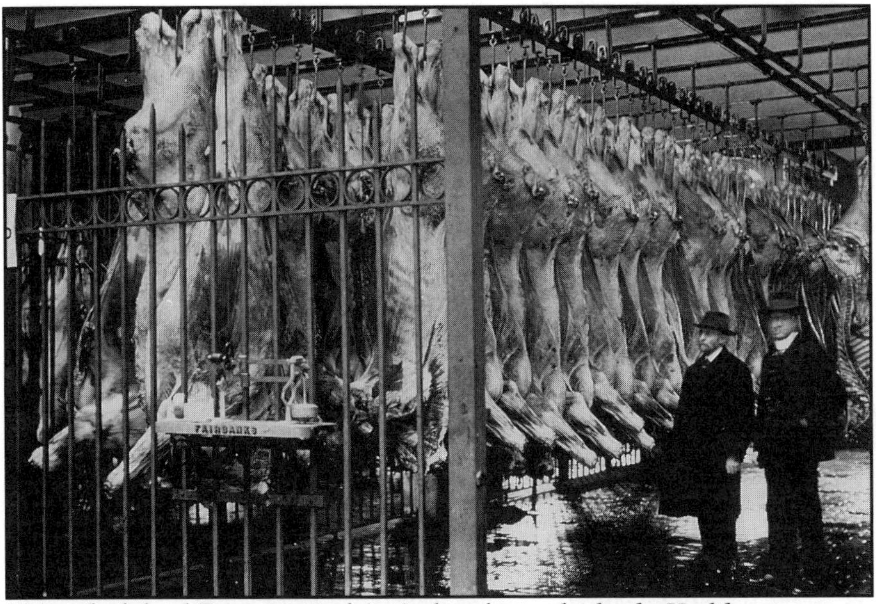

Using the federal Department of Agriculture's standards, the Health Department's veterinarians monitored the quality of Toronto's meat supplies.

requirements threatened their livelihood, Toronto's butchers rallied to create a Butchers' Association to oversee the quality and cleanliness of their businesses.[2]

When food inspection was transferred to the Medical Health Department in 1896, Dr. Charles Sheard introduced the concept of bacteriological analysis by using his annual report to warn the local board and the public about the diseases which infected the city's meat supplies. Although actinomycosis, an infectious disease affecting cattle and pigs and occasionally humans, was most prevalent in the 1890s, tuberculosis replaced it after 1900 as the most feared disease. Sheard's reading of European research and his inspectors' reports, led him to support the demand for a city-run abattoir to ensure that Torontonians were able to purchase disease-free meat.[3] His successor appointed veterinary inspectors to examine the city's meat and milk supplies — a practice which large British cities had introduced. The city's veterinarians shared inspection duties with federal Department of Agriculture staff, but neither group was large enough to control the meat trade completely. In 1914, the city opened its abattoir and many of the small slaughter-houses closed.[4]

During the First World War, the amount of food inspection declined as Health Department staff enlisted. With the return of several of the Department's veterinarians after wartime service in 1919, meat and dairy inspection began to approach their prewar levels by the mid-1920s. Under the direction of Dr. A.R.B. Richmond, the Division of Food Control expanded to a staff of twenty-four by 1935. With the growing recognition that food contamination during processing was responsible for disease out-

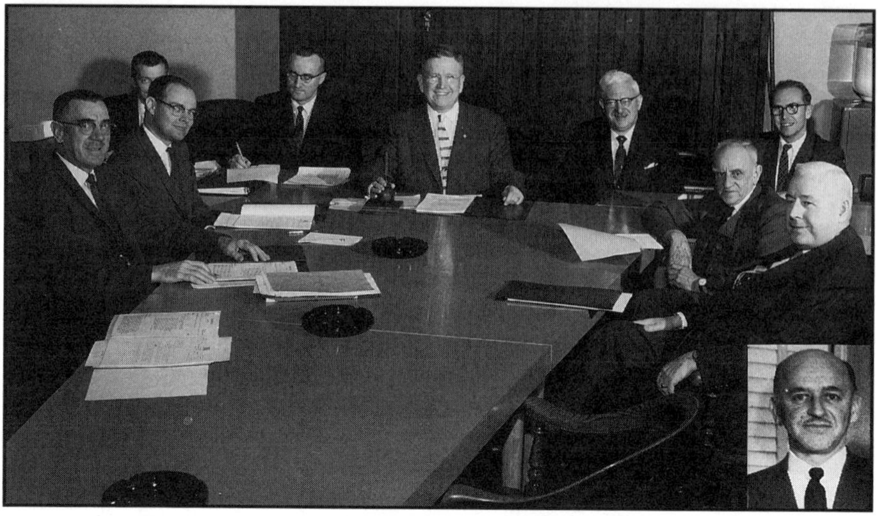

Aldermen Harold Menzies (in the striped tie) and Kenneth Ostrander (inset in right corner) expressed their worries about the Department's meat inspection practices to the medical officer, Dr. Boyd, Mayor Nathan Phillips and other members during the local board of health's meetings in 1960-61.

breaks, the Food Control staff increased their activities to include inspection of 2,621 wholesale and retail grocery, fish, fruit and vegetable, and confectionery stores, 362 bakeshops and confectionery factories, 43 poultry killing plants, 880 butcher shops, 56 meat-products plants, 64 beverage plants and 2,622 restaurants. Within the city boundaries, members of the Food Control staff were able to maintain standards and to improve the quality of the food products being consumed.[5]

To protect the meat supply, the Health Department retained jurisdiction over the abattoir until it was sold in 1960, after criticism that its director, a former inspector, was permitting inhumane slaughtering methods. A Board of Control committee investigated the charges and found them groundless but the Health Department was relieved to see this responsibility devolve into private hands.[6] Beyond the city, however, uninspected poultry killing plants still existed, and unscrupulous cattle dealers sold infected carcasses to Toronto merchants. In 1960, Alderman Kenneth Ostrander aroused public attention concerning uninspected meat sales, while in 1962, Alderman Harold Menzies provoked a major controversy over contaminated chicken.[7] Although the aldermen wanted the city to be given power to inspect outside its limits, Dr. J.M. Glenroy, the Director of Food Control, recommended a provincial inspection system instead.[8] Eventually provincial legislation was passed and the controversy died down.[9]

During the 1950s and 1960s, both Toronto and Edmonton's inspectors faced new challenges. Explaining municipal and provincial food quality and sanitation requirements to non-English-speaking immigrants was difficult but essential, because establishing trust is such an important aspect of ensuring compliance. Early in the 1970s, for example, the Chinese practice of keeping barbecued meat at room temperature, caused disagreement between the inspectors and restaurant and store owners in both cities since it contravened federal regulations which required meat to be kept chilled or heated. In Toronto, careful scientific assessment revealed that this cooking process did not pose a health threat and after lengthy negotiations a mutually satisfactory arrangement was reached. In Edmonton, the director of the inspection division opposed such a compromise and compelled the local board to follow federal guidelines rather than the merchants' wishes.[10]

"From Cow to Consumer": The Milk Campaign

For over a century, the Health Department's campaign to establish and maintain milk quality depended heavily on international techniques and standards. In the 1880s, the medical officer and his inspectors adapted the British approach and emphasized the sanitary conditions of the city's cow byres and dairies. During their visits, Toronto's inspectors found herds of cattle confined in filthy, cramped barns, being fed distillery slops instead of hay and other food. These conditions were very similar to those which inspectors uncovered in Milwaukee, New York, Hamilton and other North American cities. In 1888–9, the inspectors performed 2,563 inspections, and all dairy owners had to have a cleanliness certificate from the Department before they could apply for a city license.[11] If the sanitation standards were not met, the milk was condemned.

The difficulty in relying on subjective assessments was illustrated by a legal case in which a dairy owner whose milk had been condemned sued the medical officer and the city for damages. The dairyman, Mr. Forsyth, won his case in both the lower court and on appeal. The interesting aspect of the Appeal Court judgement, however, was that only the medical officer was liable to pay the damages of $300 because he was not a "servant of the corporation" and according to the Chief Justice, it was his error which had harmed Forsyth's reputation and business.[12] This judgement indicated the need to clarify the health officer's status and to move to the next phase of the international public health movement — bacteriological analysis — for the scientific proof that would support the inspector's activities.

In 1893, Charles Sheard did just that. Although his inspectors continued to evaluate the sanitary conditions of local dairies and farms within a forty mile radius of the city, they also collected milk samples for analysis. In the city laboratory, Shuttleworth discovered that Toronto's milk was contaminated with dirt and tuberculosis bacilli, and adulterated with water, boracic or salicylic acid, and annatto (a yellow dye.)[13] By 1909, the medical officer had concluded that municipal by-laws alone would not protect the milk supply and that a provincial milk act was imperative. From the research that he had conducted, Sheard was able to convince the local board that Toronto should adopt the milk quality standards in use in cities like Detroit, Buffalo, and Montreal because they were enforceable.[14]

In fact, Sheard was joining a crusade that had started a year earlier when the Canadian Medical Association had established a Milk Commission. This group investigated milk production practices, and urged the federal government to legislate pasteurization standards as a means of protecting Canadians against milk borne diseases like tuberculosis, diphtheria, scarlet fever, typhoid, and septic sore throat. British researchers had linked outbreaks of scarlet fever and typhoid to infected milk in the 1880s, and in 1903, two leading American pediatricians published a study that demonstrated the relationship of bad milk and cholera infantum, a gastrointestinal disease which killed thousands of children annually. For the sake of future generations, the reformers demanded government action.[15]

One of the most vocal supporters of compulsory inspection and pasteurization was Charles Hastings. He was motivated by a personal tragedy because one of his infant daughters had died of typhoid contracted through drinking contaminated milk purchased from one of the city's best dairies.[16] To spare other parents the grief which he and his wife had suffered, Hastings accepted the medical health officership when Sheard resigned in September 1910. As one of his first acts, Hastings had the city's inspectors trace the origin of the typhoid epidemic. They found that a small dairy was using contaminated well water and that one of the farmers who supplied it was recovering from a case of typhoid fever. These revelations represent a classic illustration of the mode of transmission, and encouraged Hastings to make pasteurization one of the principal goals of his years in office.[17] The episode also proved the accuracy of the milk crusaders' slogan: "You don't catch Typhoid — you eat it or drink it."[18]

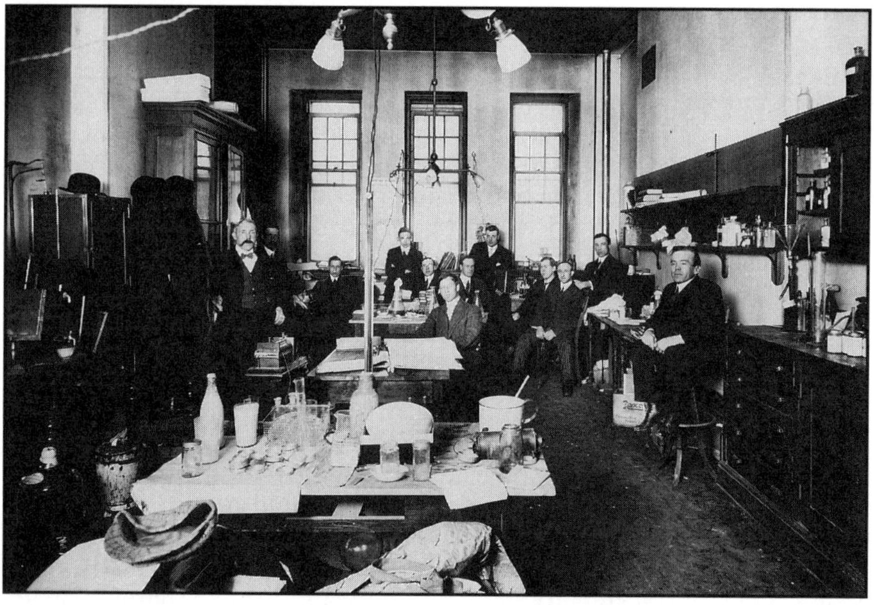

Under Charles Sheard, all the Department's analysis activities were carried out in this increasingly cramped laboratory.

DEPARTMENT OF PUBLIC HEALTH, TORONTO 5M-9-13

Owner or Lessee of Farm.................... Address.................... Inspector....................

Total Number of Cows.................... Number Milking.................... Quarts Produced....................

Breed.................... Milk Shipped to.................... By....................

			DATE		
COWS	Health	5			
	Condition	3			
	Clipped Flanks (clean)	10			
	Clean Udder	10			
	Water Supply	5			
	Feed	2	35		
STABLE	Cleanliness	12			
	Removal of Manure	4			
	Construction	5			
	Light	4			
	Ventilation	5			
	Cubic Space (500 c. ft.)	4			
	Stable Yard	6	40		
MILK HOUSE	Construction and Location	4			
	Cleanliness	5			
	Care of Utensils	4			
	Cooling Facilities	5			
	Small Mouthed Pail	7	25		
	Total		100		

Toronto's milk inspectors filled out this scorecard during their visits to the many farms which supplied city dairies.

Although the milk crusaders were disappointed that the federal government did not pass legislation requiring pasteurization, they were pleased when the Ontario government passed its Milk Act in 1911. Toronto was the first city to apply the permissive legislation but it was quickly followed by London, Guelph, Niagara Falls, Port Arthur, Stratford, and Hamilton.[19] Hastings used the opportunity to expand his staff and appointed a corps of veterinary inspectors to travel to the 2,000-2,500 farms which supplied Toronto dairies. These men were to examine the herds, the premises, and the farm workers for evidence of typhoid or tuberculosis three times a year. The 25,000 cows were not consistently tuberculin tested because the provincial law did not require this, and as Hastings discovered, trying to do so could lead to "boycott and milk famine." The most that the veterinarians could do was to prohibit infected milk from being shipped to Toronto.

In the city, the milk inspectors examined both the sanitation of the 1,425 milk stores and dairies and the quality of the product that they received from their suppliers. They used the following techniques:

> Bacterial samples are taken by removing a few cubic centimetres of milk from each can...as soon as the seals are cut, and this milk is placed in a sterile test-tube which is plugged with cotton. These samples are...examined as soon as possible. A dirt test is made by filtering one pint from each can through an absorbent

> cotton disc. If the milk contains crude dirt, it is at once condemned as unfit for human food and poured down the sewer. Sometimes the dirty milk is dyed red and returned to the shipper, and in this case a large red label is attached to the can. The farmer thus loses the milk, and if returned, his neighbors all see his condemned can at the station.[20]

The initial tests were intended to encourage farmers to maintain cleanliness and to prevent adulteration. During their inspections, the city staff also completed score cards, which assessed the cleanliness of the premises, the effectiveness of bottle sterilization procedures, and the healthfulness of employees.

Toronto's medical officer was clearly adapting methods used elsewhere. Between 1892 and 1906, twenty-seven leading American cities had set up milk commissions and during the decade before his appointment, Hastings had visited pioneers like Nathan Straus in New York City to observe milk depots in action. The Americans developed a variety of score cards, and in 1910, Edmonton's first milk and dairy inspector introduced that technique in his city. Although publication of the score card results encouraged improvements in the quality of Edmonton's milk, it did not lead to support for compulsory pasteurization.[21]

Unlike his predecessors, Hastings mounted a wide-ranging educational campaign to promote the use of available technology and thus ensure a pure milk supply. In 1911, he had introduced a monthly *Health Bulletin* to keep

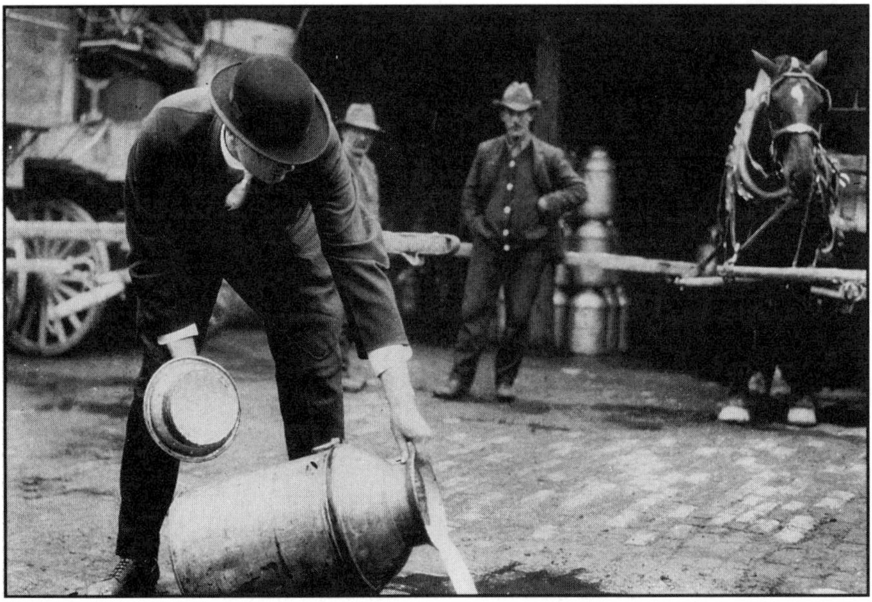

Dumping condemned milk into a city sewer effectively demonstrated the inspectors' determination to maintain high milk quality standards.

Torontonians up-to-date on the Department's work and international activities and research findings. He used this pamphlet to explain the Milk Inspection Division's work and the principle of pasteurization. Working from the inspector's score cards and the laboratory evaluations of milk samples, Hastings created a list of first class dairies whose names were

FIRST-CLASS DAIRIES.

Gratifying Increase in the Number of Best Dairies in Toronto.

The following is a list of dairies which obtained 80 marks or more out of a possible 100 at the scoring which closed on April 30, 1915. The next scoring closes on July 31, 1915, and the next list will appear in the August Bulletin.

Name. Dairy Name. Address.

Addy & Sons, Empire, 321 Rusholme Rd.
Anderson, C. F., Toronto Heights, 6 Boon Ave.
Anderson, F. G., Oakville, 6 Atkin Ave.
Ashby Bros., Beaver, 200 Riverdale Ave.
Baird, Jas., LaBeaute, 589 Dufferin St.
Barr, G. H., 583 Parliament St.
Beatty, M. H., 636 Jones Ave.
Brown, T., Lakeside, 113 Essex St.
Bunting, J. D., Beechwood, 90 Montrose Ave.
Carruthers, C. W., Western, 60 Kenwood Ave.
Caulfield & Son, 381 Roncesvalles Ave.
Chisholm Bros., Glenwill, 29 Fenwick Ave.
City Dairy Co., Spadina Crescent.
Clarke, E., Brampton, 134 Armstrong Ave.
Collins, J., Deer Park, 774 Markham St.
Cook, J., Willowdale, 287 Christie St.
Corkery, Jas. J., Downsville, 400 Euclid Ave.
Cosborne, R. D., Crescent, 670 Ontario St.
Cox, C., Runnymede, 473 Durie Ave.
Cox, R. W., Highland, Elizabeth & Park Rd. (Swansea).
Craggs, S., Westmoreland, 196 Clinton St.
Currie, J., Dovercourt, 155 Dovercourt Rd.
Dingwall, J. B., Langham Farm, 47 Gore Vale Ave.
Dockery, R. W., Acme, 21 Essex St.
Downing, H., Toronto, 108 Beaconsfield Ave.
Downing, T., Diamond, 127 Carlaw Ave.
Downing & Shortt, Ravenswood, 132 McPherson Ave.
Dunlop, J., 208 Wilton Ave.
English, T., Olive Farm, 68 Shaftesbury Ave.
Ewing & Reynolds, 718 Dufferin St.
Farmers' Dairy Co., Queen St. W.
Fayter, A. G., Royal, 246 Brock Ave.
Fitton, J., Wychwood, 64 Hendrick Ave.
Gourlie, K. R., Model Farm, 26 Brookfield Ave.
Goodman & Griffiths, Parkdale, 180 Garden Ave.
Grace, E., Yeovil, 424 Ontario St.
Hannah, W. F., Palmerston, 874 Palmerston Ave.
Heagle, J., Wheatsheaf, 89 Hallam St.
Hellowell, F., White Rose, 190 McCaul St.
Henderson, G., Fernbank, 1031 Dovercourt Rd.
High Park Dairy, 740 Dufferin St.
Hutchinson, W. A., New Jersey, 223 Osler Ave.
Legg, Mrs. E., Pine Hill, 77 Hocken Ave.
Lock, A. C., Briar Hill, 314 Dupont St.
Lock, J. H., Grimsby, 110 Robert St.
Marr, M., 16 Hamburg Ave.
Milsom, H., Leaside, 38 Soudan Ave.
Moore, J. V., Model, 199 Wilton Ave.
Muir, Wm., Beach, 19 Herbert Ave.
McCartney, W. J., Antique, 105 Millar Ave.
McKay, W. J., Canadian, 1421 Bloor St. W.
McMahon, H., Credit Valley, 103 O'Hara Ave.
Paulger, T. E., Blantyre, 1112 Queen St. E.
People's Dairy Co., 402 Parliament St.
Pett, D. A., Scarboro Farm, 17 Smith St.
Phillips, Geo., Fern Hill, 173 Prescott Ave.

Name. Dairy Name. Address.

Piper, F., Hatherleigh, 444 Soudan Ave.
Price & Sons, S., Queen St. E.
Rhodes, R., Jersey Farm, 21 Duggan Ave.
Ritchie, John, 51 Hayden St.
Roberts, T., Valley View, 835 Broadview Ave.
Robinson, F., 125 Bolton Ave.
Shaver, P., Walnut, 90 Annette St.
Smith, J. A., Cosborne Ave.
Smith, P., Cuckoo Valley, 25 Maple Grove Ave.
Smith, S. A., Alexandra, 256 Concord Ave.
Stanton, R., Richmond Hill, 1315 Davenport Rd.
Taylor, H., Cranston, 75 Bleecker St.
Tingle, J., 314 Gerrard St. E.
Warner & Sons, Linden, 376 Don Mills Rd.
Wellwood, W., Parkview, 339 Perth Ave.
White Oak Farm, 210 Mavety St.
Wilson, F., Brantford, 219 Lippincott St.
Young, J., Walmer, 159 Kendal Ave.

THE MILK JITNEY.

A dealer who brings milk to Toronto from the surrounding country has recently substituted a motor lorry for his wagon.

The milk brought to the city in this way should arrive in good condition if properly chilled before shipping.

ABOLISH THE "COMFORT."

A Bad Habit Which Should be Stopped.

There seems to be a feeling among mothers, and especially among young mothers, that when a child cries, if it is given a "comfort" to suck, everything possible has been done to soothe it. Infants acquire habits very readily, and once acquired they are difficult to break. If you rock your baby to sleep, for instance, after a few times you will find it hard to put it to sleep without rocking. The same applies to singing children to sleep. All such devices are means of focussing the babe's attention until overcome by sleep. The "comfort" of all habits is the most filthy, the most dangerous and the most unpardonable. Every nation should legislate against them and their manufacture should be prohibited.

No mother would think of taking her babe to a place where there is any infectious disease, but she overlooks the great dangers from infection to which the "comfort" exposes her child. This article is often picked up from wherever it may chance to lie, no matter in what exposed spot—it may even have been lying on the floor, or perhaps have fallen from the carriage on to the sidewalk.

Again, many mothers wet the "comfort" in their own mouths before giving it to the baby. This is especially dangerous, as the mother may be a "carrier" of some infectious disease germs, and, as the "comforts" are generally used with infants who are in a weakened condition, they are very susceptible to infection. Moreover, the child is frequently given the "comfort" to send it to sleep, and when it does so, the comfort drops from its mouth, to become a roost for swarms of flies, perhaps just come from some nearby soil napkin, or other filth. If, as is frequently the case, the

By May 1915, the Department was able to publish a lengthy list of first class Toronto dairies in the ***Health Bulletin****.*

published in the *Health Bulletin* starting in 1912. These lists not only guided consumers but also encouraged competition among the city's dairy owners. They represented the Department's move into publicity for health education purposes, a development which illustrated the close links which Hastings had with American public health officials.

One of the most well-known publicity activities which Hastings undertook was the Fly Swatting Contest of 1912. Again he derived his campaign from the American and Canadian public health movements. Colleagues like Dr. Thomas Whitelaw, Edmonton's Health Officer, and Dr. James Roberts, Hamilton's Health Officer, also conducted fly extermination campaigns in 1911 and 1912, both to eliminate a pest and to educate citizens about insect vectors. With prizes ranging from $1 to $25 offered by the *Toronto Star*, the contest was open to children and was intended to arouse their interest in protecting food and milk supplies from the ubiquitous house fly which was thought to spread typhoid and other enteric diseases. During the six weeks that the contest lasted, fly swatters became very popular and approximately 3.3 million insects were killed by enthusiastic children. The contest ended when the paper discovered that some competitors were breeding flies to increase their tallies.[22] As cars replaced horses and screens became common, the threat of fly borne contamination declined.

In spite of his initial emphasis on sanitation, Hastings's true objective was compulsory city-wide pasteurization. He used the *Health Bulletin* and public addresses to gain support. One of the most telling arguments that he put forward concerned the savings which his staff were obtaining for Torontonians. Working from an estimate that 40% of the city's milk supply had been watered before the laboratory started continuous testing, the medical officer calculated that the citizens had spent $275,000 annually on substandard milk. This amount was greater than the Health Department's budget in the early years! To make his point even more dramatically, Hastings had the Milk Control staff set up a model laboratory at the CNE in 1913. The exhibit showed visitors scientific evidence of the contaminants found in the milk supply.[23]

All of the Health Department's educational activities were designed to create community approval for pasteurization. As the only scientifically proven method of killing bacteria in milk, pasteurization was accepted by researchers and public health personnel but misunderstood or criticized by the public. Many people claimed that pasteurization destroyed the flavour and the nutritional value of milk. Numerous North American and European scientists studied the problem and concluded that the protective value of the procedure far outweighed any changes in taste.[24] Armed with this evidence, Hastings persuaded the city council to make pasteurization compulsory in 1914.

The one group who strongly opposed this measure were the milk producers. During the council debates on the issue, Hastings was warned that a large delegation of milk dealers intended to stage a protest in the council chamber. He responded by inviting them to meet in his office. During a clause by clause discussion of the by-law, the medical officer was

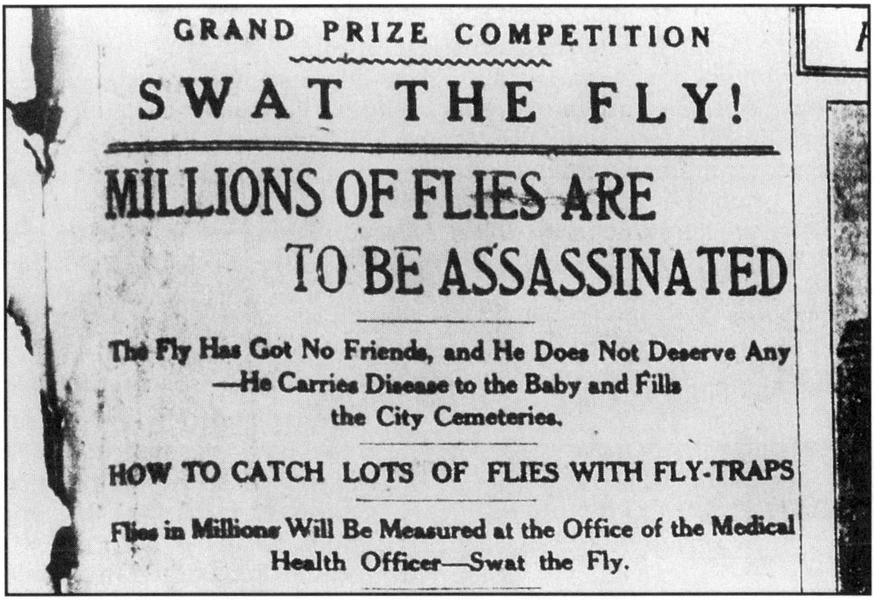
GRAND PRIZE COMPETITION

SWAT THE FLY!

MILLIONS OF FLIES ARE TO BE ASSASSINATED

The Fly Has Got No Friends, and He Does Not Deserve Any —He Carries Disease to the Baby and Fills the City Cemeteries.

HOW TO CATCH LOTS OF FLIES WITH FLY-TRAPS

Flies in Millions Will Be Measured at the Office of the Medical Health Officer—Swat the Fly.

*The **Toronto Star** sponsored the city's "Swat the Fly" Contest from June to August 1912. Designed to educate Toronto's children and eliminate a pest, the contest aroused great enthusiasm among youngsters.*

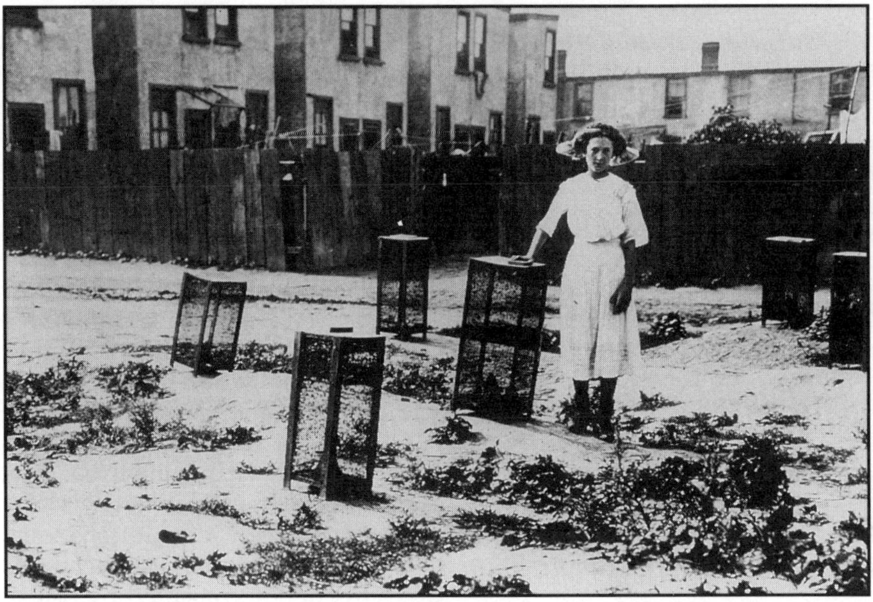

Beatrice White won first prize for killing the largest number of flies.

able to calm many of their worries. Since the most important problem seemed to be integrating the pasteurization equipment into the milk production process, Hastings agreed to a six month suspension of prosecutions to allow the producers to convert their facilities. This intelligent compromise pleased the milk dealers and they dropped their protest.[25]

Hastings continued his publicity efforts with the assistance of the Child Welfare Council of Toronto, the Canadian Public Health Association, and the National Dairy Council of Canada. Together these groups sponsored a "Milk Week" in Toronto from April 4–9, 1921. They targeted school children and homemakers, and gave the children blotters on which Mr. Milk Bottle announced that "Milk Makes Muscle," and blue buttons which said "I drink Milk." The whole community was saturated as advertisements appeared in restaurants, hotels, streetcars and department store windows. Children were asked to draw posters and make up jingles and the week ended with a play on the topic performed in Massey Hall. For adults, pamphlets, short talks at factories and offices, and public addresses by leading Canadian and American experts rounded out the campaign.[26] This effort, however, depended on the work of the sanitary inspectors in maintaining the quality of Toronto's milk supply.

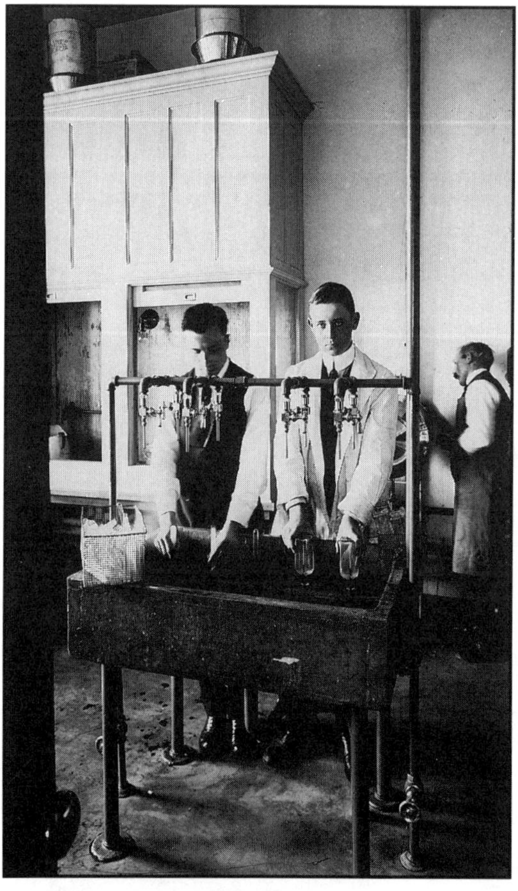

In April 1912, the Health Department opened new laboratory facilities in the city hall's attic. The milk analysis section is shown here.

With the introduction of pasteurization, the first three phases of international public health work had been melded into a coherent strategy to protect Torontonian's health. The success of the program was evident in the declining disease rate from milk borne illnesses. In contrast to Montreal which suffered a series of typhoid epidemics through the 1920s as a result of its "unsafeguarded milk supply," Toronto was able to control milk production from "cow to consumer."[27] The city's success earned it an international reputation, and Hastings was frequently consulted by British and American authorities who wanted to implement similar measures.[28]

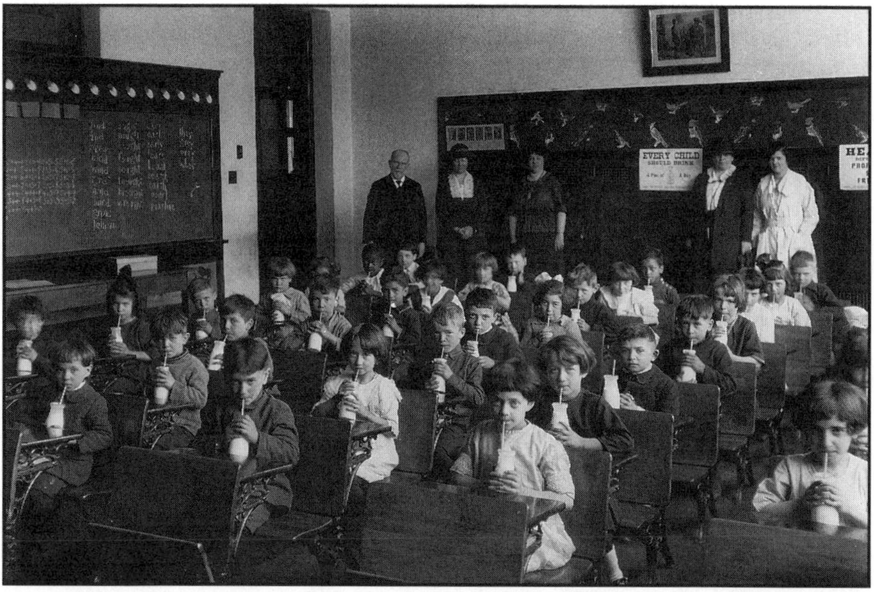

In 1923, pupils at Manning Avenue Public School participated in a milk drinking program which stressed the nutritional value of the product in their diets.

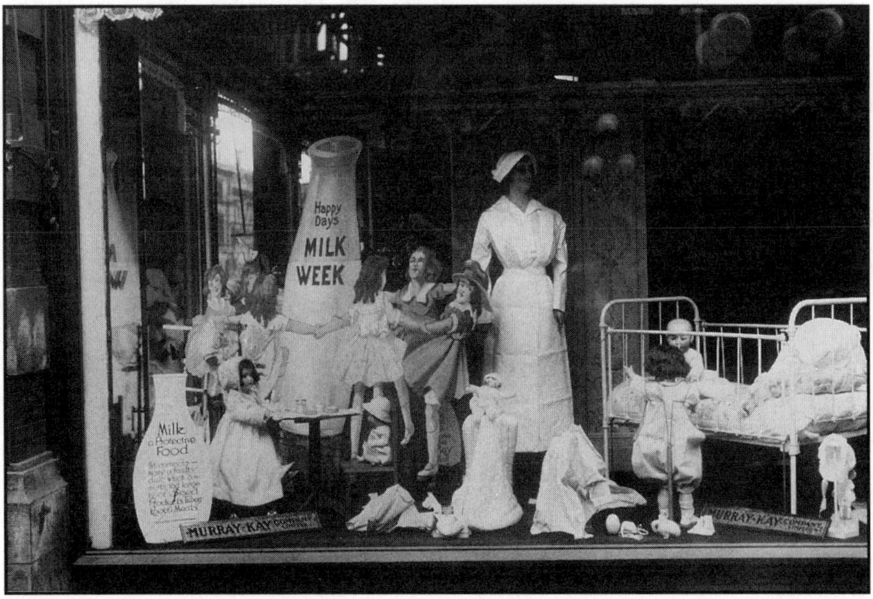

Modern advertising techniques, including commercial window displays, were used to publicize Milk Week.

In the mid-1920s, the Health Department requested that the Provincial Health Department take over farm inspection. Lack of funds prevented the province from doing this, and Toronto was left to carry on inspecting over 3,000 farms in a milk shed area stretching 300 miles from east to west and 150 miles from north to south.[29] Throughout the 1930s milk inspection on farms and in the city's dairies continued. On the farms, some producers were beginning to use refrigeration. Within the city, the Laboratory staff made 24,134 bacteriological and chemical tests of milk and milk products in 1933, and decided to introduce more tests on pasteurized samples because of growing concern about coliform contamination and adulteration.[30]

In 1938, the Hepburn government made pasteurization compulsory in Ontario. As a pioneer, Toronto's Health Department had been a source of staff for public and private groups, and by the 1940s, the milk inspection staff was drastically overburdened. Only three men examined conditions in the city's numerous dairies while five veterinarians covered rural areas. In its assessment of the inspectors' work, the Phair Committee expressed concern that the pressures of completing routine inspection prevented these men from conducting educational activities.[31] Both the *Phair Report* and the medical officer argued in favour of expanding the staff, and after the return of prosperity more inspectors were appointed. In the post-war era, they were required to have additional knowledge of milk production and analysis techniques. Technological changes in milk processing such as the introduction of tank holding and hauling, the replacement of glass bottles with plastic bottles, waxed cardboard cartons, and individual creamers in 1950s and 1960s, modified the inspectors' routine. With the amalgamation of the Food Control and Sanitation Divisions in 1974 and the introduction of computer sampling in 1975, the staff added inspecting dairies and other milk production plants to their duties.[32]

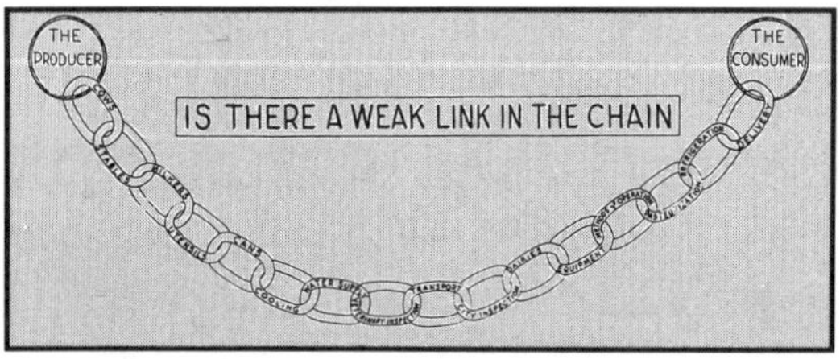

The Health Department was responsible for ensuring that there were no weak links in the chain from producer to consumer.

From Sanitation to Education: Restaurant Inspection

Since the turn of the twentieth century, Toronto's restaurants have also been inspected by Health Department staff. Starting in 1912, over two hundred restaurants serving various ethnic cuisines were examined for "cleanliness and proper equipment" under a Board of Health ordinance. Although the Health Department did not have the power to prosecute delinquent owners, it was able to influence their actions because they would not qualify for their city license without a permit from the medical officer. Hastings depended on his three full-time restaurant inspectors for this information.[33] In the 1920s, the Health Department introduced High Standard

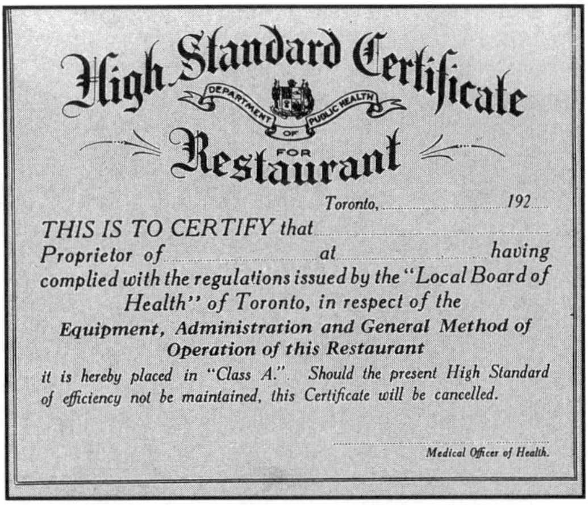
High Standard Certificate

Department of Public Health

for

Restaurant

Toronto, ... 192....

THIS IS TO CERTIFY that ....

Proprietor of .... at .... having complied with the regulations issued by the "Local Board of Health" of Toronto, in respect of the

Equipment, Administration and General Method of Operation of this Restaurant

it is hereby placed in "Class A." Should the present High Standard of efficiency not be maintained, this Certificate will be cancelled.

....

Medical Officer of Health.

High Standard Certificates were introduced in the 1920s to publicize "Class A" restaurants.

Certificates which were awarded to restaurants which conformed to the city's sanitation requirements. This publicity gimmick was intended to reward proprietors of clean restaurants and to aid the public in choosing a place to eat.

With confirmation of the role of the human disease carrier on the eve of World War I, health authorities had to reassess their focus on sanitation. Acting on the advice of the medical officer, Toronto's board of health turned its attention to food handlers. In 1923, the board passed a resolution favouring periodic inspection of food service personnel.[34] When the provincial government established its restaurant regulations, semi-annual medical inspections for waiters, waitresses, and other food handlers were included. By 1929, the restaurant inspectors were asking Toronto's 1,666 restaurant proprietors to show them the staff's medical certificates and to submit these documents to the medical officer.[35]

As the population increased, the number of restaurants also expanded. By 1935, the Department's inspectors were examining 2,622 food service premises to assess their lighting, ventilation, plumbing and general cleanliness. In the kitchen and the storage areas, the inspection staff noted dish washing procedures and the temperature of the water, the steps that the restaurant was taking to control "flies, dust and vermin" and the methods it used for the "handling and disposal of garbage." They also evaluated the health and cleanliness of the employees. This comprehensive inspection system functioned well even during the Depression. And as the Division Director, Dr. Richmond, noted in 1935, one of the more notable features was that many of the owner-operators of these restaurants came from countries with rather different standards for sanitation, yet these people "are amongst the cleanest in person and habits and the most sincere in their desire to meet all requirements."[36]

By the middle of World War II, however, the public was complaining that conditions in Toronto's restaurants had deteriorated significantly. In September 1943, a special meeting of the local board of health, Controller Robert Saunders, the health officer, the Food Control Director, and the six restaurant inspectors, was convened. Its purpose was to discuss improving sanitation, and making the provincially-required semi-annual health certificate for food handlers a legitimate exercise. During the discussion of these topics, it was clear that the health inspectors believed that their work was being undermined by inadequate support from local judges who constantly

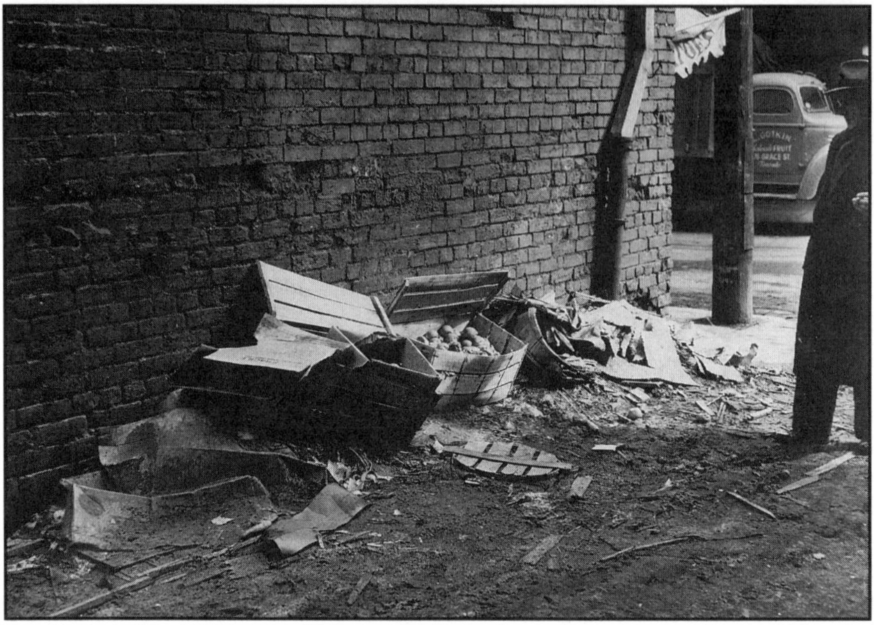

A Health Department inspector studying the type of waste disposal practices which attracted vermin and public complaints.

remanded their cases. More importantly, they also argued that most restaurant owners needed more staff and equipment than was available in wartime, and that generally, their suggestions were followed whenever feasible.

Dr. Richmond also argued on behalf of the restaurant owners, who claimed that staff shortages and their inability to raise pay rates because of federal wage controls, contributed to the problems that produced public complaints. To overcome the legal disabilities under which the Department currently struggled, the Food Control Director, his inspectors and the local board urged the province to amend its regulations to permit the medical officer to close unsanitary premises.[37] The request was vetoed by the provincial Health Department because other Ontario cities found the legislation acceptable.

Since the problem required action, the local board and the medical officer started to consult the Toronto branch of the Canadian Restaurant Association and various employees' groups in an attempt to formulate a strategy for enforcing sanitation standards.[38] Their efforts received a boost in 1946, when Robert Saunders was elected mayor. As one of the most vocal critics of unsanitary facilities, he ordered an immediate crackdown on non-conforming restaurants. To ensure that the public did not patronize these establishments, he used the morning and evening news to publicize the daily closures.[39] After he left the mayoralty to become the chairman of Ontario Hydro in 1952, the Department reverted to its traditional policy of persuasion and ceased to publicize restaurant prosecutions and closings until 1986.[40]

Mayor Saunders' other legacy to the Health Department was a rodent control division. According to the *Telegram*, Saunders spotted a large brown rat sitting in a food store window in March 1946, and decided that such "brazen" behaviour required action. He appointed A.L. Smith, one of the Department's inspectors, to head the new unit. Smith and his team started at the waterfront and moved block by block through the city, exterminating 220,000 rats by 1956.[41] In fact, the local board had been considering the rodent problem in 1945 and Saunders' action merely hastened the creation of a new sanitation activity. The council passed rodent control by-laws in 1949 and 1950 and these provided the basis for the inspectors' work on the redevelopment sites in the 1950s and 1960s, and at municipal incinerators and the CNE during the 1960s and 1970s.[42] Rodent and pest control have continued to be Departmental responsibilities, and in 1980, the inspectors received 500 complaints and made 11,391 inspections, and 7,978 re-inspections, to deal with 246 new rat infestations and 1,137 mouse infestations.[43]

Educating the Public: Food Handler Training

Vital as sanitation was, for the city's medical officer the real issue at stake in 1943 was the health and preventive knowledge of food service personnel. Given the transient nature of food industry staff, the health certificate system, which had been introduced in the 1920s, quickly became

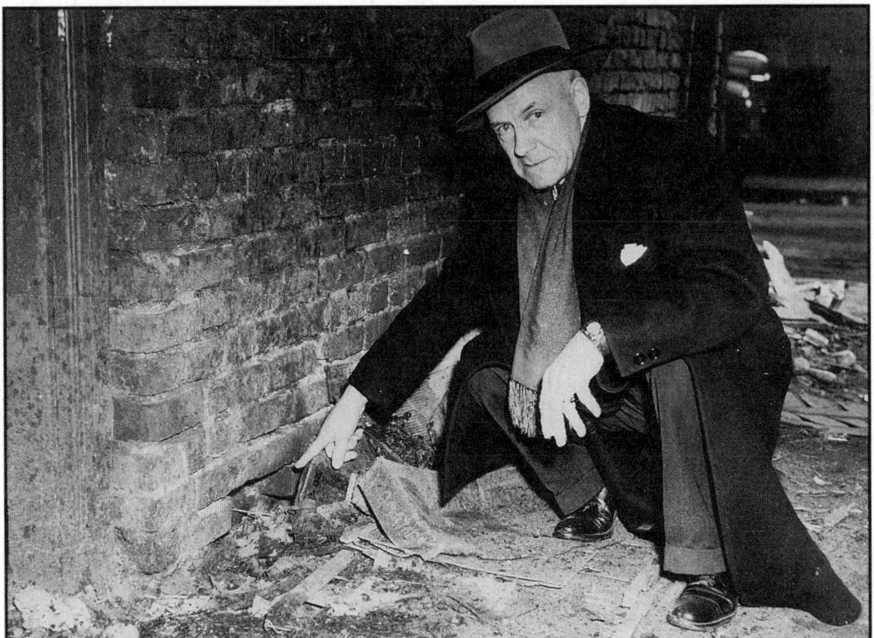

A staff inspector indicating a potential sanitation problem for the occupants of this building.

unworkable. As the population's overall health improved, the necessity for medical proof of freedom from TB and other communicable diseases ceased to be important, and by 1939, the American Public Health Association was questioning the relevance of such activities.[44] Like his American colleagues, Gordon Jackson had come to the conclusion that health education for all food handlers was the solution to the problem of occasional outbreaks of food poisoning.[45] Although the province was not willing to rescind the certificate system, both the Minister of Health and the Chief Medical Officer urged Toronto to amend the statutory by-law and introduce its own system of food handler registration and education.[46] Once again the province was depending on Toronto to pioneer a new approach to a common problem.

The medical officer responded by asking a voluntary group, the Health League of Canada, to organize short courses for food handlers. With the assistance of the food industry, the Health League introduced a food handler training program for students hired to work at the CNE in 1944. The course became an annual event for the Director of the Division and the Supervisor of Food Control because of the importance of protecting the health of the thousands of visitors who flocked to the Exhibition.[47] Of the 21 rural and urban health departments which the CPHA Study Committee on Public Health Practice surveyed in 1948, only Toronto and one other centre offered regular food handler courses.[48] During the exhibition, food control inspectors did double shifts to ensure that the lack of refrigeration for meat and other foods was not hazardous for fairgoers, and that graduates of the training course were following the lessons they had been taught. This situation improved at the end of the 1950s when permanent food concessions equipped with refrigeration were finally completed.[49]

During the 1950s and 1960s, the Food Control staff tried a variety of health education tactics. In 1960, the Department published a selection of two line poems by the medical officer, Dr. A.R.J. Boyd, the Division's Director, Dr. J.M. Glenroy, and one anonymous colleague because the 3,000 word pamphlet which they had been using had not attracted much attention. With only minor poetic license, the senior staff warned the public:

> Garbage cans placed high on racks
> Give the rodents heart attacks.
>
> When you handle other's food
> Bandages are never good.
>
> If roaches have you on the go
> Don't take chances — call a pro.
>
> Germs are not immune to slaughter
> On dishes soaked in scalding water.[50]

To take these simple facts to a wider audience, the district inspectors organized an educational campaign that targeted church groups and ethnic organizations, because church picnics, weddings, and other festive occasions were often the source of food poisoning outbreaks. The senior staff prepared sample posters which they pre-tested on local clergy. After receiving assurance that the message was straightforward and "practical" and approval from various church leaders, a combined group of fifty sanitation and food control inspectors met with women's auxiliaries and other groups in December 1964 to present their posters and give a brief talk on refrigeration. The community response was positive and the inspectors expanded their efforts to include all of the city's major ethnic groups.[51]

In 1965, a "Foodenany" featuring the musical group, the Travellers, was held to educate the young students planning to work at the CNE. This experiment in setting their education efforts to music had originated as a result of the inspectors' observations of the coffeehouses that were a part of contemporary culture. Although the performance was organized by the director of the CNE Grandstand show and strongly supported by the food industry, the experiment was not repeated because of "the evanescent nature of the folk-song enthusiasm."[52] Lack of funds was a more accurate explanation.[53]

But the Food Control inspectors continued to become more involved in health education. Starting in the mid-1970s, a program of lectures and seminars on specific issues such as food microbiology, food service sanitation, public health legislation and pest control was offered to hospital workers, students at George Brown College, and managers and staff at CNE food concessions.[54] As the Health Department's district staff discovered new needs, they altered established programs to meet them, and by 1980, had created a three hour Food Service Sanitation Certificate course to provide a basic introduction to the subject.[55]

Education alone was not sufficient to maintain food quality standards. Health Department inspectors have the power to close restaurants and other food production facilities and to order immediate clean-ups. From the 1930s to the 1950s, the Department had a fumigation section which supervised

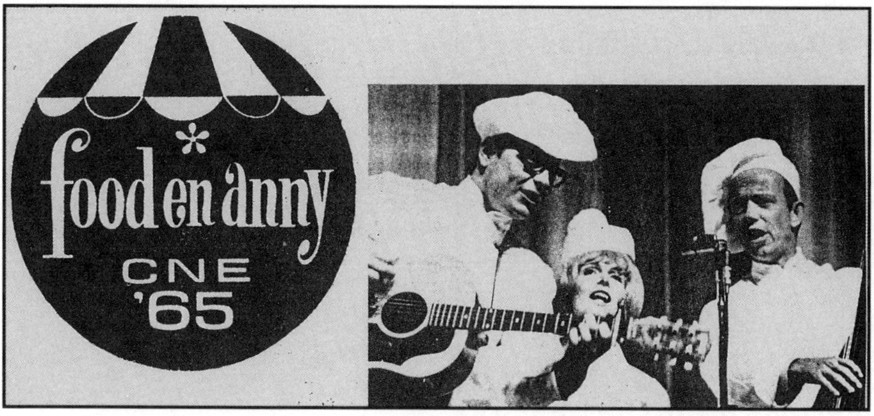

To attract young adults to the CNE's annual food handler education course in 1965, the Department and the Exhibition sponsored a performance by the Travellers, a folk singing group.

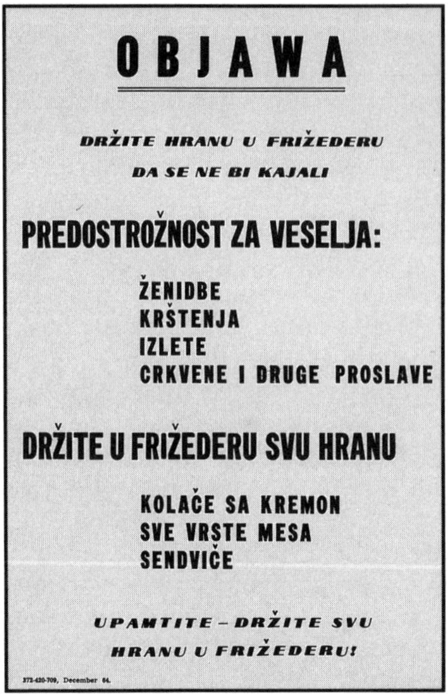

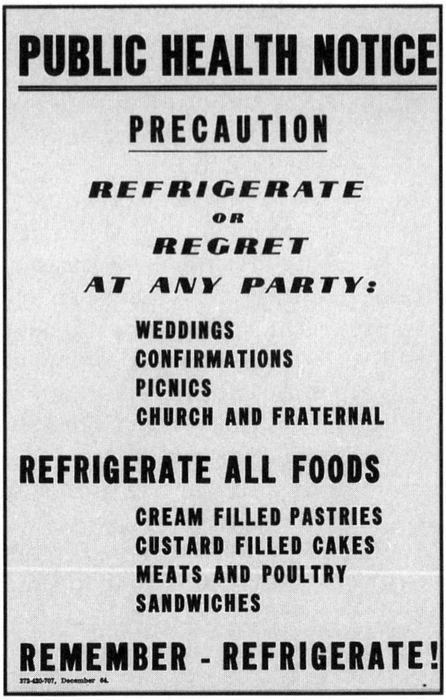

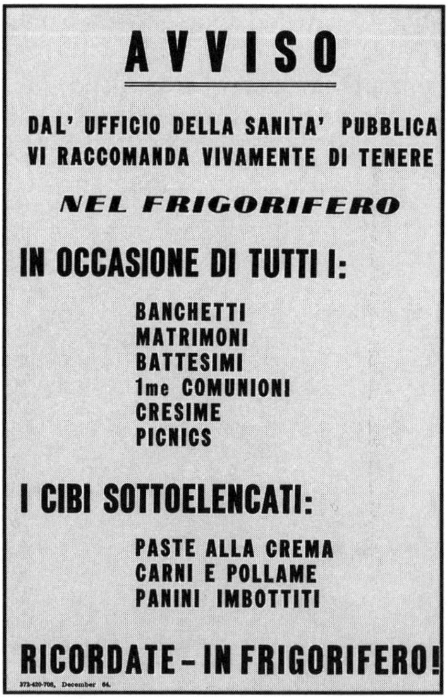

By 1964, Toronto's changing ethnic mix led the food control inspectors to have their message translated into many languages.

licensed fumigators who used cyanide gas and a variety of other chemicals to end infestations of cockroaches, rats and other types of vermin, and insects. Even the Health Department itself was not immune from infestations. In May 1956, Dr. Pequegnat sent a tongue-in-cheek letter to his executive assistant, W.S. Dunfield, who had just returned from Florida, telling him to shake the lead out "pursuant to the provisions of the Public Health Act" and rid the telephone office and stock room of silverfish. Four hours later Dunfield was able to report that he had completed his "statutory" obligation.[56] Alex McDonald, one of the staff fumigation inspectors, recalled that after fumigating a bakery, checking the premises was like walking over thousands of peanut shells in the ball park.[57] Other inspectors recall issuing orders which were obeyed only to have the premises vandalized again by customers.[58] And in 1971, inspectors in Yorkville found a man and a woman in the Mynah Bird restaurant's kitchen preparing food in the nude. The medical officer, Dr. Boyd, promptly forwarded a letter threatening prosecution under the Ontario Public Health Act if the employees were not clothed.[59]

But prosecutions were the final step. In August 1968, food control staff in the Yorkville area, which was a tourist and hippie haven at this time, became aware that an outbreak of hepatitis was occurring. This viral disease has two forms: Hepatitis A is highly infectious and can be spread through poor food handling techniques and lack of personal hygiene; Hepatitis B is transmitted through the use of contaminated needles or blood products.[60] While waiting for the results of blood tests to determine which strain was causing problems for the hippies in the neighbourhood, the food control and sanitation inspectors redoubled their already extensive efforts.

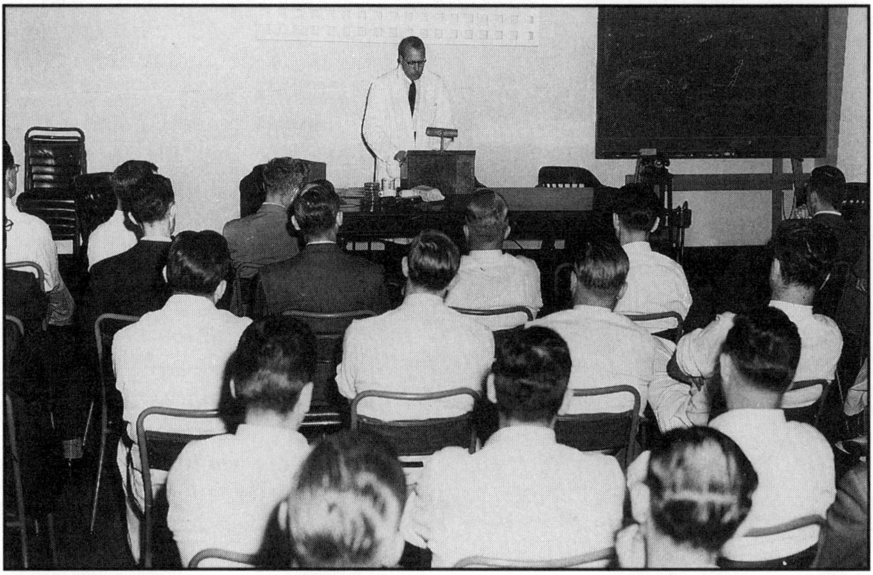

To reach a wider audience, Health Department officials spoke to groups like these supervisors of a food production plant.

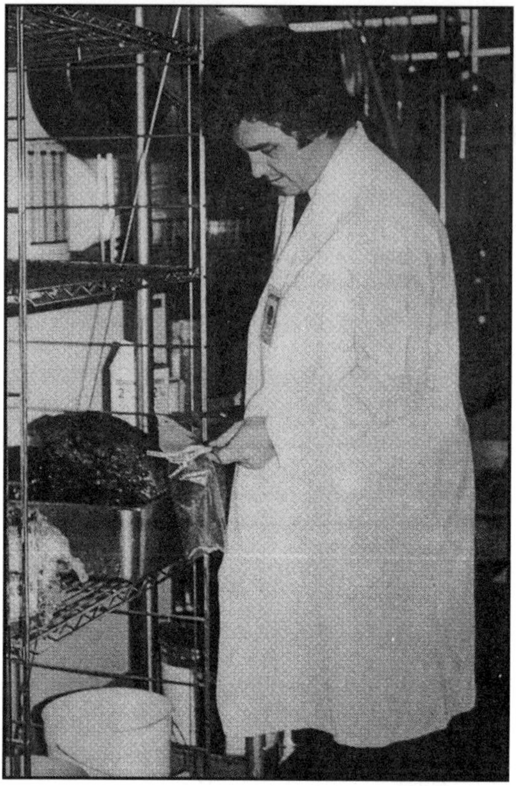

In 1976, Toronto sponsored an Olympic dinner for soccer players and dignitaries. Health Department inspectors contributed to security precautions by taking samples of the food served at this banquet, as well as all other meals served to the athletes.

Each of the numerous restaurants was inspected once or twice a day and all sanitary problems were "promptly corrected." From the inspectors' standpoint, the most impressive feature of the outbreak was the excellent co-operation that they received from the residents and business community, particularly since business declined markedly as a result of negative publicity about the "epidemic" and the Department's efforts to control it.[61] Indeed, press publicity of the whole episode reflected the wider society's fear of the hippies and their lifestyle. Ironically, the outbreak consisted of two cases of Hepatitis A and thirty cases of Hepatitis B. As the inspectors noted: "There was no evidence of spread through the food or sanitary environment."[62]

In addition to their routine inspections, food control staff investigated food poisoning outbreaks following public complaints. Through a combination of laboratory testing and detective work, they usually uncovered the offending food or food preparation problem. In 1965, 264 cases of food poisoning were traced to pastries sold by a single bakery. As a result, the inspectors visited each of the 150 homes on the baker's route to persuade the citizens to dispose of their purchases.[63] Such extensive outbreaks were rare.

Generally, small numbers of individuals suffered a variety of gastrointestinal and other ailments after eating poorly prepared or improperly stored food. In 1973, the staff studied sixty-five instances of food poisoning affecting 248 people. Forty-nine of the outbreaks were traced to restaurants, nine to retail outlets, six to home preparation problems, and the remainder to miscellaneous sources.[64] In 1975, the inspectors conducted a review of their response and investigation procedures because of growing recognition of the potential for large outbreaks as a result of conditions in senior's residences and other high risk institutional settings. Using standards set in

1966 by the International Association of Milk and Food Sanitarians, the Health Department inspectors devised a form which all department members could use to assist in tracking the source of disease outbreaks.[65]

For as the inspectors had discovered, food contamination by new parasites was becoming a problem. In 1975, giardiasis, an intestinal parasite, occurred among children in day care centres. The district public health and communicable disease inspectors were involved in trying to control the disease. They discovered that Vietnamese refugees were the human host and that these frightened immigrants resisted attempts to control their activities, especially with regard to food preparation. For the inspection staff, the rapid turnover of day care personnel, and ethnic barriers, added greatly to the difficulty of resolving this contemporary problem.[66]

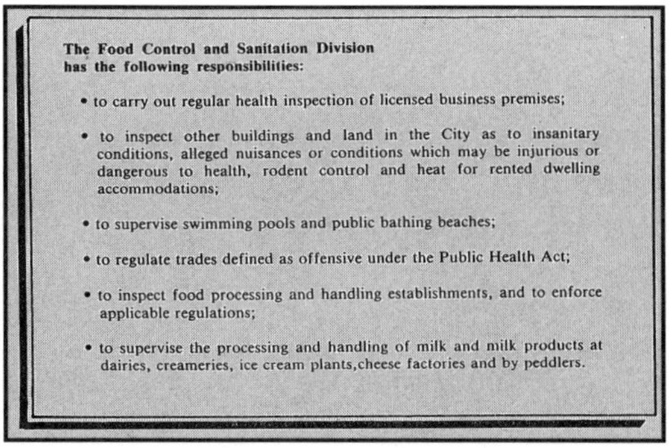
The Food Control and Sanitation Division has the following responsibilities:

- to carry out regular health inspection of licensed business premises;
- to inspect other buildings and land in the City as to insanitary conditions, alleged nuisances or conditions which may be injurious or dangerous to health, rodent control and heat for rented dwelling accommodations;
- to supervise swimming pools and public bathing beaches;
- to regulate trades defined as offensive under the Public Health Act;
- to inspect food processing and handling establishments, and to enforce applicable regulations;
- to supervise the processing and handling of milk and milk products at dairies, creameries, ice cream plants,cheese factories and by peddlers.

In 1980, the many activities which Food Control and Sanitation Division staff pursued were listed on this chart.

Nevertheless, there were successes in the 1970s. During two royal visits, the summer pedestrian malls and festivals, and Toronto's participation as a venue for soccer games during the 1976 Olympics, the Health Department's inspectors were assigned to monitor food preparation, to ensure that catering staff and chefs understood health department hygiene requirements, and to collect food samples for analysis. Their efforts ensured that visitors and residents did not suffer from food poisoning and that high standards were maintained.[67]

Conclusion

Since the early 1970s, Canadian consumers have been expressing increasing concern about chemical contamination of the food that they purchase. Indeed, the federal government's working document, *A New Perspective on Health for Canadians,* published in 1974, discussed environmental factors which affected the food chain and highlighted these as an area of future activity. The Health Department's own Health Planning Steering Committee recommended the elimination of food additives and "complete and accurate labelling" of food products in its 1978 report, *Public Health in the 1980's.* Implementing such proposals requires the support of farmers, food processors, and the public.

Will the modern activists look to the past for guidance? The success of Toronto's food inspectors in adapting to the changing focus of the international public health movement, and their ability to "educate" consumers and food producers to accept basic standards, provides a model of effective community service.

Chapter Six

Safeguarding Human Life: Fighting Smallpox and Tuberculosis

In November 1919, Charles Hastings noted:

> It is somewhat surprising that quite suddenly a certain group of the population of Toronto has become extremely sensitive and in fact antagonistic to interference with personal rights, personal liberty, but are they consistent?...In fact, practically every activity of the Board of Health and the Department of Health means depriving some of our citizens of their personal liberty and the individual right to do as they please, ofttimes compelling them to do the very things they do not want to do. That is why Departments of Health are unpopular, just in proportion to the efficiency with which they discharge their duty. Why all this interference with personal liberty and individual rights? Because British justice, properly interpreted means that when the liberty and rights of the individual are not in the interests of the welfare of the masses, the rights of the individual must yield.[1]

The medical officer made these comments in response to vociferous public opposition to compulsory vaccination during a smallpox epidemic. All of Toronto's health officers faced opposition to their disease control procedures, and all shared Hastings' belief that community needs outweighed personal concerns in this matter. But since they were functioning in a democratic society and a highly political environment, each man recognized the necessity to balance community and individual interests.

During the 1880s, William Canniff battled smallpox epidemics by creating the Department's standard disease control procedures and urging the public to be vaccinated. His successors used the germ theory to justify expanding the Department's staff and its work to include an Isolation Hospital, a Division of Communicable Diseases and Quarantine, and health education for tuberculosis sufferers and their families. In general, the Department's approach focused on persuasion and education rather than compulsion, but each aspect of the disease control system triggered a degree of public opposition. Medical colleagues, for example, criticized the Department for infringing on their practices, while the members of the Provincial Board of Health occasionally condemned their local counterparts for failing to bring the full force of the law to bear on citizens who refused to accept vaccination or other preventive measures. Mediating among these conflicting demands challenged each health officer to build on the work of his predecessors, and to adapt British and American precedents to suit Toronto's circumstances.

Their efforts to do so received reinforcement from the gradual acceptance of the germ theory of disease causation. As the public rejected the idea that contagious disease was a manifestation of divine wrath, applying the rules and regulations which provincial health legislation imposed on local authorities became easier. Opposition from practitioners also diminished after public health professionals downplayed their moral reform impulses and stressed the central role of science in defining their duties. When this shift in attitude occurred, it undercut interest in environmental influences, such as poverty and poor housing or working conditions, as factors which contributed to disease. Few health administrators noted this change in emphasis, preoccupied as they were with eradicating diseases such as smallpox and tuberculosis. Only in the late twentieth century would such concerns return to the forefront as a new generation of health activists emerged.

Creating Communicable Disease Control Procedures

In 1980, the World Health Organization certified that smallpox had been eradicated. Such news would have overjoyed medical officers in Montreal, Toronto, Charlottetown, Hamilton, Ottawa, and Edmonton, as they battled the disease between 1883 and the 1930s. These men were not aware of the viral origin of this disfiguring disease, but they gradually recognized its two main variants: *Variola major* was the virulent form which killed 20-40% of its unprotected victims, while *variola minor* was a milder disease with a death rate of approximately 1%.[2] Through the nineteenth century, epidemics of the disease swept across North America compelling health authorities to develop an effective system to control and prevent smallpox.

In 1885, when virulent smallpox erupted in Montreal, Canniff expanded his Department's role by creating Toronto's disease control procedure. He based his efforts on British and American techniques, which included notification, isolation, quarantine, and terminal fumigation, because the deadly disease spread so rapidly. The city's medical health officer was also relying on provincial legislation. According to the 1884 Public Health Act, he could expect to be notified of the disease within twenty-four hours of its diagnosis by the attending physician or the affected householder. Prompt notification was essential to limit the spread of disease, but depended on the doctor's familiarity with smallpox and the willingness of the patient's family and friends to seek medical assistance. As Canniff, Sheard and Hastings discovered, some Toronto doctors misdiagnosed smallpox as chickenpox, while others objected to the concept of notification generally.

In 1888, Canniff addressed the Canadian Medical Association on the topic. As he pointed out, lack of notification made containing disease outbreaks more difficult than was necessary. To overcome medical resistance, he sent his inspector out to have the doctors complete the blank, prestamped notification cards which his office supplied. But as he noted, his Department sometimes did not hear of the disease until he received the death certificate. Recognizing that one source of opposition lay in the lack of payment for this duty, Canniff argued in favour of a modest fee. But since community welfare required immediate notification, he informed his colleagues that to achieve this he had prosecuted three delinquent doctors in 1887.[3] His successors also prosecuted a total of five physicians, but after 1912, most doctors were willing to conform to the provincial regulations, which made notification for cholera, smallpox, diphtheria, tuberculosis, measles, mumps, erysipelas (an acute streptococcal disease), whooping cough, typhoid, chickenpox, and infantile paralysis (poliomyelitis), mandatory within twelve hours, because younger physicians understood the implications of the germ theory in the process of controlling the spread of disease.

In the 1880s, public opposition to prompt reporting was understandable. Although many Torontonians, like citizens elsewhere, believed in contagion as the source of disease, others still saw epidemics as divine retribution for sin. The idea of limiting the spread of these diseases was a novelty for workers who relied on folk remedies and could not afford medical care. But the main source of opposition to notification lay in fear of the consequences: isolation and quarantine. For many families, the thought of sending a child or spouse to city-sponsored isolation facilities was tantamount to a death sentence, yet few working class homes had sufficient space for effective isolation. Equally disturbing was the idea of being quarantined. Prior to 1900, working at seasonal jobs for a daily wage of $1.00-1.50, meant that very few people had the financial resources to sustain the fourteen or twenty-one day quarantine periods. What would the Health Department do to assist them?

In 1885, Canniff introduced the Department's procedures for isolation and quarantine. Lacking staff and wanting to be as economical as possible during the recession, the medical officer called on the City Commissioner, Emerson Coatsworth, for support. Together they visited the first home in which smallpox appeared and tried to persuade the Merricks to allow their son to be sent to the city's dilapidated smallpox hospital in the east end. The family refused, so isolation within the home was arranged and the commissioner and his staff provided groceries to the stricken household. The neighbours told the Toronto *News* that they were upset that the house had not been placarded as a warning of the danger within, although they had deduced something was wrong, as a result of observing Coatsworth's daily visits and because the laundry was hung out to dry on a Sunday![4]

The low key efforts undertaken in 1885 reflected the medical officer's initial concern about alienating public support. The appearance of new cases and the intensification of the epidemic in Montreal, where a total of 3,164 people, mainly children, died,[5] led Canniff to open the smallpox hospital. This upset nearby residents who held protest meetings and lobbied the city's aldermen to remove the facility from St. Matthew's Ward, a prime residential area in the recently annexed east end. In addition to concern about real estate values, the protesters also reflected the popular belief that smallpox was airborne and thus contaminated the neighbourhood. In British and American cities, and in Toronto during the 1849 cholera epidemic, mobs had burned down isolation facilities, so Canniff appointed a sentry in 1885-6 and again in 1888 to ensure that the patients were not harmed. Of the 26 smallpox victims in the first outbreak only three died, while in 1888 there were only eleven cases and one death.[6]

What had the medical officer learned from his experience in 1885? As a municipal appointee working under provincial regulations and civic by-laws, Canniff found himself torn between two opposing sets of values. On the one hand, Toronto's council expected him to practice restraint with city funds and not to infringe upon the citizens' civil liberties through forcible removal or confinement. On the other hand, the Provincial Board of Health expected him to prosecute physicians for misdiagnosis, automatically remove the sick to the hospital, and to conform to provincial requirements — including imposing compulsory vaccination. During the first outbreak, the medical officer tried to find a satisfactory compromise.

Canniff also used this episode to support his successful request for a contagious disease inspector. Together, the health officer and his new staff member made 491 visits to quarantined homes in 1886. As outbreaks of diphtheria, scarlet fever, and typhoid, increased during the late 1880s, the Department's inspector improved the city's disease control procedures. After notification, the inspector visited the home and the family doctor to confirm the diagnosis and make arrangements for joint supervision of the case. If he was able to persuade the family to send the disease sufferer to the city's smallpox hospital or its successor, the Riverdale Isolation Hospital, he arranged to have the city ambulance transport the individual there. The first ambulance had been donated in 1887 by philanthropist John Ross Robertson, the publisher of the *Toronto Telegram*.[7]

If the inspector failed to persuade the family to isolate the victim in the Riverdale Hospital, he then called upon the neighbours, the child's school, shopkeepers the family patronized, and other potential contacts. Unlike many Ontario centres, Toronto did not placard for diseases other than smallpox until after 1900, so the inspector's visits were an important means of alerting the public to the threat of infection. Next, he arranged for the delivery of food and fuel supplies and visited the home daily to ensure that no one was breaking quarantine. If death occurred, he supervised a quiet funeral and prompt burial. If the victim survived, the premises were fumigated, the individual was given a hygienic bath, clean clothes, and a certificate of recovery in order to return to work or school. In Toronto, terminal fumigation continued until 1944, in spite of Charles Chapin's early twentieth century research, which demonstrated that this procedure had no effect in preventing further cases of the disease. Gordon Jackson justified the Department's continued use of this outmoded activity in response to criticism of it in the *Phair Report*, by arguing that the public was conditioned to expect terminal fumigation and that "its odour and presence indirectly causes the room in nearly every instance to be cleaned with soap and water, the latter process being highly desirable and efficient."[8]

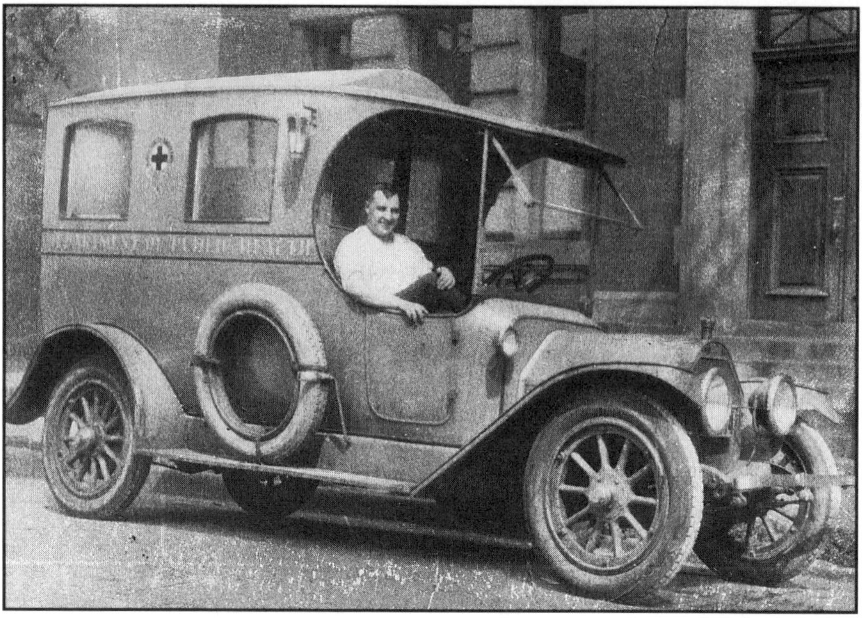

The Health Department's first motorized ambulance, a Russell Knight Model R, began service in 1914.

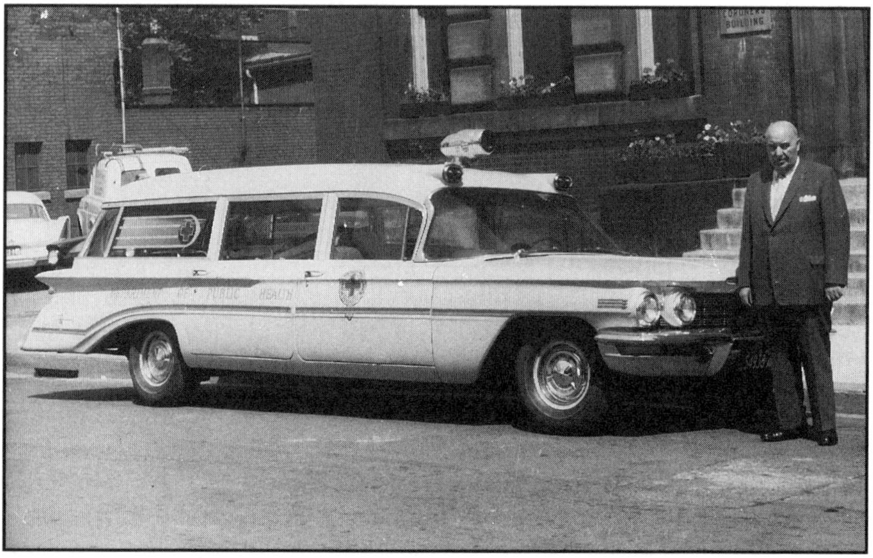

Standing beside the Department's new 1960 Oldsmobile ambulance, Thomas Virgo, the head of the Morgue and Ambulance Division since 1939, was probably reflecting on the changes which he had seen since he started driving city ambulances in 1919.

When followed rigourously, the Department's slowly evolving disease control procedures generally limited the outbreak to a single person or household. Mild or missed cases often contributed to spreading the disease, or to cases of it in widely separated parts of the city. But each aspect of the Department's disease control policy provoked opposition. Doctors disliked sharing supervision of patients with the medical officer because they feared the competition. As Charles Sheard noted, using lay inspectors alleviated much of this conflict but differences of opinion over diagnosis and quarantine measures continued.[9]

Similarly, efforts to persuade the public to enter isolation facilities were time-consuming and often frustrating. When the new Isolation Hospital opened during Norman Allen's brief period in office, the facility was located to the north of the Don Jail and consisted of a single building. Many parents refused to send their children or other family members there because of the danger of cross-infections. To respond to some of these fears, the Department got funding to build a separate wing for smallpox patients and tried to keep diphtheria and scarlet fever cases segregated. Even this did not prevent one of the health department's own inspectors from suing the city in 1910, after his child died from a cross-infection while in the Isolation Hospital.[10] By the 1930s, the Hastings Memorial Wing had been constructed on modern principles, and grateful parents were writing to the medical officer to commend the staff for their kindness and excellent care.

During the late 1880s, Canniff also pointed out to the local board of health that some people broke quarantine as a "joke." At the 1897 annual meeting of the Ontario Association of Executive Health Officers in Toronto, Sheard recounted some of his experiences to his colleagues. With placarding for example, some citizens expressed the view that "You have put that infernal placard on the door. We will defy you." In other instances, people went in and out of quarantined homes because they said they were prepared to take the risk. Several of Sheard's colleagues described similar opposition, and Guelph's Dr. Wardlaw argued in favour of standardizing quarantine periods as a means of eliminating lay and medical dissent from the health officer's pronouncements.[11]

Amendments to the provincial Public Health Act in 1912, 1923, 1931, and 1954, established standardized quarantine periods, and enabled Toronto's health officers and inspectors to refine the city's disease control measures. After 1912, placards in various colours denoted the type of disease in the stricken household. Rapid population growth expanded the inspector's workload. In 1932, a measles epidemic followed by outbreaks of whooping cough, chickenpox, and mumps, meant that the inspectors made 54,310 visits to Toronto families. Gradually, the city stopped providing this service because the amount of disease declined and the availability of antibiotics shortened the period of infection. The development of vaccines against childhood diseases such as measles, mumps, and rubella, offered an alternative to placarding and quarantine and signalled the adoption of primary prevention, rather than disease control, or secondary prevention, as the Department's preferred approach by the mid-twentieth century.

Cooperation or Compulsion?: Battling Smallpox with Vaccination

Preventing smallpox also concerned Canniff and his successors. Edward Jenner's discovery of cowpox vaccination enabled Britain, Germany, and Ontario, to pass legislation to ensure compulsory vaccination during epidemics. Was this drastic step necessary? In 1885, Canniff posted signs announcing the location of vaccination stations throughout the city and appointed vaccinators to undertake house-to-house visits in neighbourhoods in which the disease had appeared, but he would not submit to pressure from the provincial authorities for mass vaccination because he wanted to maintain public support. To publicize the benefits of the procedure, Charles Hastings, a recent medical school graduate and city vaccinator, gave two interviews to the Toronto *News* in which he used British and European statistics to prove its efficacy.[12] During the first outbreak over 9,000 people voluntarily underwent vaccination. By late 1888, the total had risen to 15,000, but the health officer had discovered that without the actual threat or presence of the disease citizens did not use the readily available preventive measure.[13]

Another factor in the lack of support for vaccination was the creation of the Toronto Anti-compulsory Vaccination League in 1888 by Dr. Alexander M. Ross. During the 1885 epidemic in Montreal, Ross had written to the *Daily Mail* specifically to warn Torontonians about the dangers of vaccination and he had now come to organize them against oppression.[14] Like his fellow critics in Britain and Germany, he believed that vaccination was "mischievous and useless" because it could sometimes cause severe pain, blindness, corrosive ulcers, abscesses, and possibly death. Furthermore, in his opinion:

> Compulsory vaccination is never attempted on the so-called better classes. It is the poor wives and children of laboring men; it is the clerks in the stores and operatives in factories and workshops; it is the workingmen and women that are threatened and driven by the hirelings of the infamous compulsory vaccination law.[15]

Ross and his supporters were justified in some of their concerns about vaccination as it was practiced in the nineteenth century. The lymph that was used to immunize the individual was occasionally contaminated with streptococcal or other organisms, and quite frequently inactive. The ivory points which were used to scarify the patient's upper arm were not always cleaned from person to person. Of equal importance was the tendency of recently vaccinated people to contaminate their wounds through ineffective bandaging or improper cleaning.[16] All these potential hazards led some citizens to avoid vaccination because they were afraid of getting an infection and being unable to work.

In 1899, Sheard used his annual report to reply to critics of vaccination. He stated that E.B. Shuttleworth had analyzed three widely marketed vaccines and that two of them were acceptable. Moreover, the medical officer claimed to have vaccinated 7,000 people with good results and therefore viewed the anti-vaccinationists as "ignorant and superstitious."[17] In 1900, the Association of Executive Health Officers discussed proper vaccination methods, sources of good quality vaccine, and the suspicion that general practitioners did not advise their patients to have their children vaccinated, and themselves revaccinated at regular intervals, because they feared patients would see this preventive service as an attempt to earn a fee.[18] While the members no doubt agreed with Dr. William Oldright of the Provincial Board of Health, that "We are one as to its [vaccination's] benefits," they probably also sympathized with Sheard's view that smallpox was "irksome and annoying" in proportion to its threat to their citizens' health.[19]

By 1900, one consequence of shoddy vaccinations was the resurgence of the Toronto Anti-Vaccination League. In 1906, the Anti-Vaccination League was able to convince the Toronto Board of Education to rescind its twelve year old rule that all children show proof of vaccination before being admitted to school. Sheard promptly entered the fray and condemned the Board of Education for pandering to the views of the 100 people who had signed the anti-vaccination petition. He was critical of their misrepresentation of his skill as a vaccinator and once again stressed the benefits.[20] A similar group in Edmonton prevented its medical officer, Dr. Whitelaw, from achieving his objective of compulsory vaccination of school children between 1908 and 1911. Only the threat of a smallpox epidemic in 1912 produced widespread vaccination in Alberta's capital.[21]

Much of the citizens' activism stemmed from opposition to compulsion. Legally, Ontario's babies had to be vaccinated for the first time at three months. Further study had indicated that revaccination should occur every five to seven years. The League opposed this and requested that the Ontario government pass legislation similar to the British law, which allowed people to reject vaccination for reasons of conscience. The Whitney government did not do so. Instead, it accepted the advice of its medical experts, and in 1914 passed a Vaccination Act that gave the medical health officer of any municipality the right to impose compulsory vaccination when the situation warranted it.[22] This law set the stage for confrontation.

In October 1919, Toronto's Health Department staff, like its counterparts in Alberta and Quebec, noticed an alarming increase in the number of cases of smallpox and chickenpox. When Hastings opened the city's vaccination stations on November 6, the Anti-Vaccination League immediately opposed him. Its members organized a protest on the steps of the city hall where they waved banners which carried slogans such as "Compulsory Vaccination German-Born — Down with Compulsion!!." A league deputation appeared before the Board of Control to explain its concerns about the quality of vaccines, the class bias of the operation, and its intense opposition to compulsion. The medical officer had been asked to attend but he left after a few minutes remarking: "I haven't got time to listen to that talk." This arrogant

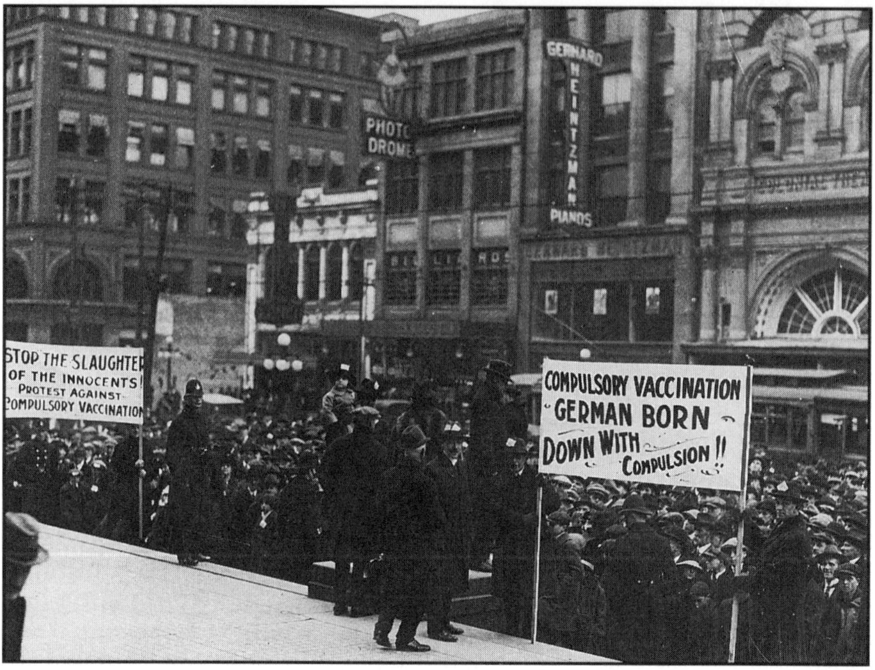

In November 1919, the Anti-Vaccination League organized a mass rally on the steps of the city hall to protest the medical officer's proposal to impose compulsory vaccination to halt the smallpox epidemic.

behaviour, and his frequent references to the success of compulsory vaccination among Canada's troops during World War I, irritated Toronto's councillors, especially Samuel McBride. With the municipal election a month away, the labour unrest of the spring and summer slowly fading from memory, and the recent defeat of the Hearst government in mind, local politicians were loath to alienate voters. As well, some members of council, including McBride, wanted to assert more control over the Health Department and its free-spending, empire-building executive officer.

During November and December, the anti-vaccination forces continued to publicize their cause through newspaper advertisements and mass rallies, one of which was attended by the Mayor, Thomas Church. Dr. J.B. Fraser, the president of the Anti-Vaccination League, told the 1200 people gathered in Massey Hall that vaccination had improved 300% in the past eleven years, but argued that there was still danger associated with the procedure. Veterans complained that compulsion was unacceptable to those who had spent four years fighting for freedom and liberty.[23]

In stark contrast to his political astuteness on other issues, Hastings did not help his cause by imposing vaccination on school children on November 10. He opted to have the students come to the city hall rather than trying to use their schools, with the result that "hordes of children" waited outside in the cold, and Health Department medical staff were overwhelmed trying to vaccinate four or five hundred a day. After the city council refused to impose compulsory vaccination early in December, the provincial health authorities threatened to get a writ of mandamus to force Toronto to do its duty. When the case was dismissed on a technicality, both sides retreated from the fight as the epidemic began to wane and concerned citizens were vaccinated.[24] Between October 1919 and March 1920, Toronto's doctors reported 2,864 cases of the disease to the Health Department, there were eleven deaths and over 200,000 people were vaccinated.[25] Although this action effectively ended the outbreak, the conflict over compulsory vaccination showed the fragile nature of public consensus about the Department's prerogatives.

During the 1920s, occasional outbursts of smallpox occurred, and in 1924 and 1928, Hastings again faced opposition from the anti-vaccinationists who had now formed the Medical Liberty League. He reiterated his belief that children should be vaccinated, but bluntly stated that adults who were anti-vaccinationists were seeking "notoriety...and their pratings were an insult to the intelligence of any sane person."[26] Why were Sheard and Hastings so vehement in their criticisms? As the one sure preventive for smallpox, vaccination was the prototype for many of medicine's claims of superiority over quackery. Opposition to vaccination was regarded by early twentieth century municipal and provincial health officers as wrong-headed and dangerous. As medical experts, these men expected to have their knowledge treated respectfully by city councils and citizens. During virulent smallpox epidemics, the public supported vaccination but in 1919, the mildness of the disease combined with organized dissent to limit council's acceptance of Hastings' advice.[27]

Like most epidemic diseases, smallpox increased and then decreased in virulence during the twentieth century. By the 1930s, it had declined to sporadic cases, and the Health Department had to organize publicity campaigns every three to four years to remind parents to have their children vaccinated. Nevertheless, the Phair Committee stated that the population immunity level was not as high as it should be, even though vaccination was available free through the city hall clinic.[28]

As the number of potential victims decreased during the 1950s, smallpox ceased to be a threat to North Americans. Nonetheless, the last case of the disease in North America occurred in Toronto in 1962, when one member of a missionary family returning from Brazil on furlough became ill. In contrast to earlier mass vaccination programs, the Health Department used the concentric ring approach. This meant that the victim and his immediate family were isolated and vaccinated, and contacts and friends were traced and revaccinated. The wider society was not required to undergo vaccination, in spite of demands for it.[29] During the late 1960s and early 1970s, medical authorities in the United States and Canada began to argue in favour of discontinuing vaccination because clinical evaluation had demonstrated that the benefits of the procedure no longer outweighed the risks. By 1975, Toronto's board of health, like Edmonton's, was able to abolish the requirement that children be vaccinated against smallpox before attending school. The battle against smallpox produced the Department's standard disease control measures and demonstrated the importance of maintaining public support for preventive procedures.

Tuberculosis: The Unending Battle

Pensively regarding the camera photographing him, the young tuberculosis victim leaves an indelible impression on the viewer. Gaunt and hollow-cheeked, he epitomizes the ravages of the "white plague." Pictures like this were used by health departments and voluntary groups to publicize their disease control and prevention work. During the first phase of the battle against tuberculosis, lay and medical reformers perceived the disease as a community problem. Poor housing, unventilated workshops, public spitting, overcrowded classrooms, and contaminated milk were singled out by social activists as factors which caused the disease.[30] Although Robert Koch identified the mycobacteria which produced tuberculosis in 1882, no effective drug treatments were available until the late 1940s. During the second phase of the battle against the disease, medical scientists focused their attention on finding a vaccine against it. Even after the vaccine was available, official health agencies at the municipal or provincial level pursued a policy of tracing disease victims and their contacts. They also assisted in placing patients in sanatoria and organized mass surveys to find new cases. Like their predecessors, they received great support from charitable groups such as the Canadian Tuberculosis Association, the National Sanitarium Association, and the Gage Institute of Toronto — all of which were formed during the 1890s and 1900s.

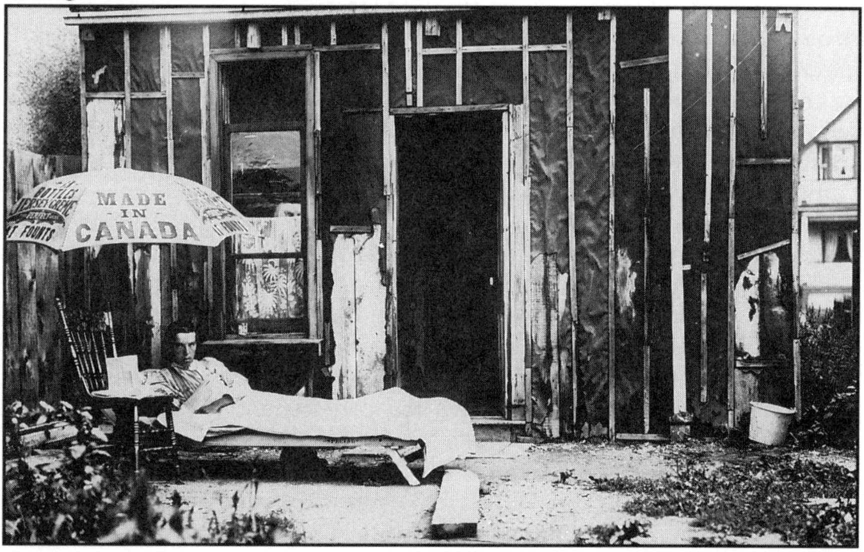

The Health Department provided the cot and umbrella which this young man used after he refused to go to a sanatarium. He died of tuberculosis shortly after this picture was taken on September 6, 1912.

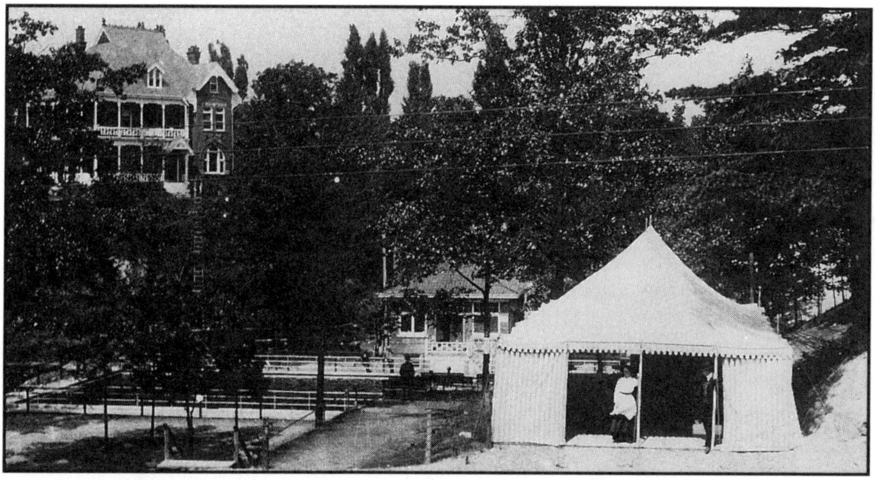

The High Park Sanitarium on Gothic Avenue cared for some of the city's tuberculosis sufferers.

At the turn of the century, private sanatoria were built in Muskoka in imitation of the institutions found in upper New York State and the American southwest. In Toronto, the local board of health requested $20,000 to construct a municipal consumptives' hospital in 1899. Both this recommendation and a proposal to hold a municipal referendum on the matter failed to pass the council.[31] Instead, Toronto's Health Department slowly integrated its anti-tuberculosis activities with those of the city's hospitals and charitable agencies during the first decade of the twentieth century.

In 1905, Dr. Harold Parsons of the Toronto General Hospital's Chest Clinic persuaded a wealthy philanthropist, Mrs. Marjory Larkin, to fund the services of a tuberculosis visiting nurse to demonstrate the benefits of education for patients and their families. Ottawa also pioneered in this work in 1905, but both Canadian cities were behind Edinburgh and New York, which had appointed tuberculosis nurses in 1887 and 1903. All of the agencies responsible for this type of health education believed, that "People who do not read or attend lectures will gather around a nurse in their own home and learn from her the gospel of preventability and curability."[32] In 1907 then, Charles Sheard who was an active member of Toronto's Anti-Tuberculosis League, convinced the board of health to hire Toronto General's TB nurse as a fulltime staff member. The city thus became responsible for both educating and assisting tuberculosis victims and their families.

Finding people suffering from the disease, however, was difficult. The social stigma attached to tuberculosis limited voluntary use of the Health Department's diagnostic facilities between 1893 and 1910, and meant that few doctors reported cases of the disease from their practices because victims were often denied life insurance coverage. In 1911, the province finally responded to decades of pressure from local medical officers and voluntary groups, and made notification mandatory. Like their counterparts in New York City who had faced similar opposition to compulsory

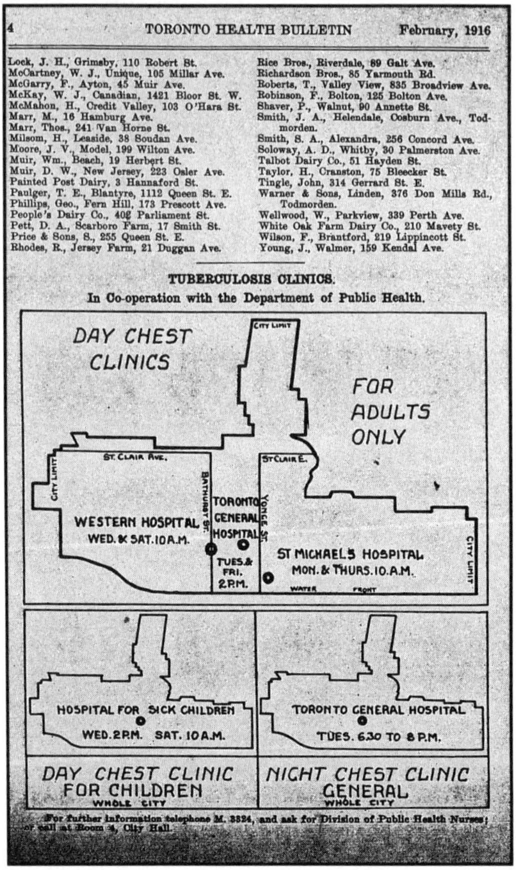
4 TORONTO HEALTH BULLETIN February, 1916

Lock, J. H., Grimsby, 110 Robert St.
McCartney, W. J., Unique, 105 Millar Ave.
McGarry, F., Ayton, 45 Muir Ave.
McKay, W. J., Canadian, 1421 Bloor St. W.
McMahon, H., Credit Valley, 103 O'Hara St.
Marr, M., 16 Hamburg Ave.
Marr, Thos., 241 Van Horne St.
Milsom, H., Leaside, 38 Soudan Ave.
Moore, J. V., Model, 199 Wilton Ave.
Muir, Wm., Beach, 19 Herbert St.
Muir, D. W., New Jersey, 223 Osler Ave.
Painted Post Dairy, 3 Hannaford St.
Paulger, T. E., Blantyre, 1112 Queen St. E.
Phillips, Geo., Fern Hill, 173 Prescott Ave.
People's Dairy Co., 402 Parliament St.
Pett, D. A., Scarboro Farm, 17 Smith St.
Price & Sons, S., 255 Queen St. E.
Rhodes, R., Jersey Farm, 21 Duggan Ave.
Rice Bros., Riverdale, 89 Galt Ave.
Richardson Bros., 85 Yarmouth Rd.
Roberts, T., Valley View, 835 Broadview Ave.
Robinson, F., Bolton, 125 Bolton Ave.
Shaver, P., Walnut, 90 Annette St.
Smith, J. A., Helendale, Cosburn Ave., Todmorden.
Smith, S. A., Alexandra, 256 Concord Ave.
Soloway, A. D., Whitby, 30 Palmerston Ave.
Talbot Dairy Co., 51 Hayden St.
Taylor, H., Cranston, 75 Bleecker St.
Tingle, John, 314 Gerrard St. E.
Warner & Sons, Linden, 376 Don Mills Rd., Todmorden.
Wellwood, W., Parkview, 339 Perth Ave.
White Oak Farm Dairy Co., 210 Mavety St.
Wilson, F., Brantford, 219 Lippincott St.
Young, J., Walmer, 159 Kendal Ave.

TUBERCULOSIS CLINICS.

In Co-operation with the Department of Public Health.

For further information telephone M. 3824, and ask for Division of Public Health Nurses; or call at Room 4, City Hall.

By February 1916, the Health Department and Toronto's teaching hospitals were providing day and evening diagnostic clinics to uncover cases of "the white plague."

reporting, Toronto's Health Department's nurses took a gradual approach to gaining doctors' support.

The medical officer was not so charitable, remarking in the November 1911 *Health Bulletin*, that "The physician who does not report cases of tuberculosis may be the direct cause of more suffering and ill-health than he can alleviate or cure in his whole lifetime of practice." He based his comment on heart-rending circumstances which his nurses uncovered during their home visits. In one instance, the nurse found a woman whose hair and bedclothes were matted with sputum, being cared for by her husband, who was also working halftime and trying to look after their three small children. The family doctor did not notify the Department about this case for three months. Hastings was furious that he had not done so earlier, as the Department provided funds for sanatorium care, education in the proper methods of sputum disposal, housekeeping assistance, and free diagnostic tests. In the medical officer's opinion, the doctor was negligent and fully responsible for the positive tuberculosis tests in two of the children. Hastings summarized his views on the matter by stating: "Our duty is to look after those whom the physician and society fail to look after."[33]

But what about immigrants? Where they the health threat that nativists in Canada and the United States feared? In December 1912, the *Health Bulletin* described an Italian boardinghouse in which a TB victim was abandoned for three days. When the nurse arrived, she found bloody sputum on the rug beside the patient. The landlord protested when told to remove and burn the rug, but by the time the nurse had finished explaining the infectious nature of the disease, he was so worried that he said "let the lady do it!" In response to a question about Toronto's tuberculosis-stricken immigrants in 1912, the Director of Public Health Nurses, Eunice Dyke, replied that

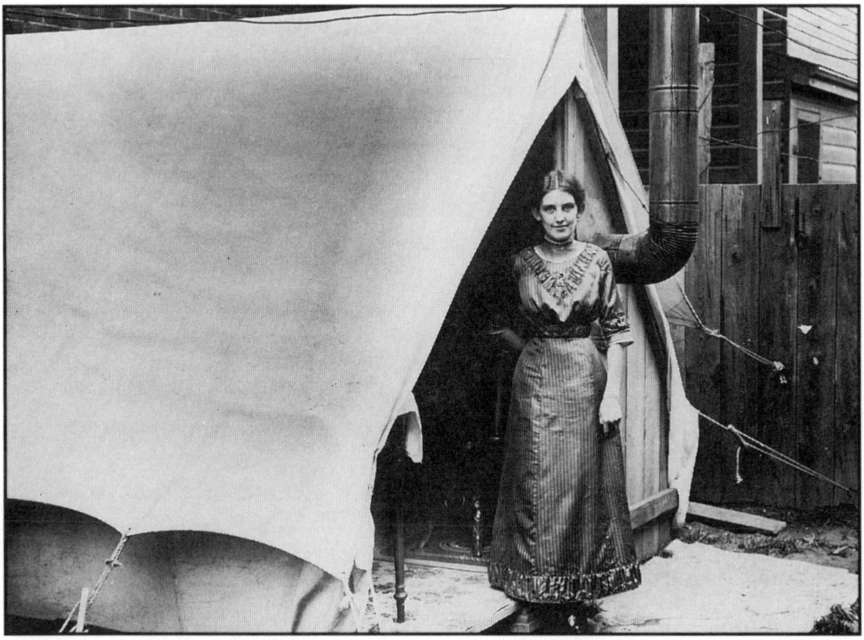

This former sanitarium patient was encouraged to live outdoors in a heated tent to complete her recovery and to protect her family from possible infection.

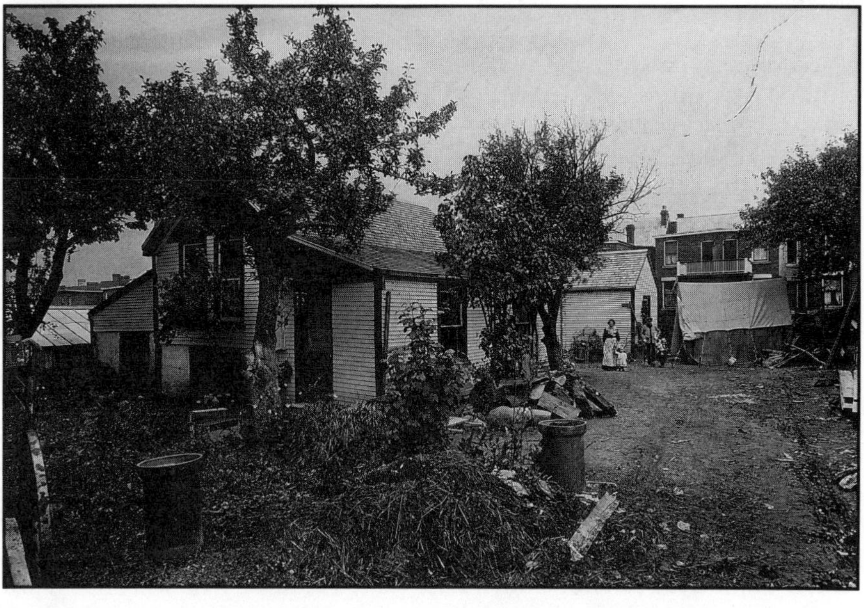

This tent at the back of his brother's market garden on Christie Street was the summer home of a TB patient who spent his winters in the Gravenhurst Sanitarium.

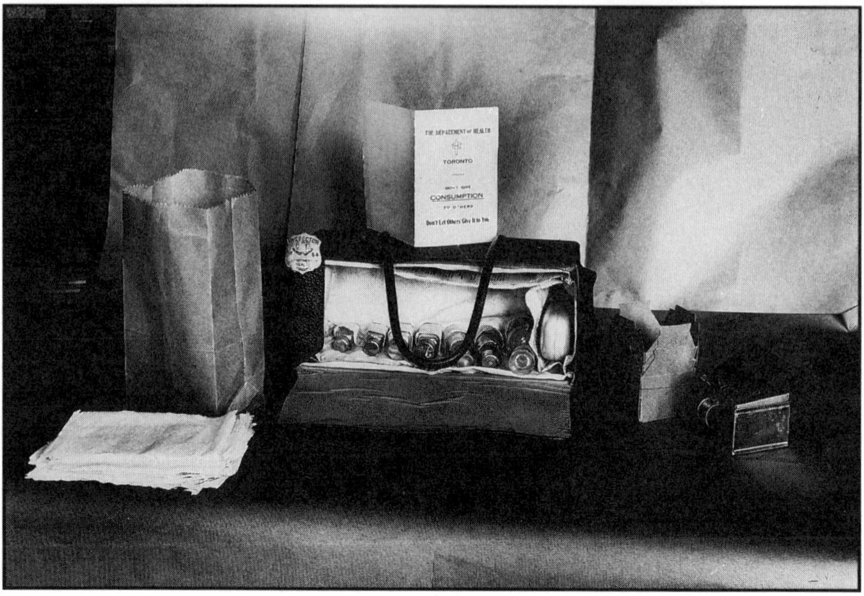

When the communicable disease control inspectors and the public health nurses visited clients with tuberculosis, they carried a black leather bag containing supplies of tissues, paper bags and sputum boxes, all of which could be burned after use. The staff also collected sputum samples and distributed educational material.

Macedonians, Italians, and "coloured", seemed to be the principal victims but that the disease was widespread in all segments of society.[34] She did not favour restricting immigration as did some of her contemporaries.

The Health Department publicized the importance of notification and received case lists from the clinics at Toronto General, St. Michael's Hospital, the Hospital for Sick Children, and the University Settlement. From 1910 to 1917, the nurses and medical inspectors of Toronto's Board of Education also reported the names of children with the disease. All of these sources of information were essential because the infection rate for close contacts of TB cases is 50 to 65%.[35] Researchers in Framingham Massachusetts surveyed their town and discovered nine active and nine inactive cases of TB for every death from the disease.[36]

Canadian and American public health administrators responded to these revelations by creating case-finding and case-supervision procedures. Once a positive diagnosis had been made, the Health Department arranged for sanatorium treatment at the Toronto Free Hospital, the Muskoka Free Hospital, or the Queen Alexandra Sanatorium in London. With the family doctor's approval, public health nurses visited patients who were not able to obtain sanatoria beds and helped them adjust to their disease. Rest, fresh air, and good food were the standard treatment. Disinfection of the premises by the Division of Communicable Disease Control fumigator, free sputum cups, and paper handkerchiefs, were provided by the Department. The nurses arranged for further assistance from other charitable groups because the city did not offer financial support to tuberculosis victims as it did to people quarantined for other diseases.

In contrast to its leading role in the control of smallpox, the Department became a team player in the battle against tuberculosis. The Canadian Tuberculosis Association provided much of the literature which the nurses distributed during home visits. The IODE Preventorium accommodated tubercular children, while the Hospital for Sick Children's Heather Club, and the Samaritan Club, looked after the needs of victims in their homes. According to Dyke and Hastings, the Department's role was to co-ordinate all this activity.

Prevention or Cure?: A New Approach to Tuberculosis

During the 1920s, the messianic fervour of the first phase of the anti-tuberculosis crusade faded. It was replaced by joint government and charitable agency activity aimed at prevention. In 1924 the Provincial Health Department established a travelling X-ray clinic. Based in Toronto, this free clinic supplemented the diagnostic services provided by the Gage Institute and the hospitals. The purpose was to conduct the mass screening activities which health administrators believed would uncover new cases more quickly. In the 1920s, many states and provinces carried out mass screening and tuberculin testing. That same decade, the French introduced the BCG vaccine against tuberculosis but it was not widely used in Canada until after the Second World War. During the interwar years, the focus here remained on early detection, prompt reporting, treatment of the victim, and health education for family and friends, financed through the sale of Christmas Seals (starting in 1927).

In Ontario, the Depression aroused concern about the burgeoning costs of sanatoria care. Although the province had been paying 75 cents a day for poverty-stricken sanatoria patients since 1920, municipalities had to fund their own indigent patients at the rate of $1.50 a day. Such costs were impossible for bankrupt municipalities and even cities like Toronto, which escaped financial collapse, looked for assistance. In 1933, the province created a Division of Tuberculosis Prevention to oversee curative and preventive activities in an effort to eliminate duplication and cut costs. Prevention was cheaper than treatment, which often took several years and then required rehabilitation services. Between 1935 and 1940, the province increased the number of travelling diagnostic clinics to six, based in Toronto, Ottawa, Belleville, Timmins, North Bay, and Fort William.[37]

In 1938, the Hepburn government amended the Sanatoria for Consumptives Act to provide full provincial funding for the care of indigents in all these institutions. But municipalities were still required to pay for patients' transportation to and from the sanatorium, and for his or her pneumothorax surgery and after care. In Toronto, the Department of Health supervised the medical aspects of post-sanatorium care, while the Department of Public

Welfare assessed the applicants' financial status.[38] By the 1940s, Toronto's tuberculosis control program required the efforts of the diagnostician, laboratory technicians, communicable disease inspectors, district and hospital social service nurses, and the supervisor of communicable disease nursing. The discovery of three active cases of the disease among secondary students at Bloor Collegiate demonstrated the necessity for further efforts in 1940, but questions of cost and the availability of staff led the Department to turn to non-profit agencies and volunteer chest specialists for assistance.

In its evaluation of Toronto's Health Department, the Phair Committee criticized the city for its failure to appoint a doctor to head its tuberculosis control program fulltime, the laboratory staff for failing to conduct cultural examinations and animal inoculation tests for the disease, the public health nurses for taking on too much responsibility for directing the program, and the hospitals for continuing to charge a fee for X-rays and other diagnostic activities. These criticisms were based on the APHA guidelines for effective tuberculosis programs.[39]

Jackson responded by noting that he had been asking to hire a medical supervisor for the tuberculosis control programme for five years, and that although the board of health had supported him, finding an available expert would be difficult during the war. He defended his laboratory technicians by pointing out that they did not have the facilities to do TB cultures. Moreover, the division had been threatened with extinction since 1933, as a result of budget cutbacks and the Board of Control's desire to eliminate city services by transferring the task to the provincial laboratories. And he pointedly defended the nursing staff by reminding Phair of the Division's international reputation. Finally, the medical officer argued that while he would like the hospitals to offer free x-ray service, he could not order them to do so.[40] Underlying the apparent municipal-provincial conflict was a shared determination to eradicate tuberculosis in the post-war world.

With advice from the province, Jackson organized a series of meetings with the city's hospitals to discuss purchasing miniature X-ray equipment in order to conduct mass screening of high school students, civic employees, firemen, policemen, and hospital admissions. This project failed to receive the necessary support from the city's hospitals and the Health Department turned instead to the Gage Institute.[41] In 1949, that clinic uncovered 370 active cases of the disease while the hospital chest clinics found 290. In response, the Department created a separate Tuberculosis Division and appointed a fulltime medical director to administer it; by doing so, Toronto was responding to the Phair Committee's efforts to initiate medical direction of tuberculosis prevention. By 1951, the local board of health was discussing a new concern — the potential health threat from immigrants and displaced persons with active or inactive cases of TB. The province and the city tried to maintain contact with these new arrivals, but their rapid movement from place to place seeking work made this a frustrating task.

During the Second World War, European and American researchers developed drugs which cured tuberculosis. Streptomycin, para-aminosalicylic acid, and isoniazid, were all in use by the 1950s. These drugs changed

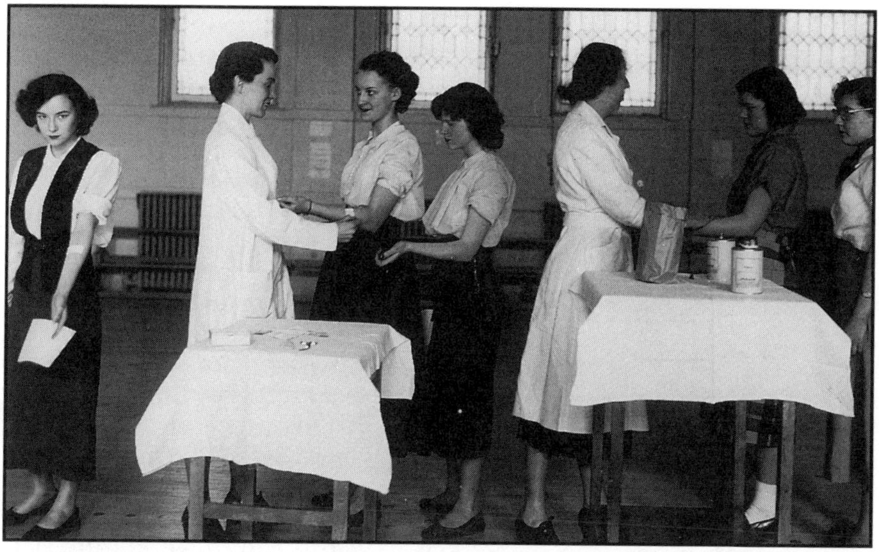

Concern about the spread of tuberculosis in the late 1940s led to a mass screening effort among Toronto high school students using tuberculin tests .

the Health Department's duties because they could be given either in hospital or in the home. One former nurse recalled that when she joined the Department in 1943, people diagnosed with tuberculosis were sent away to sanatoria within a day or two. Their families and friends were examined to find other cases, and the whole process required diligent detective work to trace the source of the infection. The adoption of drug therapy did not eliminate the necessity for uncovering contacts and new cases, but it did shorten the length of time that each client was treated and ended the abrupt breakup of families. Like their counterparts in Edmonton, Toronto's staff found dealing with recovering TB victims a challenge, because the speed with which the antibiotics stopped the coughing and fever which characterized active cases led many TB sufferers to conclude that they were cured and to stop taking their medication. As sanatoria around Ontario began to close because the antibiotics were apparently so effective, medical writers and the public assumed that another scourge had been beaten. Merging the TB Control Division with the Division of Communicable Disease Control in 1967, indicated that the Health Department's senior administrators also believed that a separate campaign was no longer necessary.

In 1967, Torontonians were surprised to learn that the city's death rate from tuberculosis was 4.3 per 100,000, compared to a provincial rate of 2.2 per 100,000 in 1965. Even more unexpected, its case rate was 44.9 per 100,000, in contrast to the provincial rate of 20.9. Were these statistics overstating the amount of tuberculosis? To find out, the new director of Communicable Disease Control coordinated a four year tuberculosis case-finding survey of all citizens, with the assistance of the Ontario Health Department, the Ontario Tuberculosis Association, the Gage Institute, and citizen's groups.

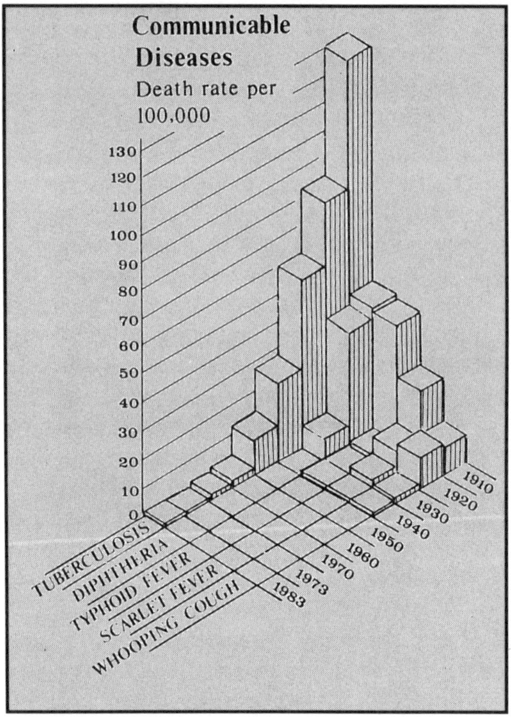

By 1983, the nineteenth century killer diseases, including tuberculosis, had disappeared as threats to Torontonians' health.

The Communicable Disease Control and Epidemiology Division has the following responsibilities:

- to carry out epidemiological investigation of reported and suspected cases of communicable and parasitic diseases;
- to arrange examination and treatment of all such cases, and hospitalization where necessary;
- to interview for contacts of communicable disease cases;
- to follow-up cases and contacts;
- to act as liaison with hospital clinics for tuberculosis and other respiratory diseases;
- to provide promotional, consultative, advisory and educational services in communicable, parasitic and respiratory disease, and to enforce all Acts relating to such diseases.

By 1980, many of the long-established duties of the Communicable Disease Control and Epidemiology Division were being refocused in new directions, including health promotion and educational consultation.

Using Mantoux tests and X-rays on positive reactors, the Department systematically examined the population.[42] New or reactivated cases of tuberculosis now received treatment with ethambutol and rifampin from their family doctors and the Department introduced a chemotherapeutic preventive program for children, young adults, and reactivated cases.

Through the 1970s, rates began to decline toward the provincial level, but the arrival of refugees from Latin America, Vietnam, Cambodia and other war-torn third world countries, prompted the Department to intensify its case finding activities. Children in grades one and eight were automatically tuberculin tested but in 1979-80, all new Canadian students were examined in the Toronto schools. Three active cases of the disease were discovered.[43] In 1981, tuberculosis cases and deaths were at an all time low but an assessment of the Department's statistics demonstrated what the staff had long realized: tuberculosis in the late twentieth century is predominantly a disease of the poor, the alcoholic, the diabetic, and the elderly.[44] The long crusade against the "white plague" illustrated that narrowing the vision of the reformers — from the social to the biological causes of the disease — initially appeared to lower the morbidity and mortality rates from the disease, particularly after the introduction of chemotherapeutic measures in the late 1940s. The resurgence of the disease and its appearance among immigrants and native Canadians, however, brings social and environmental variables back to centre stage.

Conclusion

At the end of his November 1919 report to the local board of health, Charles Hastings observed that:

> It must be apparent to every citizen that Boards of Health and Departments of Health have one object, and one only in view, and that is the most efficient way of safeguarding human life and controlling disease, and in doing so, require to act in the light of the most advanced knowledge obtainable.[45]

The medical officer was highlighting the combination of humanitarianism and faith in expertise which guided him and his predecessors in their battles against smallpox and other communicable diseases. To do so, they had to educate citizens to accept supervision of their families during epidemics. Beginning with visits by quarantine inspectors, the department's strategy for controlling the spread of contagious disease evolved to include the work of the Ambulance Division, the Isolation Hospital, and the diagnostic service provided by the city laboratory. The Department's procedures for controlling the spread of contagious diseases were the first step in eradicating them.

Preventing disease was more difficult. Although vaccination protected people against smallpox, public opposition to the measure frustrated officials such as Canniff, Sheard and Hastings. Until citizens were convinced that the quality of the vaccine was sufficiently high to prohibit side effects, vocal opponents continued to flourish. By the beginning of the twentieth century, some health experts believed that health education would be a more effective means of preventing disease than imposing regulations, because they argued that if the public understood the scientific foundation for health rules, they would be more likely to follow them. Through their work with TB victims, their families, and community groups, the Department's public health nurses educated Torontonians in basic principles of disease causation, prevention and control.

During its first half century, Toronto's Health Department established disease control procedures and health education activities, which contributed to "safeguarding human life" from epidemic diseases such as smallpox and endemic diseases such as tuberculosis. The development of antibiotics in the 1930s and 1940s made many of the established activities obsolete. As a result, health departments throughout the English-speaking world had to review their policies and procedures and focus on primary prevention.

Chapter Seven

Discovery and Application: The Triumph of Prevention

> The role of the public health agency is to make available the proven results of research to the public as early as community preventive action becomes practicable.[1]

A century ago, the bacteriological revolution that was just beginning in European laboratories laid the foundation for the preceding statement. During the 1880s, the germ theory of disease causation was proven, as French and German scientists discovered the bacteria which caused many different illnesses. Since identification alone did not provide either a cure or preventive measures, local health officers in Europe and North America continued to practice the disease control procedures that had developed in response to gastrointestinal diseases. These scientific discoveries did, however, justify the establishment of diagnostic laboratories, and refinements to quarantine procedures based on the concept of human disease carriers.

As medical science became more sophisticated, researchers in "immunology, virology, genetics, cytology, biochemistry and molecular biology" began to create vaccines against childhood killers, and a new era in prevention opened.[2] Instead of relying on secondary and tertiary prevention, that is, controlling the disease and rehabilitating its victim, primary prevention, which attempts to avert the disease, was now possible. Ironically, public health administrators learned that as they eradicated one childhood scourge, such as diphtheria, another, like poliomyelitis, became prominent. As medical professionals, they supported the research model, and organized public participation in clinical trials designed to test new techniques for controlling or preventing communicable diseases. Toronto's Health Department was a frequent contributor to research studies because it had close ties to the University of Toronto School of Hygiene and the Connaught Laboratories.

As the following case studies illustrate, Toronto's Health Department moved from secondary and tertiary measures against diphtheria and poliomyelitis, to primary prevention during the twentieth century. To alert the public to the Department's control policies and preventive measures, the health officers established contact with science writers for newspapers, magazines, radio stations, and later television. Their publicity efforts ensured the success of mass immunization campaigns. By the 1970s, the decline in communicable diseases and the decline in public demand for Department-sponsored immunization, enabled the city's staff to begin to look at new health concerns, and to question the relevance of the medical research model to contemporary health problems.

Be Wise — Immunize!: Eliminating Diphtheria

For nineteenth and early twentieth century medical officers in North America, diphtheria was one of the most significant childhood diseases. The cyclical epidemics, which sometimes killed several children in the same family within hours, struck fear into parents and medical practitioners because so little could be done as the child struggled for life. Diphtheria bacteria produced a false membrane which could suffocate its victims if it grew over the larynx. If death did not intervene, the disease produced a toxin which spread through the body causing damage to muscles, nerves, and occasionally heart failure.[3] Since tracheotomies had a limited success rate, practitioners and public health activists turned to accepted disease control measures to prevent the disease from spreading. European researchers uncovered the bacteria which caused the disease, developed treatment for it, and ultimately produced a primary preventive, namely, immunization with diphtheria toxoid. Toronto's health officers, who adapted these discoveries to the city's needs, required an understanding of the germ theory of disease, public support and funding, and the ability to co-ordinate the activities of researchers, staff members and voluntary organizations.

The process began in 1886, when William Canniff discovered that the 214 cases of diphtheria in 1885 had increased to 625 cases, many of which were not reported to his office. Like most of his contemporaries, Canniff believed that an insanitary environment caused the disease but he also recommended complete isolation of the victim. Since many Torontonians were unable to do this, he pushed for the construction of a public isolation hospital. When the hospital finally opened in 1892, it provided facilities for citizens suffering from diphtheria, scarlet fever and other contagious diseases. By 1900, the facility was full of patients stricken during an epidemic, and Toronto's death rate from diphtheria represented one-third of the province's mortality from the disease, although the city only contained one-tenth of its population.[4] In New York, Milwaukee, and Hamilton, the disease took a fearful toll as well. Could medical science find a way to control or prevent this fearful malady?

Proving the Germ Theory: Developing Diagnostic Techniques

In 1883–4, two German researchers, Edwin Klebs and Friedrich Loeffler, identified the *cornyebacterium diphtheriae* which caused the disease. Their discovery sparked a competition between the Pasteur Institute in Paris and the Koch Institute in Berlin to discover a vaccine against diphtheria. The Klebs-Loeffler discovery also provided a new tool in the war against communicable diseases: laboratory analysis for diagnostic purposes. As a result, the state of Michigan and the city of Providence each established a bacteriological laboratory in 1888. Ontario's Provincial Board of Health followed in 1890, and New York City's Health Department in 1892. These facilities enabled state, provincial, and municipal health authorities to play a leadership role in the adoption of the practical aspects of the germ theory, and led them to modify their previous emphasis on environmental and social causes of disease. As well, many of the laboratories combined public service with a commitment to research, and gradually became internationally recognized for their contributions. These facilities and laboratories attached to university medical schools pioneered the medical research model of scientific discovery.

After his appointment as Toronto's medical health officer, Charles Sheard established a system for laboratory analysis of all suspected diphtheria cases. Like New York City, Milwaukee and Hamilton, Toronto's Health Department created a chain of culture stations in the city's drugstores. Here doctors could pick up culture kits containing throat swabs which were delivered to the city laboratory after being used. This innovation was not universally appreciated because it threatened the control of private practitioners over their patients. As Sheard ruefully informed his professional peers in the Executive Health Officers Association, one Toronto doctor told him that "he could diagnose diphtheria before bacteriology was ever known and he could diagnose it after" without using the Health Department's Laboratory or accepting its findings. In fact, this man challenged the medical officer to take him to court for allowing children to return to school in spite of positive tests.[5]

In addition to demonstrating one individual's opposition to medical advances, the episode also raised the issue of human diphtheria carriers. The concept of apparently healthy people infecting others was suggested by Robert Koch in 1892, and confirmed by William Park and Arthur Beebe of New York City's Bacteriological Laboratory in 1893–4. Although this discovery explained the many unknown first cases which caused epidemics, what policies were health departments to pursue in dealing with apparently healthy carriers? In Ontario, the provincial authorities defined quarantine periods for healthy and convalescent carriers. One consequence of these regulations was lengthy periods of quarantine for young carriers. In a 1948 radio talk, two members of the Women Elector's Association recalled that as children, one spent six weeks and the other, four months in the Riverdale Isolation Hospital, until they no longer tested positive for the diphtheria bacillus.

Cure or Prevention?: From Diphtheria Antitoxin to Toxoid

Since 1884, French researchers had been searching for a vaccine to cure or prevent diphtheria, using Louis Pasteur's discovery of rabies vaccine as a model. In 1893, Emile Roux of the Pasteur Institute announced that he and a colleague, Alexandre Yersin, had isolated an antitoxin from the blood of horses infected with diphtheria. This biological product had been used in the diphtheria wards of Paris hospitals with amazing results. Children stricken with the disease had responded to the treatment, and its use on contacts of disease victims appeared to confer limited immunity. The scientific community at the International Congress on Hygiene and Demography in Budapest listened to Roux with interest, but with certain reservations. Did antitoxin really work or would it prove to be another failure like Koch's tuberculin? Clearly more research was required, but the modern clinical trial with its experimental and control groups was not yet widely accepted.

Nevertheless, careful research studies were done in New York City because Hermann Biggs, the city Health Commissioner, visited the Pasteur Institute and returned to New York with samples of antitoxin for clinical use. He also encouraged William Park to produce the city's own supplies, to ensure that doctors could treat the needy as well as those who could afford to pay the high cost of the antitoxin.[6] Starting in 1895, Sheard, too, began to use small amounts of antitoxin to treat diphtheria cases in Toronto's Isolation Hospital. As medical officers and practitioners throughout Ontario tested antitoxin, they, like their colleagues in Europe and the United States, learned that large doses of the vaccine given within twenty-four hours of the onset of the disease produced the best results. The antitoxin treatment was discussed at the Ontario Medical Association's meetings in 1895, 1896, 1903, and 1904. In 1895, Sheard expressed ambivalence about its effectiveness, but by 1904, he agreed with the colleague who remarked: "It [antitoxin] was now fully established as the proper treatment."[7] Nevertheless, as Toronto's medical officer pointed out, healthy carriers were a significant factor in spreading the disease.

The use of bacteriological diagnosis and antitoxin provided a means of controlling epidemics as long as parents and doctors reported cases of the disease, agreed to allow the victim to be isolated, and accepted quarantine for themselves and other family members and boarders. Middle class children stricken with contagious diseases were confined to their bedrooms with a disinfectant-soaked sheet hanging in the doorway. Human contact was restricted to their mothers, or nurses and doctors, or clergymen, all of whom had to wash thoroughly with disinfectant after they left the room. The invalid's dishes, utensils and other household items were sterilized, books and toys were burned, and bedclothes were boiled once the disease had run its course.[8] The cost and difficulty of isolating a diphtheria victim led many families to send their children to the Isolation Hospital, where expert medical and nursing care was available twenty-four hours a day and supplies of antitoxin were on hand.

But what about prevention? Would a modified form of antitoxin immunize susceptible individuals? How could susceptibility be established? In 1907 an American researcher, Theobald Smith, suggested that a toxin-antitoxin combination would create an effective toxoid. His work provided William Park and Emil Behring with the impetus for further research into toxoid preparation. In 1913, a Hungarian-born researcher, Dr. Bela Schick, announced in New York City that he had developed a test to determine which children were immune to the disease, and thus would not require toxoid immunization.[9] These developments laid the foundation for primary rather than secondary prevention of this disease.

Research and Service in Canada: Creating Connaught Laboratories

The achievement of Park's researchers attracted interest from people committed to the new science of bacteriology. One of the visitors to the New York facility was Dr. John FitzGerald, a Toronto graduate who had studied at the Pasteur Institute, the University of Freiburg, and the Lister Institute. As a proponent of the "new public health," FitzGerald wanted to establish an antitoxin laboratory at the University of Toronto.[10] With the assistance of Professor John Amyot, of the Faculty of Medicine's fledgling Department of Hygiene, FitzGerald achieved his goal in 1913. One year later, the Provincial Board of Health began to distribute the product at cost to municipalities and practitioners. In 1916, as a result of the demand for vaccines and sera which the First World War had prompted, the Antitoxin Laboratories expanded, courtesy of a generous donation from Colonel Albert Gooderham, and were renamed the Connaught Laboratories. The new facility began to produce biological products for all of Canada as well as the armed services, and became one of the leading centres for research in bacteriology, virology and immunology.

In 1916, the Ontario government also agreed to provide antitoxin free to all doctors and health departments who requested it. In Toronto, supplies of antitoxin could be picked up from the city's six hospitals, the Department of Public Health, or any one of the fifty-four drugstores in which culture stations were located.[11] In spite of the existence of this treatment, the death rate from diphtheria did not decline as quickly as Charles Hastings expected. In the *Health Bulletins,* he reminded his readers that the peak months for diphtheria were October to December, and that all parents should be suspicious of colds and sore throats. In stressing this, he was echoing the warnings of his predecessors who had identified the school as a major source of infection. The medical officer also urged the public to forego folk remedies like turpentine, sulphur and onions, and instead, to consult their family doctors or district medical staff for prompt diagnosis and treatment.[12]

Reorganizing the Department's Disease Control System

In 1910-11, Hastings reorganized the Health Department's disease control procedures. First, he created a Division of Communicable Disease Control and Quarantine, to supervise patients in their homes and to fumigate the premises after the disease had run its course. By 1915, this section of the Department consisted of a chief inspector, ten staff inspectors, and three disinfectors. They too shared the crowded main office in the city hall, but most of their work was in the field. For the poor, the inspectors arranged coal and groceries, and in 1913, Hastings convinced the councillors to pay working mothers $1.00 a day to stay home with their sick children. The departmental diagnostician assisted the Communicable Diseases staff by visiting families without physicians, to diagnose cases of communicable disease.

His efforts were supported by the Division of Laboratories, which grew from a single bacteriologist in 1910 to a staff of 12, including a full-time epidemiologist, by 1915. These men and women worked in cramped facilities in the attic of the city hall. There were separate rooms for milk testing, sample preparation, serological, tuberculosis and diphtheria testing, and offices for the diagnostician and the clerical staff. On the wall of the laboratory, an 8' by 6' chart illustrated the bacteria which the staff were seeking as they conducted their tests.[13] When diphtheria throat swabs arrived, they were cultured immediately and a diagnosis was phoned to the attending physician by 10:30 a.m. the following day. If the test result was positive, the case was also reported to the Communicable Disease Division staff. Since the Department was aware of the hardship which quarantine imposed, Hastings announced in 1913 that if laboratory tests indicated that diphtheria contacts did not have the disease and were not carriers, they would be allowed to go back to work.[14]

In spite of these control measures, the number of cases of disease increased as non-immunized children were exposed to the bacteria. In 1920, there were 2,258 cases of diphtheria and 224 deaths in Toronto. Hastings was horrified and exhorted parents to contact the Department for help and antitoxin. As he had during the previous decade, the medical officer stressed the importance of prevention. In contrast to New York and Edmonton, however, Toronto did not undertake mass immunization of school children with the toxin-antitoxin mixture.[15] Instead, one district which was suffering a diphtheria outbreak in 1926, was chosen on the advice of the Connaught

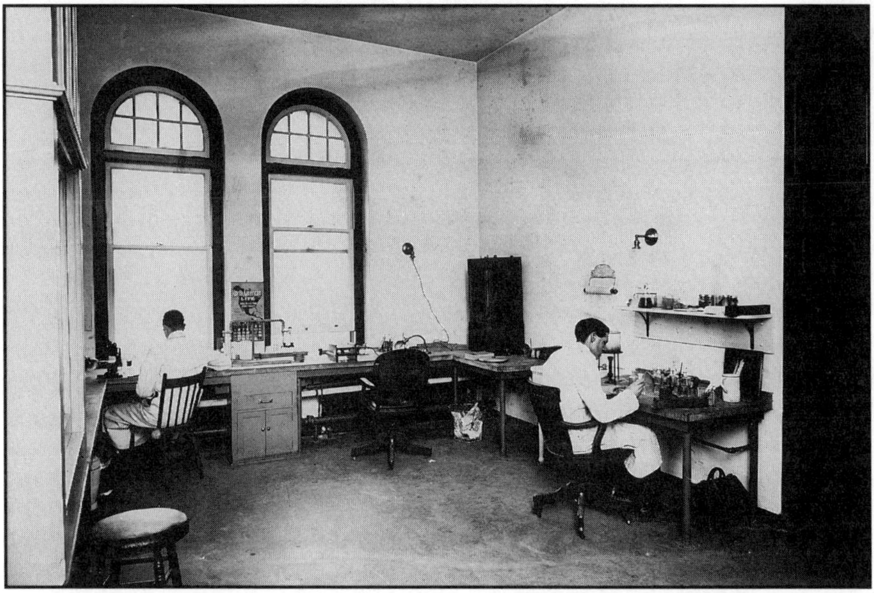

The laboratory staff member on the right is examining communicable disease samples delivered in the black bag beneath his desk. Other samples arrived in the culture kits which Toronto doctors picked up from local drugstores.

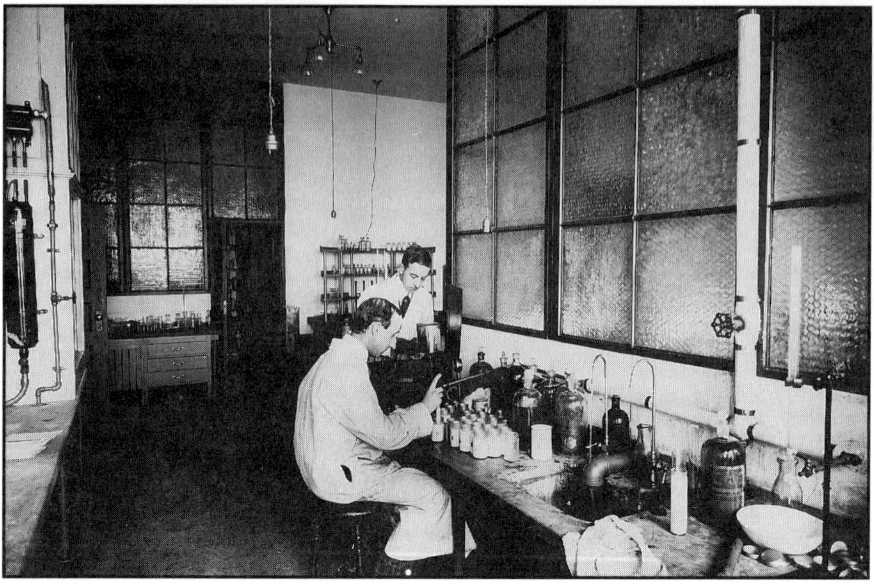

More spacious quarters were a necessity since the Laboratory Division's workload increased significantly as a result of the city's population growth and physician's use of the free service.

Laboratories as the site of a small field trial of Gaston Ramon's recently-developed toxoid. The trial was co-ordinated by the district's public health nurses, who arranged to have consent forms taken home by the children who were to be immunized. Each child's "shot" was recorded on his or her school health record, and the Health Department's Statistical Services Division tabulated the results for the newly-opened School of Hygiene's researchers.

In 1927, Toronto, Hamilton, Brantford, and Windsor, participated in Connaught's campaign to immunize their school children using the Schick test and two doses of toxoid.[16] By 1928, Toronto parents were asking to have the program expanded to include pre-school children. Opposition from the city's doctors who objected to the infringement on their services, led to the project's cancellation in 1929, on the assumption that general practitioners would provide immunization.[17]

Toronto's Toxoid Campaigns, 1931–1945

A sharp increase in the number of cases and deaths from diphtheria in 1930, led the new medical officer, Gordon Jackson, to reintroduce the toxoid campaign in September. He immediately faced criticism from the Academy of Medicine, who suggested that the system in use in Detroit, where private doctors were paid a fee by the city for immunization work, should be tried in Toronto. Jackson and his deputy medical officer, Leon Pequegnat, visited the American city and returned to inform their colleagues, that Toronto's city solicitor indicated that the Health Department would be liable for damages from any suits arising from such a system. As if this were not sufficient reason, Jackson also told the members that, although he too was a doctor, as a civic official he could not recommend such a change simply for the sake of the profession. Needless to say, Jackson's comments did not endear him to struggling doctors during the Depression.[18] His views, however, did indicate the extent to which professional administrators identified with the political needs of the system in which they worked.

In 1931, a toxoid campaign for pre-schoolers was introduced in seven of the twenty-five child health centres which the Health Department directed. In contrast to the ongoing immunization program in the schools, which relied on the children taking permission forms home to their parents, the public health nurses offered personal counselling about the importance of immunization in the child health centres. Jackson's most striking innovation, however, was creating a Toronto Diphtheria Committee consisting of prominent citizens and "representatives of educational boards, the Board of Health, the church, the newspapers, broadcasting stations and advertising agencies," with the assistance of the Toronto branch of the Canadian Social Hygiene Council. Drawing on American advertising techniques and campaign tactics, this group supervised an annual Toxoid Week during the 1930s and 1940s. Through posters, billboards, newspaper stories and editorials and educational material provided to teachers and ministers, provincial and city public health professionals, the mayors, the chairmen of the local board of health and their supporters saturated the community with information about the clinics.

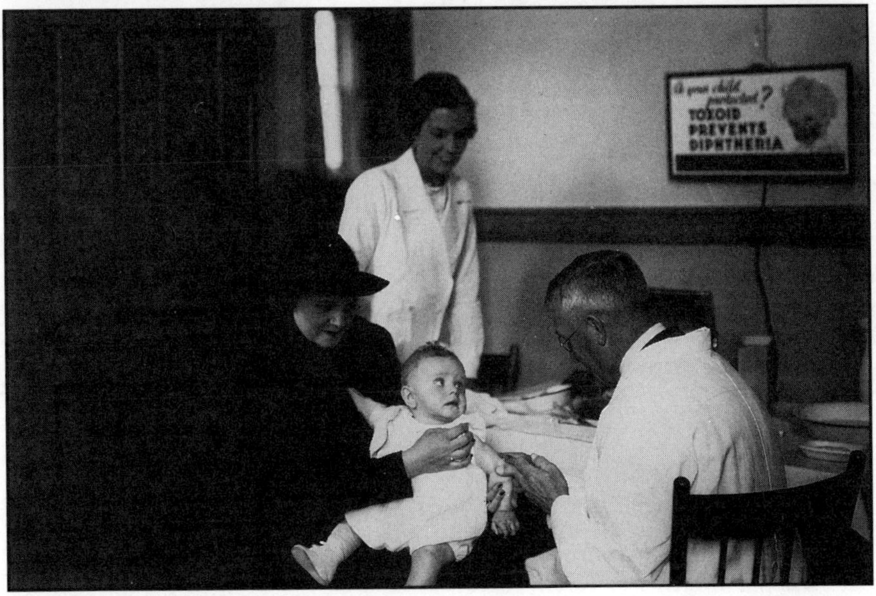

The Health Department's doctors immunized Toronto babies against diphtheria during their visits to child health centres in the 1940s.

In addition to "spot" radio announcements, a fifteen minute drama on diphtheria prevention attracted public attention. Both Bell Telephone and Toronto Hydro included messages about the immunization programs in their monthly bills, while TTC streetcars carried advertisements for the toxoid clinics. Such sustained advertising ensured high immunization levels and in 1934, 1937 and 1940, Toronto was one of the few cities[19] in the world which did not have any deaths from diphtheria. In 1937, for example, Quebec City's medical officer reported 55 deaths and 458 cases of the disease by mid-November.[20] Toronto's Diphtheria Committee celebrated the city's first year with no cases and no deaths in 1940, by holding a testimonial dinner for the medical officer and presenting him with a silver cigarette case. Toronto's successful campaign attracted national and international attention; Montreal held its first toxoid week in 1941, and the British government used Toronto's example during its diphtheria eradication campaign in the 1940s.[21]

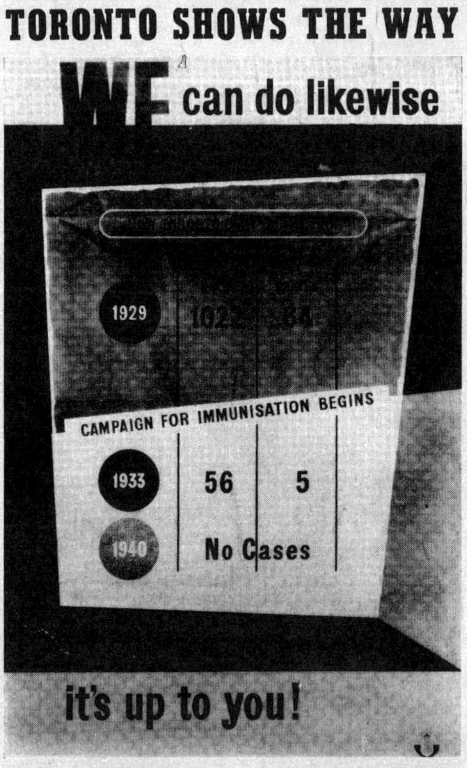

Reproduced above is a poster used by the Ministry of Health, London, England, during its recent Diphtheria Immunisation Campaign. An official of the ministry declared: "I have read the report of Toxoid Week held in Toronto under the joint auspices of the Diphtheria Committee of the Health League of Canada and the Toronto Department of Health. You will see from this copy of one of our posters that we urge the people in this country to emulate the example of Toronto."

This British poster illustrates the international influence of Toronto's Toxoid Campaign.

By 1942 Jackson was bemoaning the lack of interest that parents were displaying about immunizing their babies. He was also worried because diphtheria was reappearing; there had been 20 cases and two deaths in 1941, and 40 cases and six deaths in the first four months of 1942. To alert doctors to their responsibilities, a short article in the Academy of Medicine's *Bulletin* reminded them of the importance of taking throat swabs and making prompt use of antitoxin for close contacts.[22] Both the chairman of the local board of health and the province's Deputy Health Minister expressed concern that the toxoid week had become ineffective. Responding to their suggestion that a more dynamic approach was required, Jackson stated that he and his deputy did not see any need for drastic change, since approximately 60% of the population had been immunized. Neither of the city officials believed that the increased costs of a more adventurous advertising campaign would truly assist in increasing toxoid use.

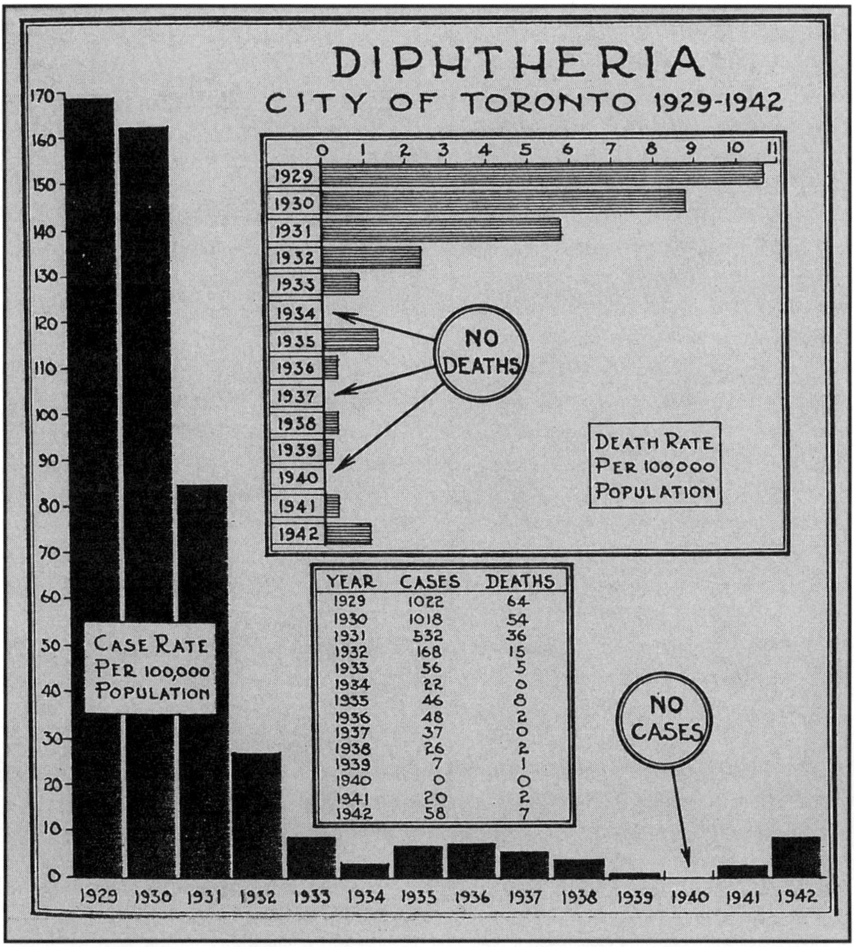

This 1942 graph illustrates the rapid decline in the diphtheria cases and deaths as a result of community-wide immunization.

Immunization Services in the Post-war Era

As toxoid became recognized as a preventive with minimal side effects, researchers at the Connaught Laboratories investigated combinations of vaccines and, in 1949, the DPT or diphtheria, pertussis (whooping cough) and tetanus sequence of immunization shots was introduced in Toronto's child health centres. In its assessment of public health practice in Canada a year later, however, the CPHA study committee recommended careful evaluation of the use of public health professionals in immunization programs. The committee members argued that such duties should be carried out by general practitioners, except in remote areas or in cities with large

BOOK-MARK

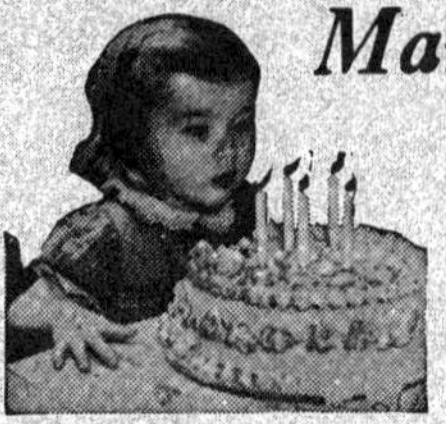

Mark this!

TOXOID PREVENTS DIPHTHERIA

DIPHTHERIA

doesn't wait for "school age".

Every child between six months of age and five years is at the age when he is most likely to take diphtheria. And during this time he is much more likely to **die** if he catches it! Nearly two-thirds of all diphtheria deaths occur among little children — **under five.**

Toxoid will protect your child against this disease. If he has not been given Toxoid or immunized against diphtheria — see your doctor at once.

WHOOPING COUGH

causes more deaths among infants under one year of age than diphtheria, smallpox, and scarlet fever combined!

Many cases occur in infants of six months of age or less, while the largest proportion occurs between the ages of one year and three years.

Whooping Cough vaccine protects children against Whooping Cough. If your child has not been protected, see your doctor at once.

It is now possible to protect against diphtheria and whooping cough at the same time. Consult your doctor.

No father or mother can afford to neglect taking these precautionary steps. See your doctor at once — or take your child to the nearest child health centre — (See list on reverse side). These centres are operated for your convenience — yet health authorities report that thousands of Toronto children are not receiving this protection. PARENTS, DO NOT DELAY! ACT NOW!

HEALTH LEAGUE OF CANADA

111 Avenue Road, Toronto

(Over)

CHILD HEALTH CENTRES

Operated by Department of Public Health. **Children over 6 months and under 6 years** of age who have never been given Toxoid may be immunized at any of these centres.
Time: The centres are open at 2 p.m.

EAST OF DON RIVER

Kimbourne United Church, Wolverleigh & Woodington — Fri.
Baptist Church, 114 Pape Ave. — Wed.
Kew Beach United Church, 140 Wineva Ave. — Thurs.
Riverdale Presbyterian Church, 662 Pape Ave. — Tues.
St. Matthew's Church, 135 First Ave. — Wed.
Rhodes Ave. United Church Hall, 1456 Gerrard St. E. — Tues.

FROM YONGE ST. TO DON RIVER

Kemp House, 18 Gifford St. — Tues.
Metropolitan Church House, 57 Shuter — Thurs.
St. Enoch's Church, Winchester & Metcalfe Sts. — Thurs.

FROM YONGE ST. TO BATHURST ST.

Hospital for Sick Children, College St. — Wed.
Church of the Redeemer, 166 Bloor W. — Wed.
St. Christopher House, 67 Wales Ave. — Wed.
University Settlement, 23 Grange Road 1.30 p.m. — Tues.

WEST FROM BATHURST, BELOW BLOOR

Bonar Presbyterian Church Hall, 349 Lansdowne Ave. — Wed.
Parkdale Presbyterian Church, 250 Dunn Ave. — Tues.
St. Matthias Church Parish Hall, 45 Bellwoods Ave. — Thurs.

WEST FROM BATHURST, ABOVE BLOOR

St. Cyprian's Church Parish Hall, Manning & Follis Aves. — Tues.
Perth Ave. United Church, Wallace and Perth Aves. — Tues.
St. Chad's Church, 1689 Dufferin St. — Thurs.
Y.W.C.A. St. John's Rd. & Dundas W. — Wed.
Westmoreland United Church, Westmoreland & Hallam — Fri.

NORTH TORONTO

St. Leonard's Church, Wanless Ave. and Yonge St. — Fri.
Manor Rd. United Church, Manor Rd. and Forman Ave. — Fri.

For children of all ages — Riverdale Isolation Hospital—Wednesday, 3 p.m.; Saturday, 10 a.m.

UNDER SUPERVISION OF CHURCHES

PROTESTANT—

St. John's Clinic, St. John's Garrison Church, 54 Portland St. Saturdays, 9.00-12.00 a.m. Wednesdays, 9.00-12.00 a.m. Supervision of Dr. G. A. Davis, 12 Belsize Dr.

CATHOLIC—

Our Lady's Child Health Centre, St. Mary's Parish House, Bathurst and Adelaide Sts. Thursdays, 2.00-4.00 p.m.

St. Basil's Child Health Centre, St. Basil's Parish House, St. Joseph Street. Fridays, 2.00-4.00 p.m. Supervision of Dr. W. T. G. Knowlton.

St. Gerrard's Child Health Centre, 131 McCaul St. Thursdays, 9.30-11.00 a.m. Supervision of Dr. M. A. Scandiffio.

St. Paul's Child Health Centre, St. Paul's Parish Hall, Power and Queen Street East. Tuesdays, 2.00-4.00 p.m. Supervision of Dr. A. Brady.

St. Michael's Hall, Bond St. (above Shuter). Tuesdays, 2.00-4.00 p.m. Supervision of Dr. Wm. O'Brien.

HEALTH LEAGUE OF CANADA

111 Avenue Road, Toronto

(Over)

The Health League of Canada used this bookmark to publicize the benefits of diphtheria and whooping cough immunization. Although parents were urged to use their family doctor, the bookmark also listed city clinics.

numbers of indigent citizens.[23] Toronto, however, continued to provide immunization services for its pre-school and school-age children to ensure maximum levels of population immunity.

In 1960, the deputy medical officer, George Moss, reported to his colleagues that Connaught-sponsored research indicated that Torontonians no longer had the diphtheria bacillus in their throats. Impressive as this achievement was, he expressed concern because of the discovery of a large number of subclinical cases and carriers in London, England and actual outbreaks of the disease in Winnipeg and Detroit.[24] Two years later, his fears were realized when several cases of diphtheria occurred among Italian immigrant children. Although the Toronto Department tried to keep the story quiet, the provincial authorities named the family for the *Telegram* which promptly called the stricken household for a "scoop" on life under quarantine.[25]

In 1963, Moss used the press to warn the public about the potential for an outbreak of a virulent strain of diphtheria, as a result of the death of a two year old, and the discovery of 24 carriers. He urged parents to ensure that their babies were vaccinated, and encouraged them to use the fourteen immunization centres which the public health nurses and Medical Services Division staff provided.[26] During the 1970s, as the public adapted to government-sponsored medical insurance plans, Toronto's Health Department gradually curbed its activities because families turned to their general practitioners for this service. In 1977, however, the Medical Services staff were concerned about the fragmentation in service, and the decline in immunization levels among pre-school and kindergarten students. The doctors recommended an extensive publicity effort and suggested assessing the community's immunization status. They also advocated requiring proof of immunization prior to school admission, and in 1984, the Ontario government passed legislation that fulfilled their objectives.[27]

Conquering Polio: Medical Science Triumphant

Carefree hours swimming, playing with friends, and visiting the CNE were a summer pleasure which Toronto's children took for granted. But during the polio epidemics of the 1930s and 1950s, these simple pastimes caused parents great anxiety because of the threat of infection. Did children with a slight fever, sore throat, stiff neck muscles, no energy and perhaps an upset stomach, have the frightening disease — or were they just under the weather? For concerned families, the warnings that Toronto's newspapers published meant close attention to even the slightest symptom, as they sought to protect their children against infection. Infantile paralysis, as poliomyelitis was known, was probably endemic in North America, especially prior to the sanitation improvements that occurred between 1880 and 1920. In 1916, the disease became epidemic in the United States; there were 29,000 cases and 9,000 deaths.[28] New York City was particularly hard hit, and this led Hastings to issue warnings through the press about the importance of immediate medical attention.

Unlike diphtheria, polio is a filterable virus. Although this was demonstrated by Viennese immunologist Karl Landsteiner and his assistant, Erwin Popper, in 1908, efforts to create an effective diagnostic test were unsuccessful. Similar difficulties arose concerning preventive measures. New York had tried to quarantine cases and required all patients to be isolated, but the many unrecognized cases defeated these efforts. Treatment consisted of a convalescent serum derived from blood provided by survivors. Even the focus of the disease within the body was debated. In 1910, Dr. Simon Flexner argued that it was spread through the nasal passages, while a Swedish research team reported to an international conference in Washington in 1912 that it was found in the "contents and walls of the small intestine."[29]

The confusion surrounding polio's epidemiology, progress in the human body, prevention, treatment, and cure challenged immunologists, virologists, orthopedic surgeons, and public health experts. In Toronto, sporadic outbreaks led the medical officer to summarize existing knowledge for the public in the *Health Bulletin* in September 1926, and to warn the local board of health about a possible epidemic in July 1929. In 1926, the public learned about the seasonal variation, the lack of a diagnostic test, the direct human contagion from mild cases or carriers, and the vulnerability of young children. Three years later, the board was reminded about Winnipeg's severe epidemic in 1928, and told that convalescent serum was produced by the Connaught Laboratories, purchased by the Ontario Health Department and distributed by Toronto's Health Department.[30]

Toronto had the opportunity to develop its disease control procedures during polio epidemics in 1930, 1934, and 1937. On August 12, 1930, the *Toronto Star* began to publicize a possible polio epidemic based on provincial reports. Toronto's medical officer, Gordon Jackson, wanted the population to be "alert but not scared" by this advance notification. As the number of cases rose, doctors and parents questioned the Department about the wisdom of opening the schools in September. Both Jackson and Pequegnat argued that the medical inspection their staff provided would protect the healthy while bringing prompt assistance to the sick. Children suspected of having polio were isolated either in their homes or the Isolation Hospital and treated with convalescent serum. By the end of the epidemic, 263 cases and 20 deaths had been recorded.[31]

New York City suffered another polio epidemic in 1931. This outbreak enabled researchers from Harvard to evaluate the effectiveness of convalescent serum. Their findings challenged it as an effective therapy against the disease.[32] The Ontario Health Department's advisors, however, continued to support the production and distribution of the serum because they believed that it offered some protection. In 1934, when Toronto faced its next bout with the disease, Jackson remarked sadly: "No sooner had diphtheria been conquered and almost cast into oblivion than this new horror appears on the horizon." He told the local board that the citizens and the press had rallied gallantly to combat the disease, which had appeared in sixteen different schools and then spread throughout the city. The Department's disinfectors and nurses were kept very busy, while support staff in the central office maintained meticulous records and shared in the growing sense of tension until the epidemic peaked. Jackson also explicitly compared the tools which he had to fight diphtheria — toxoid and antitoxin — with the lack of weapons against this "mysterious and dreadful ailment."[33] In 1935, researchers in New York and Philadelphia introduced vaccines against polio. Lacking the knowledge that there were three strains of the virus, these products, in fact, caused the disease in some of the children who were immunized. This failure left public health administrators feeling vulnerable and led them to concentrate on treatment and rehabilitation.[34]

After a slow start in June 1937, Toronto's worst epidemic of the decade began in earnest in August. It peaked the week of September 11 when 133 new cases of the disease were reported. By September 20, the Department had 280 cases in hospital, 100 at home, 96 homes were quarantined for active cases, and 188 homes were quarantined for contacts.[35] The communicable disease inspectors relied on notification from doctors, parents, and concerned neighbours. In contrast to earlier epidemics, the breadwinner was not allowed to go to work because of the perceived virulence of the disease.

The 1937 epidemic was also memorable for the public health nurses who visited stricken homes three times a week. Since the dental staff were not providing service to school children during the outbreak, they volunteered to drive the nurses to their many appointments. As in earlier outbreaks, district nurses occasionally found tragic situations, such as the little girl who suffered numerous bug bites while strapped to her bed.[36] This type of discovery, and the effects of the Depression, meant that the nurses had to coordinate public and private charitable activities. The city, the Toronto Red Cross and the provincial authorities supplied home nursing services, beds, mattresses, splints, and special foods. Charitable organizations such as the Rotary and the Kinsmen provided games, toys, reading material, trips to the Orthopedic Hospital, and other types of assistance.

By the time the outbreak was over there had been 768 cases and 40 deaths. Many more of the victims were left paralysed. The rest of the province had experienced similar increases in paralysed cases, which led the Hepburn government to create an Orthopedic Hospital in Toronto to treat victims. Like many of his medical colleagues, Jackson stressed the importance of prompt rehabilitation efforts and maintaining a strong mental attitude among patients. Although he did not define their activities as tertiary prevention, the Department hired two physiotherapists who taught selected staff, parents and grandparents how to exercise children's paralysed limbs.

In contrast to the conflict which the diphtheria immunization effort had provoked within the medical community, the 1937 polio epidemic produced unity. On September 1, Jackson attended a two hour meeting with the Academy of Medicine's council, and together they drafted a press release intended to reassure citizens that all possible measures were being taken. These included asking the Public and Separate Schools Boards to keep the city's schools closed until the medical community agreed it was safe to open them.

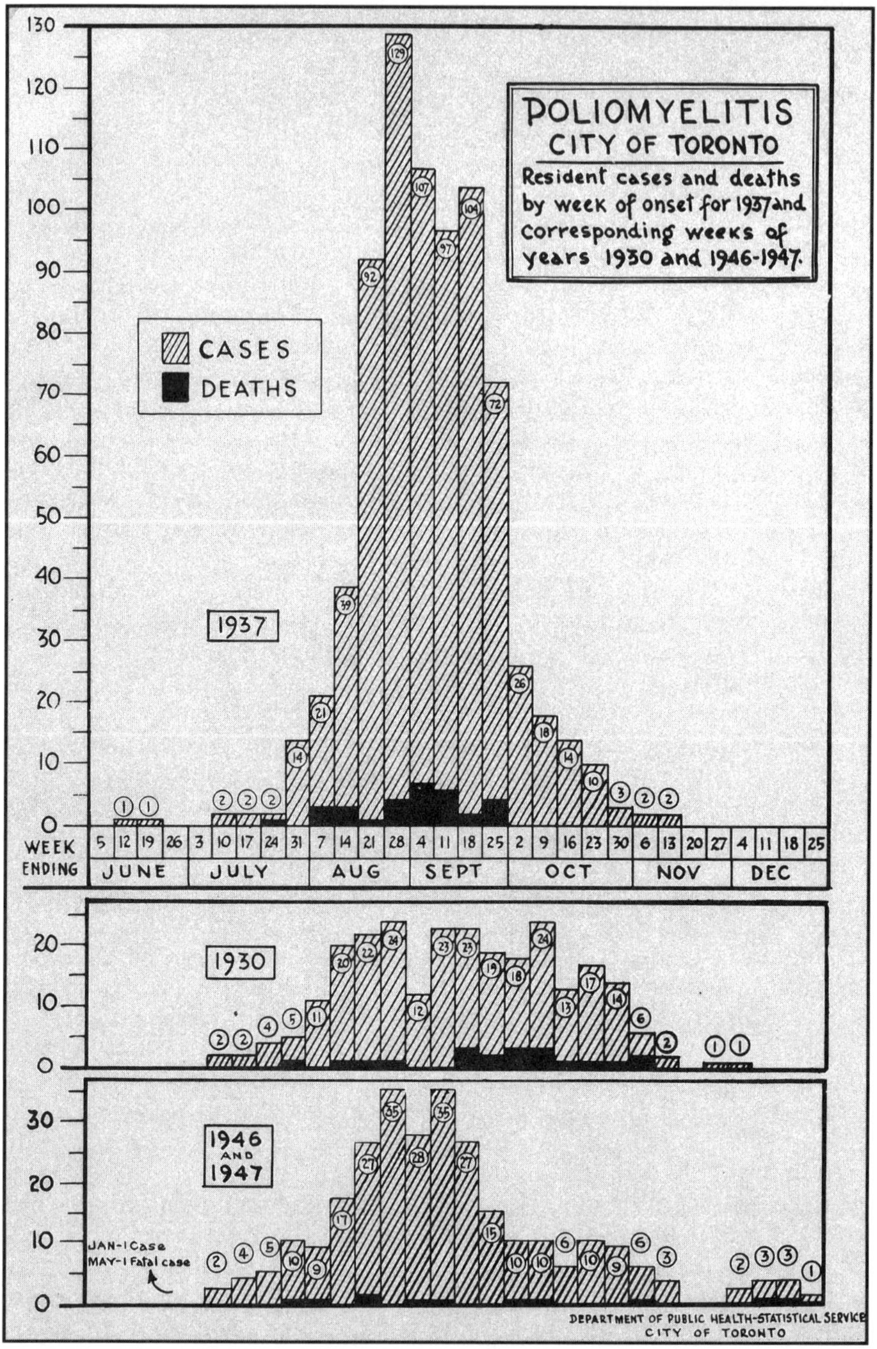

This graph clearly indicates the seasonal nature of polio outbreaks and the large number of cases which Toronto experienced in 1937 in comparison to other years.

By the second week in October, the public health experts announced that the epidemic had peaked in late September and that the city's schools could be opened. To obtain enough nurses to examine the elementary pupils while the district medical officers inspected the secondary school students, the Division of Public Health Nursing called on the services of former members. Married public health nurses and those who now worked for the VON, the St. Elizabeth Visiting Nurses, the Neighbourhood Worker's Association, the Toronto Red Cross, and the University's School of Nursing, quickly volunteered. After two and a half weeks, all the children in Toronto's 94 public schools and its 32 separate schools had been assessed, and the volunteers returned to their regular duties. A few new cases of the disease were uncovered through this mass screening but its major impact was to reassure concerned parents that the epidemic was over.

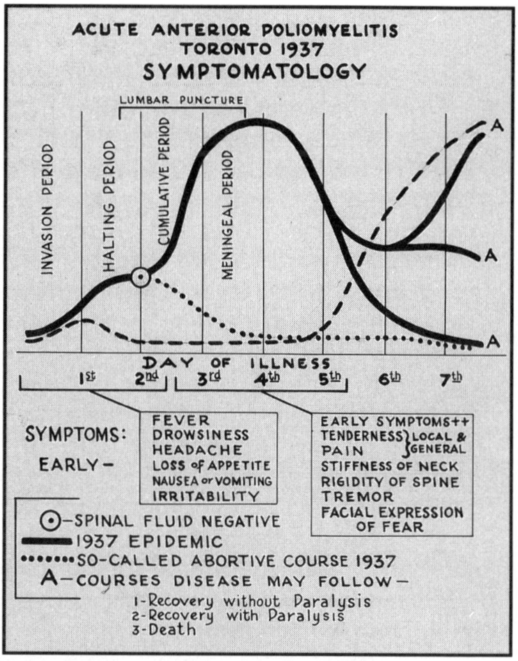

Prepared with data supplied by the Departmental Diagnostician, this chart illustrates the staff's interest in contributing to the research process.

Advancing Knowledge: Clinical Experiments and New Vaccines

In addition to their work in the field, the Isolation Hospital, the diagnostic clinics, and the Hospital Social Service section, the public health nurses assisted a research team from the Hospital for Sick Children (HSC), the Connaught Laboratories, and the School of Hygiene. Like their colleagues in London, Ontario, the researchers wanted to learn whether zinc-sulphate nasal spray would prevent polio and if it was an effective public health measure. Through newspaper advertisements, the experimenters received more than 6,000 applications for 5,000 places. Health Department nurses supervised the clinical trials at Toronto General and HSC; they also interviewed the children in their homes to test for loss of smell, and used other children on whom they called, to develop a control group. The results of the spraying were unimpressive. Children who had received the spray were just as likely to get polio as those who had not been sprayed. Equally important, the spraying required the services of expert otolaryngologists and was time consuming and expensive.[37] This clinical trial had been funded by the Ontario Health Department, and represented the way that the close ties between the research community, provincial experts, and local health administrators were used to advance medical knowledge.

As American researchers also found zinc sulphate spray useless, the research focus shifted to finding an effective vaccine. Support for the campaign originated in the White House where F.D. Roosevelt, himself a polio casualty, assisted with the organization of the National Foundation for Infant Paralysis in 1937. Through the March of Dimes, ordinary citizens contributed to the research funds which enabled scientists at various American universities to discover the three strains of poliovirus, and prove that the disease lodged in the alimentary tract before attacking the central nervous system. In 1950, Dr. Jonas Salk, a University of Pittsburgh researcher funded by the National Foundation, announced that he had created a killed-virus vaccine for each of the three types of viruses. The challenge lay in mass producing the viruses and killing them with formalin.

Widespread polio outbreaks in North America in 1951 and 1953 added urgency to the research process. Public fears were high. In 1951, when journalist Scott Young told the admissions nurse at the Hospital for Sick Children that he had brought his five year old son, Neil, to be tested for polio, two women standing nearby moved hurriedly away. Little Neil was given a painful lumbar puncture which confirmed the disease, and admitted to the hospital for a week of care in the isolation ward. His family was sent home to Omemee and quarantined.[38] Part of the fear stemmed from the increasing number of adult cases. In 1951, Toronto had 376 cases with 16 deaths, while in 1953, there were 271 cases and 12 fatalities.[39]

During the early 1950s, Connaught Laboratories played a large role in producing polio viruses and became the sole Canadian producer of the Salk vaccine for the national Department of Health and Welfare. An extensive clinical trial, which included forty-four American states, two Canadian provinces and Finland, began in 1954. On April 12, 1955, exactly ten years after Roosevelt's death, the National Foundation announced that the Salk vaccine was effective and that mass immunization using commercial preparations would begin immediately in the United States.[40]

In Canada, the federal government also arranged for immunization programs, but they were administered by local health departments because of shortages in the vaccine. In Toronto, the campaign was limited to children in grades one, two, and three, because research had demonstrated that they were the most susceptible age group. In the spring of 1955, Connie Gray, the Assistant Superintendent of Public Health Nursing, organized vaccination teams consisting of two doctors, three nurses, and two to four volunteers, to immunize thousands of youngsters. After the students' consent forms had been signed, the immunization teams travelled from school to school with their vials of vaccine, needles, syringes, and sterilizing equipment. Long lines of baby boom children were quickly given the three shots which were expected to confer immunity from the three strains of the poliovirus.

But tragedy struck in the United States. Cases of polio occurring within three weeks of vaccination put the reputation of the vaccine in jeopardy. The

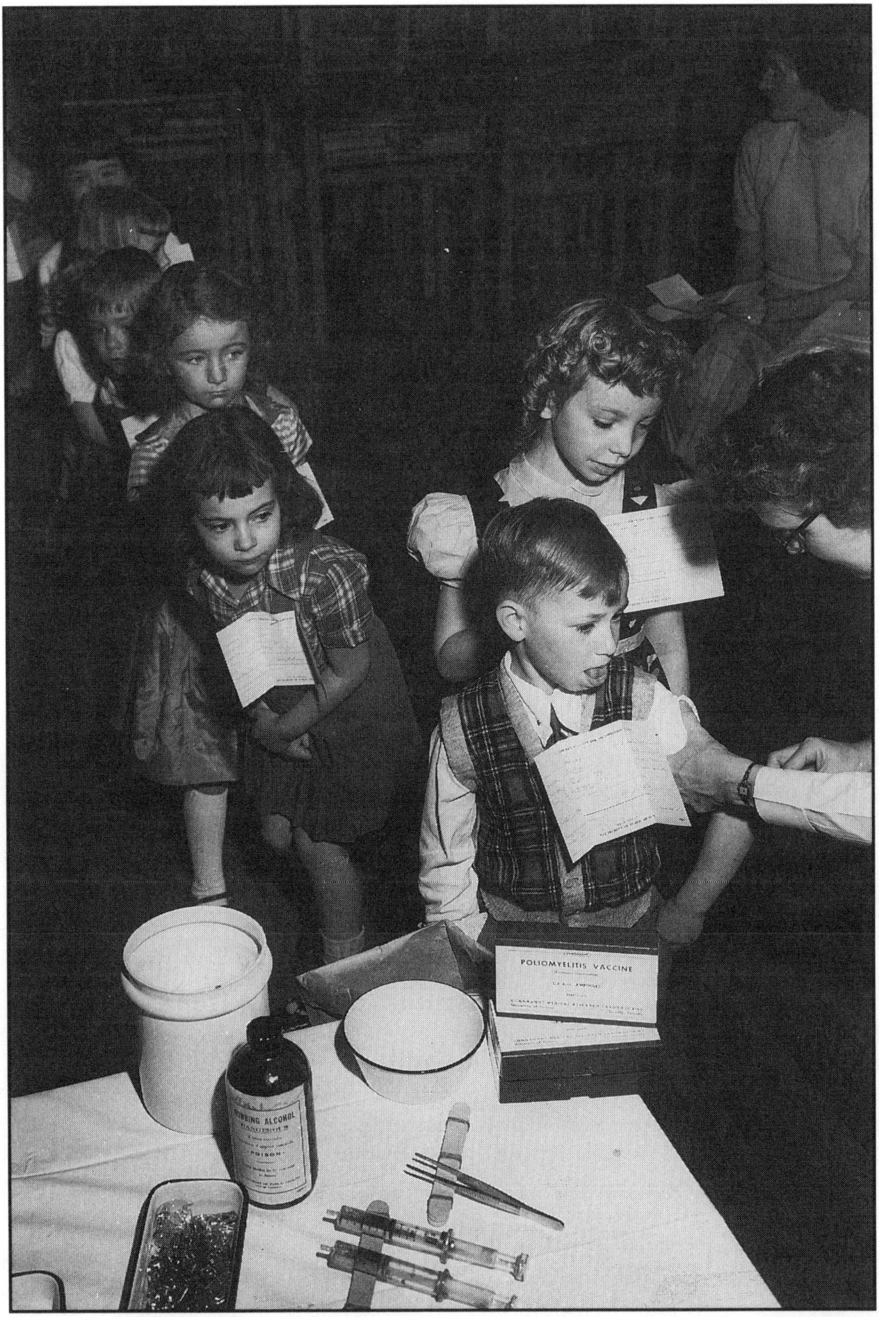

Apprehensive but intrigued, Toronto school children await their turn to be immmunized with Salk vaccine.

American Surgeon-General immediately stopped the program while investigators probed its source. Quickly, the outbreaks were traced to lots of the vaccine produced by the Cutter Laboratory in Berkeley, California. By May 14, vaccination resumed in the United States.[41] Since the vaccine in Canada was triple tested by Connaught, the Provincial Virus Laboratory, and the federal Department of Health and Welfare, Paul Martin, the Minister of National Health and Welfare, decided that immunization would continue here.[42] There were no cases of polio among those who received the more than two million doses of the vaccine in Canada, and by September 13, 1955, the *Toronto Telegram* was editorializing that the "Polio Vaccine Proves Itself."[43]

With the decline in the number of communicable disease cases, the city began to question the necessity for continuing to support the Riverdale Isolation Hospital. During the 1940s, the provincial deputy health minister had suggested converting one building into a convalescent hospital. Polio epidemics in 1946 and 1949, as well as in the early 1950s, added to the discussion, because the local board of health got into an acrimonious debate with the provincial health department about payment for non-resident patients. In 1953, the needs of senior citizens for a chronic care facility, and concern about alternate accommodation for convalescent patients, coincided with the creation of Metropolitan Toronto. From 1954 to 1956, the city and Metro shared jurisdiction over the facility but in 1957, it became Metro's responsibility.

By 1957, Toronto's polio immunization program had been expanded to include all of the city's elementary and secondary schools, and parents wanted this preventive measure extended to pre-schoolers. That year, the child health centres offered polio immunization to children who did not have family doctors. As cases of the disease declined among children, adults became its victims. The Canadian March of Dimes and various other groups, including Local 79 of Toronto's municipal employees' union, asked the local board of health to extend protective immunization to adults who could not afford it. This request irritated the president of the Ontario Medical Association who attended a business luncheon to discuss the matter. He pointed out that doctors would provide service to all patients who requested the vaccine, regardless of ability to pay, since they received free supplies from provincial authorities. Other politicians and citizen's groups attending the meeting argued that such programs were the Health Department's responsibility.[44]

Although he warned the board of health that organizing adult clinics because of an outbreak in Montreal was futile since immunity was not immediate after vaccination, the medical officer, Dr. Boyd, responded to the board's request and opened four adult evening clinics in September. Based in the city's high schools, aided by volunteers and supplies from the March of Dimes, the effort to immunize using combined polio and tetanus vaccine was a disappointment. Only the lunchtime clinic at City Hall really attracted large numbers because, as Boyd had predicted, adults were slipshod about completing the three doses of the Salk vaccine.[45] Between 1959 and 1961,

The Health League provided this brochure which answered common questions about polio immunization to interested Health Departments, doctors and citizens.

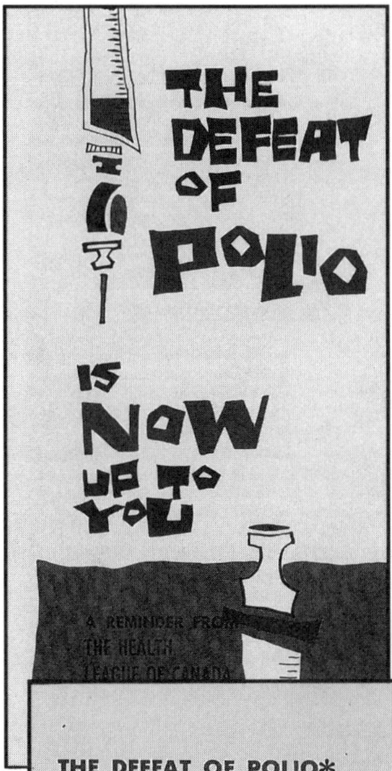

THE DEFEAT OF POLIO*

is in your doctor's hands. But the final, conclusive step in achieving this victory is in *your* hands. If the dread killer and crippler is to be listed with smallpox, diphtheria, tetanus and other once-invincible maladies, *you must be vaccinated.* Vaccination is your protection. So be wise, immunize . . . soon!

Here are the answers to your questions about poliomyelitis vaccine:

Q. WHAT IS POLIOMYELITIS VACCINE?

The vaccine is polio virus, grown in the laboratory, then killed and made safe so that it is effective in causing the body to build defences against the disease.

Q. WHO SHOULD BE VACCINATED?

Everyone. Although poliomyelitis attacks are still most prevalent and serious in the one to 21 age group and among pregnant women, no one is exempt.

Q. WHERE ARE VACCINE INJECTIONS AVAILABLE?

Consult your family doctor or local health department.

Q. HOW MANY INJECTIONS ARE REQUIRED?

Three doses are needed, with a month's interval between the first and second, and not less than seven months' interval before the third.

Q. WHEN DOES PROTECTION BEGIN?

Body defences begin to form seven to 10 days following the first injection and increase sharply after the second. The third dose raises these defences to the desired high level. A booster injection two or three years later enables the defences to remain at that level.

Q. HOW COMMON IS POLIOMYELITIS IN CANADA?

The disease, once called infantile paralysis, has been known in Canada for some years. However, there has been a steady increase in the number of cases since 1946.

***HERE'S CONCLUSIVE EVIDENCE**

In 1956 a control test was run on 1,800,000 vaccinated and unvaccinated children in Ontario under 18 years of age. Among the 840,000 who had received one or more inoculations there were five cases of paralytic polio. Among the 960,000 who were unvaccinated, 71 attacks were recorded.

No case of paralytic polio has occurred in any child in Canada who has received all three inoculations!

In a recent severe polio epidemic in Chicago during which 1,850 paralytic attacks were recorded, *no child who had received all three injections contracted polio!*

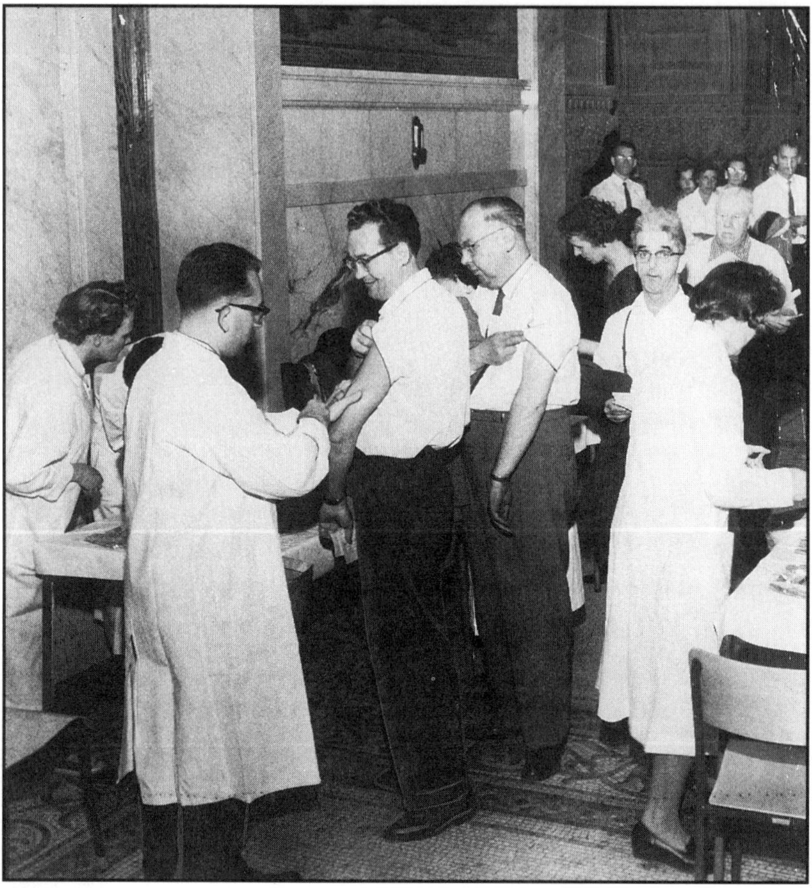

In 1959, Health Department staff immunized adults with the Salk vaccine in the city hall rotunda.

only 52,000 of Toronto's 465,000 adults over twenty, completed the three shots.[46]

The Health Department, however, worried about unprotected adults and was willing to launch another mass campaign when the next vaccine, the Sabin live oral vaccine, was announced. In contrast to the killed-virus Salk vaccine, the Sabin used small numbers of live viruses in a sweet syrup to take the viruses directly to the alimentary canal, where they multiplied and produced antibodies which circulated in the bloodstream.[47] Once again the Connaught Laboratories produced much of the vaccine used in Canada. All the health departments in Metropolitan Toronto and York County agreed to coordinate their immunization programs to ensure maximum public awareness and immunization.[48]

After receiving federal approval in March, the vaccine was launched on a week's notice, with great fanfare and publicity in May 1962, to counter any potential summer epidemics. Still, concern about possible side effects prompted the various health officers to publicize not just the benefits, but also contraindications to the vaccine's usage. Radio and television broadcasts, advertisements, and news reports, supplemented the traditional reliance on newspapers and posters. The effectiveness of the publicity produced a run on Toronto's fourteen clinics, which led the *Telegram* to caption its photos of the opening on May 15 as "1–Jam up 2–Line up 3–Drink up!." Nonetheless, the deputy medical officer, Dr. Moss, expressed disappointment that only 27,820 Torontonians were immunized on the first day, because the staff had been prepared to serve three to five times that number.[49]

In Toronto, mass immunization with these two vaccines has eliminated the threat of disease, except for those whose religious beliefs prohibit use of such preventive measures. In 1978, some young members of the Dutch Reformed Church returned to Toronto suffering from polio after a visit to Holland. Although several cases of paralysis resulted, the bulk of the population was unaffected, except for the pressure on vaccine supplies which occurred when people realized that their immunization was not up-to-date.

The eradication of polio as a threat to Torontonians' health illustrated how medical science in conjunction with preventive services moved from control and rehabilitation to primary prevention. During the 1920s and 1930s, Toronto's Health Department staff relied on traditional measures to prevent and control the spread of the disease. They followed the progress of research in Canada and the United States and often modelled their procedures on those in use in cities like New York and Edmonton.[50] In 1955 and 1962, the Department staff created immunization programs which introduced the Salk and Sabin vaccines to widespread use. By assisting with research studies carried out by Connaught Laboratories and the School of Hygiene, the doctors and nurses contributed invaluable data which ensured the safety and effectiveness of the vaccines. When the polio vaccine was added to the DPT preparation to create a quadruple antigen, medical science indeed had triumphed over significant childhood killers.

Conclusion

In 1960, George Moss told his colleagues in the Ontario Public Health Association that "Discovery, without application, has but little value."[51] Toronto's deputy medical officer was reminding his colleagues of the important role which local health departments played as the link between the research community and the public. These ties had developed during the 1920s and 1930s, when Toronto had served as one of several centres for clinical trials of diphtheria toxoid and polio convalescent serum, and thus contributed to the advance of medical science while continuing to safeguard its citizens' health. This process influenced the Department's disease control procedures and tied it closely to the medical model, because it shifted attention away from poverty and other social and environmental factors in disease and disease control.

By the 1950s, however, Toronto's medical officers recognized that the battle against many of the age-old bacterial and viral diseases was being won and that new challenges were on the horizon. The sporadic cases of diphtheria and smallpox that occurred in the following decade, and the resurgence of tuberculosis, suggested that victory was not complete, and that Toronto would have to remain vigilant because of the possibility of importing contagious diseases. Nevertheless, the disease control and prevention activities of the inspectors, the public health nurses, the medical directors and the senior administrators, like those of the food control and sanitation inspectors, had contributed to lengthening Torontonian's life-spans, and protected them from the hazards which had taken such a toll in the nineteenth century. The impact of their work was apparent in the declining importance of communicable diseases as sources of morbidity and mortality in the city. Instead, chronic diseases and environmental problems became the leading killers after 1945. This trend challenged the Department to redefine its disease control procedures, to differentiate more clearly among primary, secondary and tertiary prevention, and to evaluate the appropriateness of the medical research model as a tool for dealing with these new health threats.

Chapter Eight

Modernizing Motherhood: Health Education

"Education is the means by which probably nine-tenths of permanent efficient public health work is accomplished."[1] This bold declaration by Charles Hastings summed up the Victorian social reformers' belief, that "educating" the public held the key to modernizing society and lowering Canada's high infant and maternal mortality rates. But what type of education should be used? What social values were being introduced, in addition to information about babies' growth patterns and the environmental factors which threatened their health? Was education being used as an alternative to an attack on poverty?

As they had with sanitation measures and disease control procedures, Toronto's health reformers turned to the programs and rhetoric which health crusaders in Britain and the United States used for inspiration in their educational work. Under Hastings's dynamic direction, Toronto's Health Department imitated London, New York City, Boston, Montreal, and Hamilton, when it took over existing programs such as volunteer-run milk depots and baby clinics. The right of a public agency to provide these services provoked controversy and opposition from doctors and some taxpayers, but in the early years, the reformers were able to overcome these objections. By transforming the volunteer activities into basic services which the Department provided, Hastings and his nursing director, Eunice Dyke, were establishing a pattern which their successors emulated. External groups identified a health concern, created a demonstration project, and then surrendered the responsibility to local health authorities.

This pattern functioned well during the creative and economically prosperous years of Hastings's administration. During the Great Depression, however, lack of funds and the shift to behavioural science and professionalism altered the staff's approach to women and children's services. Using material produced by the Department's medical consultants, the Canadian Public Health Association, the Child Welfare Council, the Red Cross, the federal and provincial maternal and child health bureaus, and other Canadian and American health organizations, the staff helped popularize the latest discoveries in medical research and child psychology. Such activities contributed to standardizing child rearing practices, and when added to other sources of information, such as articles in newspapers and magazines, modernized motherhood.

The Department's strategies for reaching women changed over time. Initially, home visits and the child health centres were the foundation for the educational efforts because they fostered personal contact and enabled the nurses to see their clients in their own environment. By the late 1940s, group activities were becoming more accepted because of the lack of nursing staff and the growing number of new mothers in the post-war years. Like their colleagues in the Medical Services Division, the public health nurses participated in a variety of clinical trials and experiments to test the effectiveness of specific community health education services between 1950 and the 1980s. Gradually, they became aware of significant social developments which were making their long-established programs obsolete. Through the 1950s, the number of working women increased, and many were compelled to return to the work force after the birth of their children, as a result of economic necessity. The large number of babies born during the decade, however, provided a significant clientele for the child health centres, and masked the underlying social changes which would irrevocably alter the Department's approach to this type of educational activity.

The arrival of large numbers of non-English-speaking immigrants also posed a challenge. Would the Department be able to hire multilingual nurses as it had during the first wave of immigration prior to 1914? Did the immigrant women who attended the Department's child health centres fully understand the advice and literature which they received? And how could the staff communicate their knowledge without threatening the cultural values of the newcomers? As Toronto was transformed from a predominantly British and Protestant city to a multicultural metropolis, the Health Department became one of the major contact points between the host society and immigrants. In contrast to the prewar period when assimilation was the dominant philosophy, the post-war decades saw a growing respect for the beliefs and practices of immigrants, which resulted in the introduction of transcultural nursing education courses during the 1960s.

These social changes occurred as the public health movement entered a period of crisis and self-examination. During the 1950s, some public health administrators and nursing educators began to question whether the services that were being provided were relevant to society's needs. As the number of senior citizens increased and chronic diseases became the most important causes of mortality, these experts argued in favour of revising existing programs and modifying the focus on women and children. In the 1960s, the slow process of dismantling the services and programs which were an entrenched aspect of the Department's activities, began in response to growing interest in evaluating the effectiveness and efficiency of publicly-funded agencies.

By the 1970s, the impact of the women's movement and multiculturalism prompted growing disenchantment with their role and concern about the long-standing emphasis on traditional forms of health education among the Department's nurses. Younger staff also began to ask whether home visits to all newborns could be curtailed in favour of visiting high risk infants, and if the Department's prenatal classes could be reoriented to reach immigrant groups. Senior administrators were aware of the growing interest in program evaluation and health promotion. As a result of these factors, the service component which had evolved since 1910 was dismantled in an effort to focus attention on primary prevention and health advocacy.

Saving the City's Babies

In 1910, the first of Dr. Helen MacMurchy's three reports on infant mortality in Ontario shocked Torontonians into the realization that their city had the same problem as London, New York, Milwaukee, and Montreal, because 131 out of every 1,000 live babies died before they were a year old. Although parents and physicians were expected to report births to the city clerk, who then reported to the Health Department's statistician, under-reporting was widespread until 1920 and hence official data were unreliable. But the grim figures reiterated in 1911 and 1912 prompted an immediate response from charitable groups and led to calls for public efforts to halt "the slaughter of the innocents."[2] Drawing on the international child saving movement for models, concerned reformers identified three key factors in infant deaths: poverty, maternal ignorance, and diarrheal disease from improper feeding. The solutions which French, British, and American doctors and lay reformers had developed for these problems were to create milk depots, to provide expert medical advice through baby clinics, and to send health visitors into homes to teach women how to care for their babies.[3]

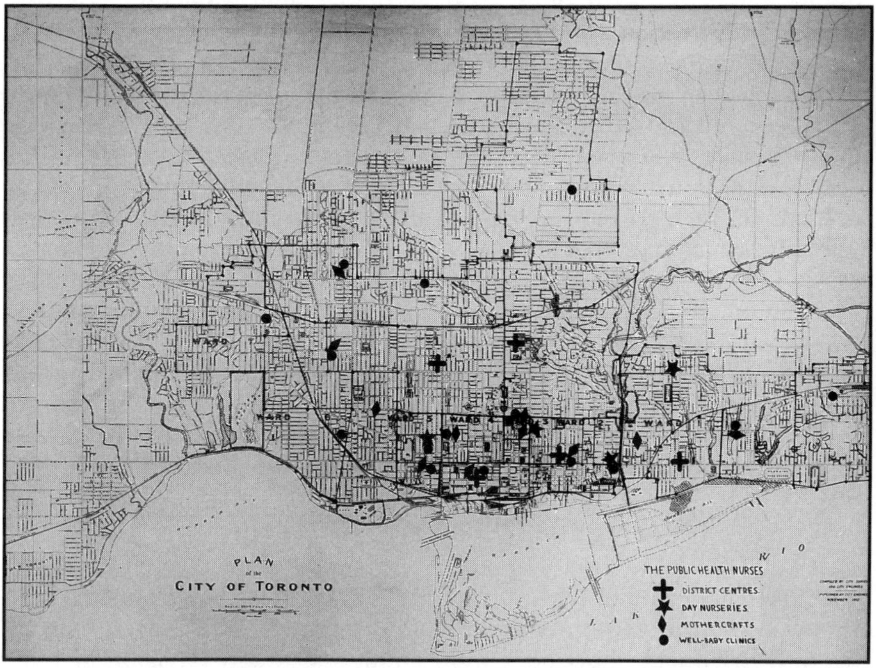

Depending on their location, Toronto women could seek assistance from the Department's public health nurses, or the staff at the day nurseries, mothercraft centres and well baby clinics run by voluntary groups.

A variety of voluntary groups in Toronto copied these models and set up a system of milk depots and well baby clinics at the Evangelia and University Settlements, St. Christopher House, and the Fred Victor Mission. Several women's groups, churches, and Women's College Hospital, also joined the Hospital for Sick Children (HSC) in providing pasteurized milk to less affluent Toronto children. Most of these groups depended on part-time medical staff and philanthropists for funding. Such community-based charitable efforts were the prototype for future expansions of health education and service activities, but in 1912–13, the basic objective was to provide pasteurized milk and train Toronto's mothers in proper infant feeding techniques.

Prior to his appointment, Hastings had been deeply involved in publicizing child health problems. His experience as an obstetrician and his social gospel beliefs led to a rapid expansion of the Department's child saving work. One of his first steps was to appoint three nurses to advise mothers on infant feeding in July and August 1912, because more babies died of gastro-intestinal problems during the summer months. Recognizing that this duplicated other activists' efforts, Hastings organized a meeting at which the summer work was divided between these welfare agencies and the Department, to ensure that all needy families received assistance. Pure milk production was centralized at the Hospital for Sick Children, and the Department's nurses visited the home to see that the mother understood how to protect the health of her child and the quality of the milk. This laid the foundation for systematic birth registration visits and gave the nurses a chance to develop a district clientele.[4]

Among many medical experts there was a widespread belief that most women did not know how to care for their infants, since they relied on their female relatives and neighbours for advice and guidance. To overcome this presumed maternal reliance on folklore, many of the settlements and several hospitals set up well baby clinics. At these weekly meetings, women had their babies examined by volunteer doctors and were given instructions on how to improve or maintain the child's growth rate. In 1913 the medical volunteers at several of the clinics asked Toronto's medical officer about forming an association of clinics "in cooperation with the city." Hastings turned them down because he believed that the Hospital for Sick Children should co-ordinate such services. By September that year, he had changed his mind because the lack of nurses and "somewhat irregular" clinic attendance by medical staff had failed to halt the rising infant death rate.[5]

Creating the Division of Child Hygiene

After Hastings and his statistician demonstrated the weakness of the existing system, most of the voluntary groups transferred their nurses to the Health Department, more staff were hired, and a new Division of Child Hygiene was created in 1914. After some conflict with existing clinic medical directors, the administrative relationship was clarified in 1915 when Dr. Alan Brown of the Hospital for Sick Children became the division's part-time medical director. His appointment reflected Hastings's determination to integrate medical expertise into the preventive services which the Department provided. Like its relationship with the University of Toronto's Faculty of Medicine, the links with the Hospital for Sick Children benefited the Health Department by providing access to medical research and outpatient services. In return, the Department's clinics were used to test new immunization procedures and preventive measures.

For Alan Brown, soon to be recognized as Canada's leading pediatrician, this position provided an ideal opportunity to offer extensive training to potential specialists while at the same time educating Toronto's women in modern child rearing practices.[6] To ensure that there was a standardized approach to the activities of each clinic, Brown held training sessions for doctors at the Hospital for Sick Children and personally chose the volunteer physicians. As late as 1949, the chief of pediatrics at the Medical Faculty and the physician-in-chief of HSC were responsible for staffing the clinics and assisting with policy formation.

In the early years, great emphasis was placed on breast feeding because a recent epidemiological study at Toronto General Hospital had corroborated British and American authorities' arguments that mother's milk protected the baby from gastrointestinal disease.[7] Using American publicity material, Hastings reiterated this message in the *Health Bulletins* which also listed clinic locations and times. The Department's growing corps of nurses reinforced the doctors' advice when they weighed the babies during the weekly afternoon clinics. Assisted by community volunteers who arranged the clinic facilities and provided snacks, the public health nurses provided counselling and maintained records of the child's progress. The nurses' work was fundamentally educational, but if health problems were noticed, they did district follow-up work to ensure that the baby received care or treatment.

Tact and diplomacy were necessary for both the doctors and nurses who staffed the clinics. The work that they were doing was seen as infringing on

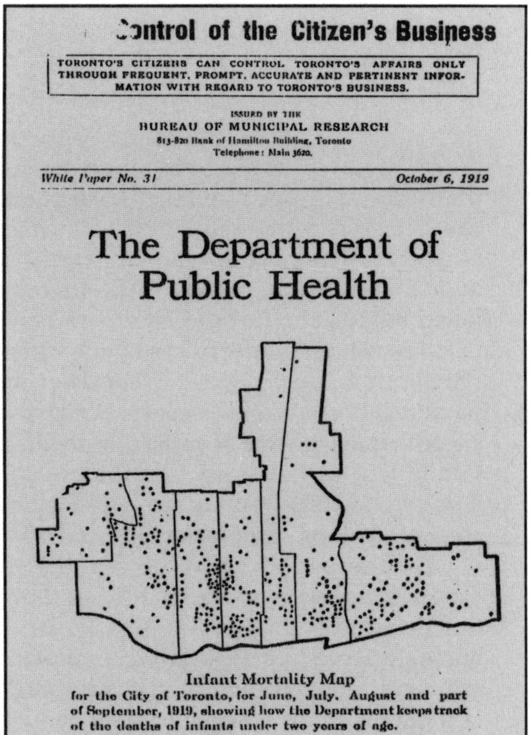

The Health Department used pin maps to indicate districts with high infant mortality.

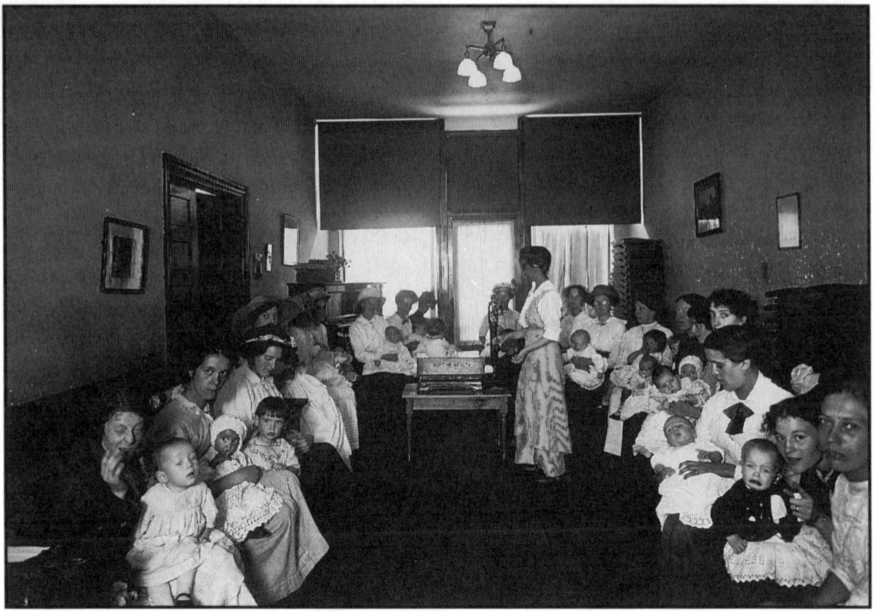

One of the public health nurses is weighing a baby in the Department's portable scales while other mothers and their infants wait their turn at the Riverdale Settlement.

the prerogatives of local practitioners. To forestall conflict, the nurses asked physicians if they wanted the Department staff to visit new mothers, and the clinic doctors sent form letters to their colleagues informing them of their patients' attendance at the clinic and requesting permission to provide advice and immunization. These attempts to overcome medical opposition failed because in Toronto like New York, Oxford, and Montreal, practitioners resented public services which were available to the entire community. They wanted public agencies to relieve them of care for the poor but to leave paying patients to their exclusive ministrations. Muted criticism of Hastings' expansionary efforts appeared in medical journals, and in the creation of a Public Health Relations Committee at Toronto's Academy of Medicine.[8] During the 1920s, public support for this municipal service was strong in spite of doctors' reservations.

For the public health nurses, the well baby clinics were merely one aspect of a larger educational program. In their home visits, they initially functioned as educators and social workers. In their role as teachers, the nurses offered practical advice about household sanitation, refrigerating milk and food supplies, and the importance of screens to prevent fly contamination. They warned women about the dangers of "summer diarrhea" and the necessity for prompt medical attention to prevent dehydration. As well, the nurses stressed that siblings or adults with colds or other contagious disease should not be allowed to handle the baby. To fulfil Eunice

Dyke's belief that hands-on demonstration was more effective than verbal or written instruction, nurses during the 1910s and 1920s showed new mothers how to bathe their babies or prepare their bottles.[9]

When home visiting started, the nurses quickly realized that many parents were unable to adopt their suggestions because they could not afford to buy high quality milk or the ice to cool it. Since the Department did not intend to expand its mandate to include direct relief efforts, poverty-stricken families were assisted through referrals to the Neighbourhood Workers' Association, an umbrella group for city charities. From 1921 to 1931, the Health Department served as the city's relief agency and many staff nurses were concerned when the Department of Public Welfare was created. Although they feared the loss of contact with city social workers, the nurses found that sharing office space with their municipal colleagues and representatives of community groups, enabled them to continue to provide prompt referrals. The nurses and their supervisors thus served as a source of information for both clients and other agencies.

In Toronto, religious and cultural differences affected the Department's maternal and child programs in the decade prior to and during World War I. To deal with their ethnic population, cities like New York pioneered the use multilingual nurses and translated their health pamphlets into other languages. Toronto copied these efforts and in 1915 and 1916, the Department

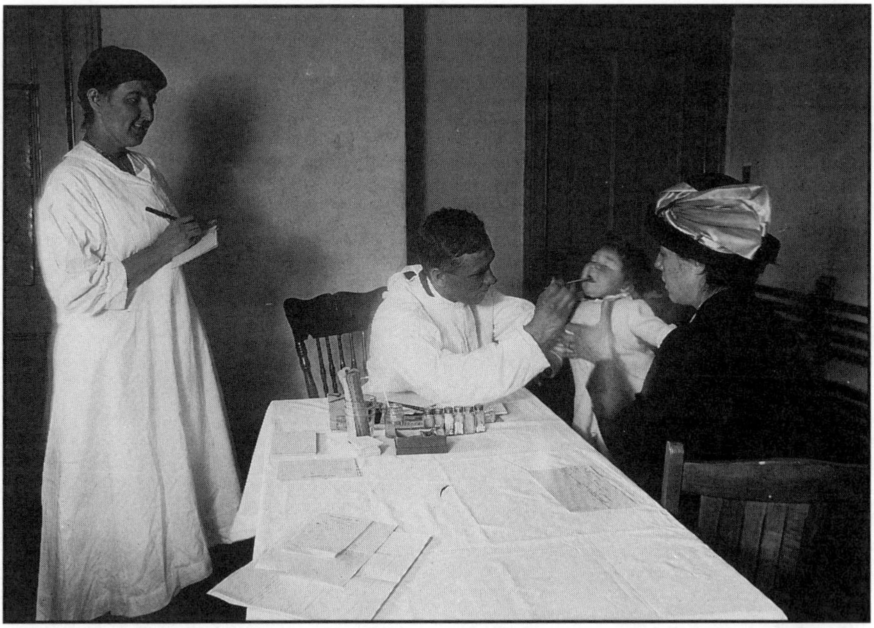

At least once a year, babies were examined by the Department's doctors or a medical volunteer. The nurse pictured at the St. Christopher House Clinic, like her colleagues in the other districts, used the information provided during the examination as the basis for home visits.

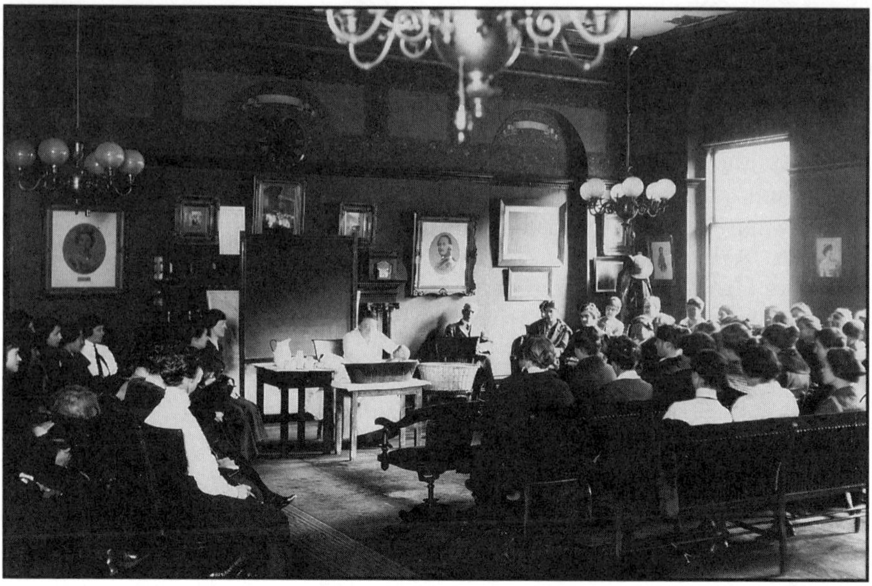

To prepare nurses for their home demonstrations, staff training sessions such as the baby bathing pictured in March 1919 were used.

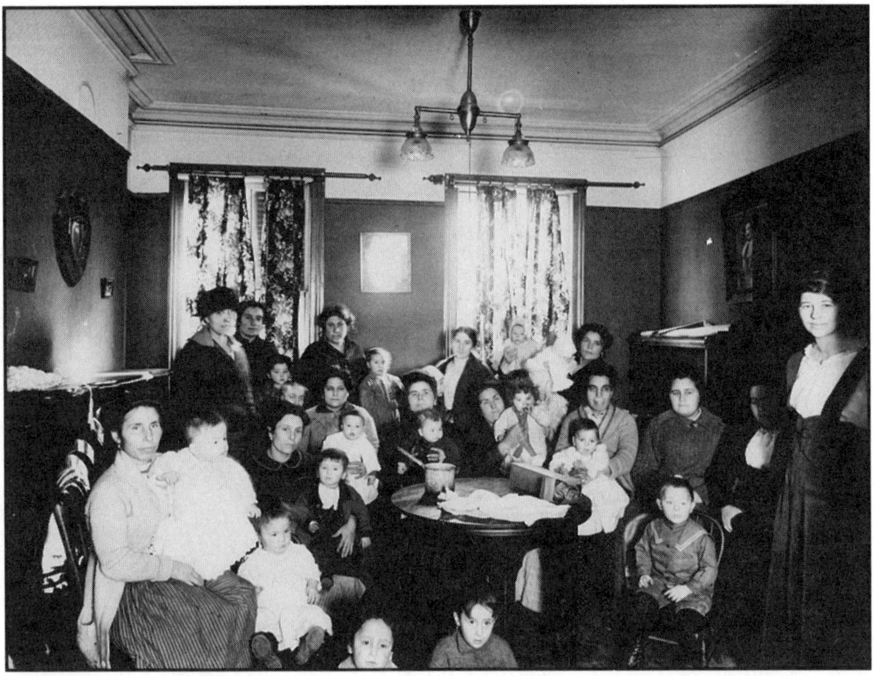

The members of this Italian mothercraft group were photographed with their children in January 1915.

hired two "language" nurses, Matilda Simoni and Zara Price, to serve the city's Italian, Polish, and Russian citizens. In 1920, Parashka Stamenova joined the staff to work with the Macedonian community. This initial attempt to serve a multicultural population in its own languages did not survive post-war tensions or the decline of immigration in the 1920s. Simoni resigned in 1921, but Price and Stamenova remained on staff in spite of city employment policies which called for the removal of "aliens" in 1925 unless they became citizens.[10] By using nurses from the same cultural background as the clients that they were serving, the Department was acting simultaneously as an agent of assimilation and a buffer against the pain of acculturation. Given the widespread belief in the superiority of the British-Canadian way of life, few health reformers were unduly concerned with the psychic cost of the advice that they were giving the first group of immigrants.

Changing Theories: Modernizing Childhood

During the 1920s and 1930s, the content of all the nurses' home visits and clinic consultations changed. As pediatricians and child psychologists achieved public recognition as experts in infant health and behaviour, magazines, newspaper columns, and the advice literature prepared by the city, the province, and the federal health department, began to stress the importance of routine and training in child management. The interplay between experts and their clients illustrated the shift from didactic teaching to behavioural advice and from traditional to modern child rearing practices.[11] For Canadians, the best known example of this approach was the professional effort to raise the Dionne quintuplets in Northern Ontario. From 1934 onward, *Chatelaine* and other women's magazines joined newspapers and professional journals in describing the combined efforts of Drs. Allan Roy Dafoe, Alan Brown, and William Blatz, of the St. George's Child Study Institute, to prescribe a regimen for the little girls.

Such widespread publicity made the public health nurses' educational work easier. By 1935, the nurses were reporting that more women were asking for advice about training problems, not just the physical aspects of their baby's care. As a result, the nurses changed their teaching techniques to encourage greater participation by the mothers that they counselled. To do this, the staff stopped didactic presentations and gave women charts to complete, on which they listed the sleeping, eating, and behavioural problems which their children developed.[12] This marked the transition from the humanitarian focus of the first generation of nurse educators to the professional orientation of their successors. In large measure, this development occurred because the infant mortality rate in Toronto had declined by fifty per cent by the middle of the 1920s, and the research results of behavioural psychologists were achieving public acceptance. When allied with the increasing social work component of public health nursing education, these factors contributed to a subtle but significant change in the approach of Toronto's nurses to their role as agents of modernization.

Expanding Services: The Fight for Pre-school Clinics

Although service in the well baby clinics was initially offered for infants under one year, the Department soon recognized that little was being done for pre-school children. By 1922, the network of twenty-one clinics had become child health centres, and Hastings was using the Department's monthly *Health Bulletin* to urge parents to bring their pre-school children for free examinations. He justified the expansion of service by arguing that many correctable physical problems were evident in kindergarten and grade one students, and that these should be looked after before the child started school. His comments led the executive of the Child Welfare Council and Toronto's Home and School Council to ask the Academy of Medicine if it supported pre-school examination by Health Department doctors and nurses. Not surprisingly, the doctors responded negatively to this extension of state medicine. While the members of the Public Health Relations Committee urged their colleagues to pay greater attention to pre-school clients, Toronto's doctors, like their American counterparts, were too busy with curative activities to do preventive counselling and immunization.[13]

In large measure, practitioners' concern stemmed from the increasing use of the child health centres. In 1916, 822 clinics with an attendance of 13,715 babies, or an average of 17 per clinic were held. By 1928, 1,667 clinics staffed by one doctor, two public health nurses and several volunteers provided 47,096 children with free medical advice. For contemporaries, the clinics and home visits were a success, because Toronto's infant mortality rate declined from 132.2 per 1,000 live births in 1910, to 63 in 1923, and by 1924, 75% of its mothers were breast feeding their children.[14] Toronto, however, was not unique. In Britain, the United States and other Canadian centres, the infant death rate had been declining since 1900. Better sanitation, pure water supplies, and pasteurized milk all played a role in lowering the toll.

Nevertheless, the popular perception that health education had contributed to the decline led to increasing support for extending such service to the pre-school population. In 1929 and 1930, the Home and School Club, the Board of Education, and the Health Department, decided to hold pre-school examination and toxoid clinics for the two to six age group in several schools on Saturday mornings. These clinics did not survive long under Depression conditions. In spite of this setback, public demand for the expansion of services continued. In 1933, a deputation from the Local Council of Women, the Child Welfare Council of Toronto, the Home and School Council, the Community Health Association, and the municipal chapter of the IODE, presented a list of projected health needs based on information culled from the medical officer's monthly reports from 1929 to 1933. These women argued that the Department's staff had found 16,887 pre-schoolers with health problems in 1930–31, a 30% increase from 1929. They feared that a similar increase had occurred as the Depression worsened in 1932 and urged the Board of Control to increase the Health Department's appropriations to allow it to expand its child health services.[15]

Although he appreciated the spirit in which the suggestions were made, Jackson pointed out that his shrunken nursing staff had done their job by finding the defects. He did not think city finances would permit any expansion at this time. In adopting this position, the medical officer was identifying with other civic administrators and conforming to the politicians' interest in limiting expenditures.[16] Like health officers in Britain and the United States, Jackson substituted health education for service during the depths of the Depression.[17]

Continued pressure from the women's groups secured the opening of five pre-school centres in 1936, but the Board of Control cut the request for continued funding from 1937 until 1942, in spite of clear public demand for the service. During that period, both Alan Brown and the Phair Committee condemned the lack of specific services for the pre-school child. The medical officer responded to these criticisms by explaining that in addition to lack of funds, his staff had discovered that using existing child health centres was more effective, as most parents could not afford the time to make two trips to separate clinics.[18]

In 1952, a national health grant from the federal government enabled the Department to create an alternative to a network of city clinics by introducing a trial system of pre-school registration in the Hillcrest demonstration area. To ensure medical support, the new health officer, Dr. Pequegnat, sent a letter to all local practitioners asking them to complete the child health inventory card which his staff distributed to mothers during the preregistra-

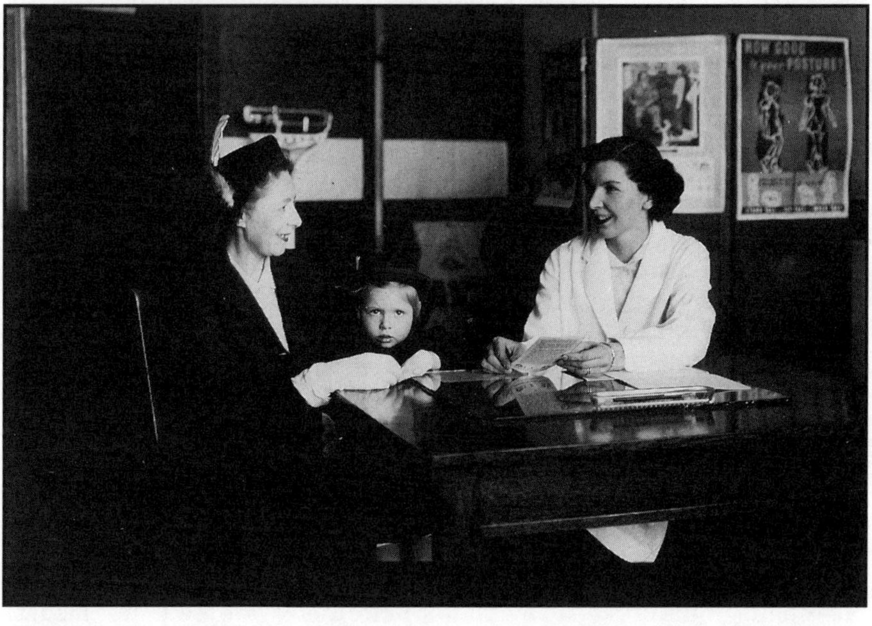

This serious pre-schooler was photographed with her mother and the district nurse to illustrate an article describing pre-school registration, published in the 1952 ***Health Bulletin.***

tion meeting. He followed this with an address to the Toronto Academy of Medicine in which he emphasized each doctor's responsibility for preschoolers' health, and pointed out that a thorough physical examination, immunization and behavioural assessment before they entered kindergarten would cut down the amount of service that the school doctor had to provide. In effect, Pequegnat was trying to broaden the range of services which general practitioners offered to include preventive work.[19] By suggesting this approach, the medical officer was conforming to the contemporary view that prevention and cure formed part of the spectrum of health care. He was also being realistic because the Ontario Health Survey had demonstrated a lack of public health personnel, and as a veteran of the squabbles with the profession during the 1930s and 1940s, Pequegnat wanted to ensure co-operation not conflict. The pre-registration program proved so successful that it was implemented in all of the Department's districts, and by the end of the 1950s, the majority of children were examined by their family physicians prior to entering kindergarten.

From Baby Boom to Bust: The Decline of the Child Health Centres

The post-war era brought new challenges to the public health nurses and medical staff in the child health centres. Most of the clinics were held in church basements, community centres, settlements, and other rented premises. Even though the women and children only attended monthly, the district clinics, which were held three or four afternoons a week, became very busy during the baby boom between 1947 and 1963. For many war brides and new mothers, these sessions provided a chance to share their experiences with others like themselves. Former nurses recall a pleasant family-style atmosphere developing in spite of the often long waits to see the doctor or the nurse. To keep the 35 to 72 children who attended each clinic happy while their mothers were consulting with the nurses, play stations were introduced in 1955. But as the nurses ruefully noted, the toys which the volunteers provided when the clinics re-opened in September always seemed to disappear by the following spring.

There was, of course, a class and ethnic dimension to this service. Although the clinic at Glenview Presbyterian church in North Toronto was well attended, most women in that district preferred to visit their family physicians for pediatric checkups. Many women from the less affluent districts like the East End and Riverdale, attended the clinics because they did not have family doctors until medicare was introduced. But as a former district supervisor observed: "Mind you, sometimes, it is the poorer people who don't take advantage of what is in the community."

Equally striking was the rapidity with which Italian, Portuguese, and Greek immigrants flocked to the clinics. Since there were few ethnic medical practitioners in their communities during the 1950s, they willingly used city services. Through the 1950s, concerned nurses in the heavily immigrant-populated districts began to take night courses at the University of Toronto

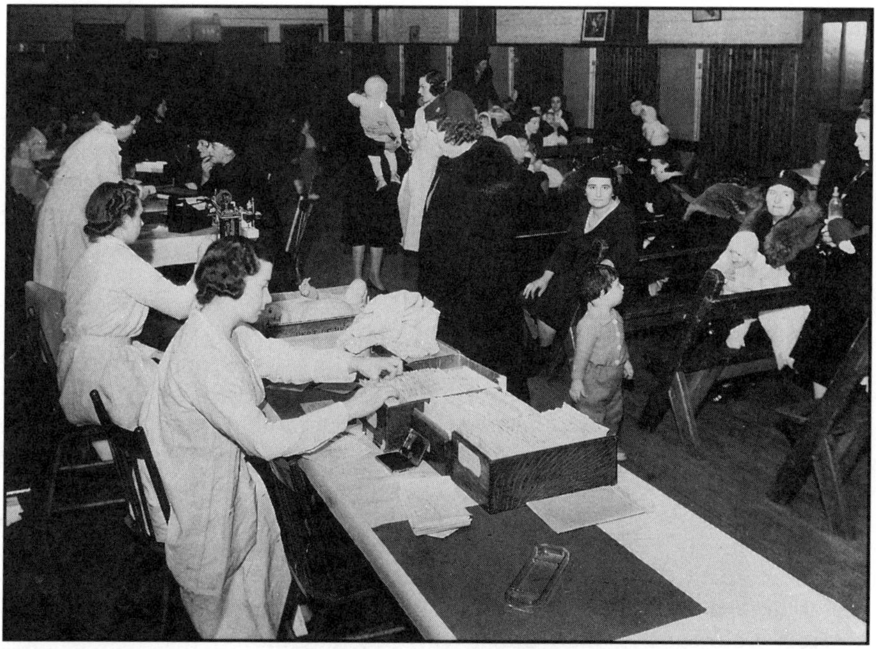

This child health centre held in a church basement in the late 1940s shows how busy the staff were responding to the demand for their services.

in order to be able to communicate at a basic level with their new clients. By 1958, Eileen Cryderman, the Director of Public Health Nursing, reported to Dr. Boyd that her division needed more staff and more clinics. The doctors and the nurses working in the Parkdale, Riverdale, and Hillcrest districts had informed her, that the addition of immunization to their duties and the rapid increase in the number of newborns, limited their time for counselling women about their pre-school children. From the staff's perspective, the difficulty was compounded by the slow process of translation. Although the Department's few bilingual nurses assisted their colleagues at the child health centres and on home visits, hiring additional multilingual staff was difficult because they were few in number and other agencies were also seeking their services.

The situation attracted the attention of the local board of health, and in his report on the matter, Boyd noted that 46% of the babies born in 1957 had attended child health centres. Repeat visits, however, were slowly declining because of the two to three month waiting periods for appointments. The medical officer recommended opening three new child health centres and five immunization centres, to attract more newborns and to have time to carry out more pre-school assessments. By 1961, Toronto had thirty-one clinics operating just as the baby boom began to end.

Had the boom turned to bust? In 1959, Dr. Gordon Martin, the Director of the Ontario Health Department's Public Health Administration Branch, and a colleague, conducted a survey of maternal and child health programs in the province. All of Ontario's thirty-three health units and its fourteen local health departments devoted roughly two-thirds of their staff time to these activities. But Martin concluded that there was still friction between practitioners and health department staff about the use of child health centres for educational and immunization services. He also noted a growing interest among health professionals in modifying the topics, which they discussed with parents, to include more recent research material on problems such as accidents.[20]

But were modifications to the content of the discussions sufficient? In 1961, R.B. Freeman published a brief article called "Measuring the effectiveness of public health nursing services;" it was a forerunner of the spate of evaluation procedures that were developed during the following decade.[21] Questioning the status quo became the norm in the 1960s. For Toronto's nursing directors, the rapid decline in attendance at the child health centres demanded a careful survey of client's reactions and an attempt to redefine the centres' activities.

In 1962, senior nursing staff proposed some potentially radical solutions to the child health centres' problems. In contrast to their predecessors who had stressed the importance of community coverage, they suggested focused work in high birth rate areas. As well, they questioned the appropriateness of clinic visits for women with several children, and instead, sug-

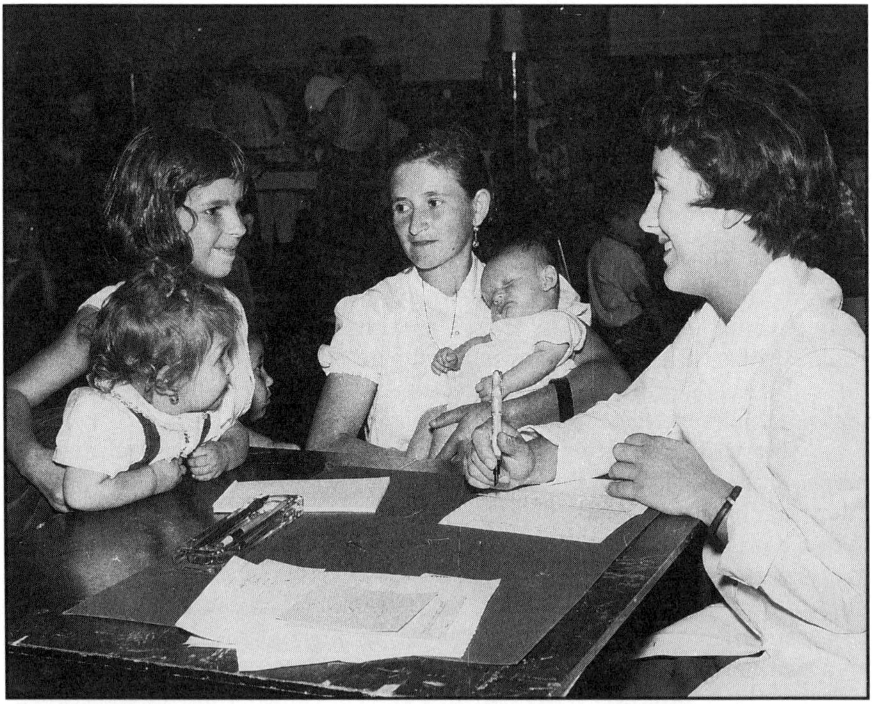

During the 1950s and 1960s, immigrant children often translated the nurse's advice for their parents and neighbours.

REGISTER OF CHILDREN

Date of Admission	NAME	Sex	Date of Birth	Name and Address of Agency or Persons from whom Received	Name and Telephone Number of Physician to be Called in Case of Illness	Date on which Removed	Name and Address of Agency or Persons by whom Removed

Baby boarding house operators were expected to keep a register of their clients and submit it to the Health Department's inspection staff.

gested home visits to discuss books like Eric Erikson's *Childhood and Society*. Above all, the report's authors stressed that the Department had to recognize that many women would be returning to work, and that their concerns centred around finding appropriate care for their babies.[22] Although the Health Department had been responsible for inspecting maternity boarding homes since 1897 and had added day nurseries and play schools to its roster of activities during the First World War, the nurses were aware of a shortage of registered facilities for infants. Even the Department of Public Welfare and City of Toronto day nurseries did not take children who were less than two years old.

As more Toronto women rejected the social convention that dictated that married women did not work, the need to modify the Department's maternal health education programs grew. During the 1960s, female participation rates in the work force increased to the point that 80% of women in their child bearing years were working by 1971. This socioeconomic change spelled the end of the child health centres because women no longer were able to visit them in the afternoons, and the majority turned to their family doctors for immunization and advice.

In spite of growing questions about the effectiveness of the child health centres, some new duties were added to its services. In 1961, mental retardation was described in the *Annual Statement* as a "gray plague" that had been increasing since 1946 as a result of the rising birth rate and the increasing survival of afflicted babies. Sixty years of experience had led scientists to conclude that the chief causes of mental retardation were birth injuries, mongolism (today known as Down's syndrome), congenital anomalies, infectious diseases and metabolic diseases. To prevent or minimize birth defects, Mental Health division staff recommended good prenatal care and education about phenylketonuria (PKU). Since this metabolic disease could be treated effectively if discovered early, a system of routine PKU testing was introduced in the child health centres for all infants under six weeks.[23] By providing this type of primary prevention, Toronto's Department was joining an international effort which included health authorities in cities like Oxford, which began routine testing in 1968.[24] Today, genetic counselling is available to parents with a family history of mental or physical problems, but the causes of many cases of mental retardation remain unknown.

During the 1970s, Toronto's birth rate, like that of all industrial cities, plummeted as women practiced family planning and were integrated into the workforce on a permanent basis. As attendance continued to decline, the child health centres were closed and by 1980, there were only five clinics left. Two of them closed during the year. Through the 1970s, friction between the Nursing and Medical Services divisions increased, because the nurses wanted to reallocate staff to other community functions while the doctors expressed concern about lack of follow-up for clinic clients.[25] And a philosophical change in nursing education from training in health education to an emphasis on community action for health promotion, exacerbated relations between the two groups as they tried to divide the Department's services and programs into primary, secondary, and tertiary forms of prevention. With decentralization, all the child health centres were closed and home visits were restricted to high risk babies, as the nurses refocused their health education efforts on health advocacy.

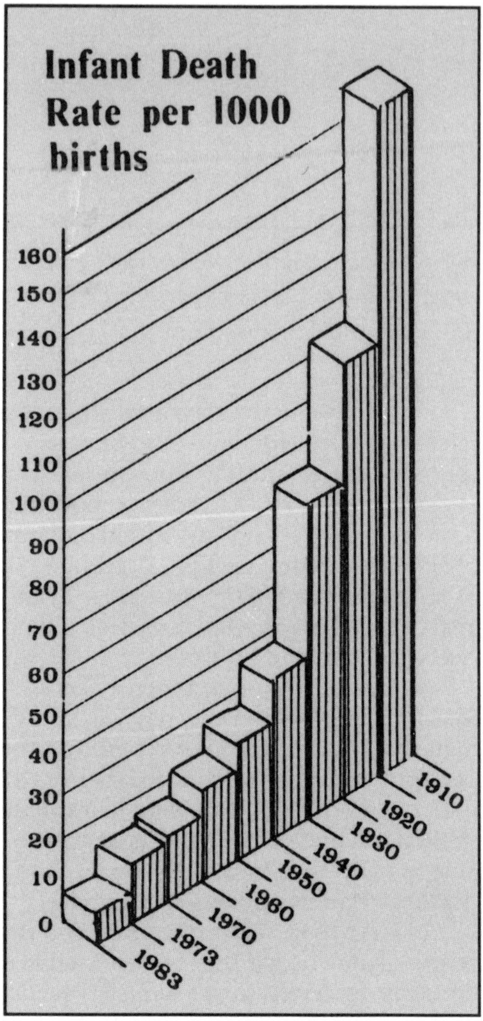

By 1983, Toronto's infant mortality rate was a fraction of its size in 1910.

Combating Maternal Mortality

"Departments of public health...must realize that they are nation builders" whose "work begin[s] with conception and end[s] with the grave."[26] As an ardent imperialist, Hastings shared the concern of many of his Canadian and British contemporaries about high infant and maternal mortality rates among the poor. For the social reformers, the high rejection rate for Boer War and First World War recruits demonstrated the long-term effects of maternal and child poverty. In Britain, the National League for Health, Maternity and

Child Welfare created London's first antenatal centre in 1915, and after permissive legislation was passed in 1918, clinics offering antenatal care were opened in hospitals and by local health authorities.[27]

Toronto's reformers also began to respond to the problem at this time. In 1913, the Department's nurses started to keep "sporadic" records of pregnant women that they visited, and with the opening of prenatal clinics at the Toronto General and St. Michael's Hospitals, were able to recommend expert medical assistance for the poor. For more affluent women, the nurses provided general advice on "bodily care, proper food, dress and housing" and urged them to turn to their family physicians for regular examinations.[28] Both groups were warned not to use midwives, and the Department's nurses were expected to report any cases in which they suspected these women had assisted, because midwifery was illegal.[29] To ensure that women received more appropriate advice, the Department prepared a brochure called *Pre-natal Care — Advice to the Expectant Mother.* Distributed first in 1922, the pamphlet was updated in 1927 under the direction of the professor of Obstetrics and Gynaecology at the University of Toronto.[30]

Like their counterparts in England and Chicago, few Toronto women sought prenatal medical care because pregnancy was still seen as a private matter. Most women asked their mothers, relatives, neighbours, and friends, for advice on the physical and psychological changes which occurred during pregnancy. If they could afford it, women engaged medical assistance for their confinements but most still expected to give birth at home. Hospital lying-in wards were for the poor, while the private patient's pavilion at Toronto General or private maternity hospitals catered to a more affluent

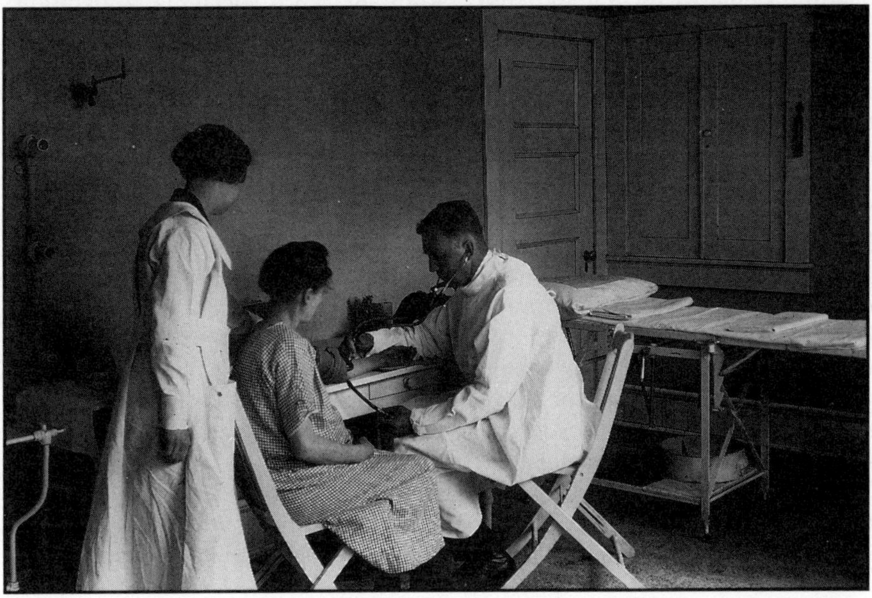

Taken in June 1924, this picture shows a prenatal clinic at the Evangelia Settlement.

clientele.[31] Persuading the city's women to adopt medical supervision of their pregnancies remained a challenge for the nurses during the 1920s, as five city-run prenatal clinics were added to the seven located in Toronto's hospitals.

During this decade, the problem of maternal mortality became a prominent topic among public health professionals as they contemplated the lessons of the Great War. In Britain, Dr. Janet Campbell reported on the growing number of maternal deaths in spite of educational efforts and clinic services. In 1924, Canada's Dominion Health Council asked Dr. Helen MacMurchy to study the problem in this country, and her preliminary findings led the Canadian Medical Association to press for a full study. When her report was released in 1928, Canadians were horrified to learn that we had the fourth worst maternal mortality rate among leading industrial nations. Only the United States, Scotland and Belgium lost more mothers. But were such losses preventable? MacMurchy, like Campbell, argued that lack of adequate care during the prenatal period and at confinement contributed to the sepsis, hemorrhage, and eclampsia, which killed new mothers.[32]

Saving the City's Mothers: The Maternal Welfare Service

Combating maternal mortality demanded public action because according to Gordon Jackson, "the passing of a mother is particularly devastating in that it leaves in its wake an irreparable trail of pain and suffering, a broken home and too often a scattered family." Echoing concerned women's groups, Toronto's health officer feared that delinquency and "social maladjustment" was the price paid for lack of health education and medical service for expectant women.[33] In 1931, Toronto was one of many Canadian cities which became involved in the crusade against maternal mortality. On Mother's Day, a well-publicized mass rally was held in the Eaton Auditorium to discuss the problem. Sponsored by the Local Council of Women and the Child Welfare Council, the meeting had the support of the Department of Public Health, the Academy of Medicine, the Victorian Order of Nurses, the St. Elizabeth Visiting Nurses, the Neighbourhood Worker's Association and several other charitable agencies. The delegates prepared a resolution asking for the creation of a committee to investigate "*All* causal factors." The Health Department was nominated as the project's leader because the reformers believed that maternal mortality was not simply a medical problem, and wanted the medical, social, and educational issues examined. By adopting this request, the local board of health became involved in an on-going effort to lower Toronto's maternal mortality rate.

With Medical Officer Gordon Jackson at its head, the Advisory Committee on Maternal Welfare established subcommittees, which undertook a detailed two year study of the causes of the problem. In its final report, the committee recommended the creation of a home based relief scheme that would ensure all needy mothers of adequate pre- and postnatal care. Introduced on September 1, 1933, the maternal welfare service had cared for 4,500 patients by 1939. Only seven of these women died. This meant that the plan had a mortality rate of 1.6 per 1,000 live births in comparison to the general city rate of 5.4 per 1,000.[34] Throughout the 1930s, the scheme was funded on an annual basis, which led local women's groups to keep a close watch on city politicians and the Health Department. Their lobbying activities and the lack of medical opposition ensured that the program would continue. In contrast to their reaction to other Department programs, the doctors accepted the maternal welfare service because it was restricted to indigent patients, and if physicians participated, the city paid them a minimal fee for their efforts.[35]

Pioneering in Prenatal Education

During the 1930s, Toronto's Visiting Homemakers Association became concerned about the adequacy of the relief diet provided by the city. With the assistance of researchers from the Department of Public Health Nutrition in the School of Hygiene, they conducted a series of surveys to determine food consumption levels. In most homes, women fed their husbands and children first, even when they were pregnant. These revelations, and pressure from the Phair Committee to develop more effective prenatal activities, led the Health Department nurses to join the VON, the St. Elizabeth Visiting Nurses Association, and the Visiting Homemakers, in designing and introducing prenatal classes sponsored by the Welfare Council of the Community Chest in 1944.[36] Although most North American health departments agreed that educating women about pregnancy and childbirth

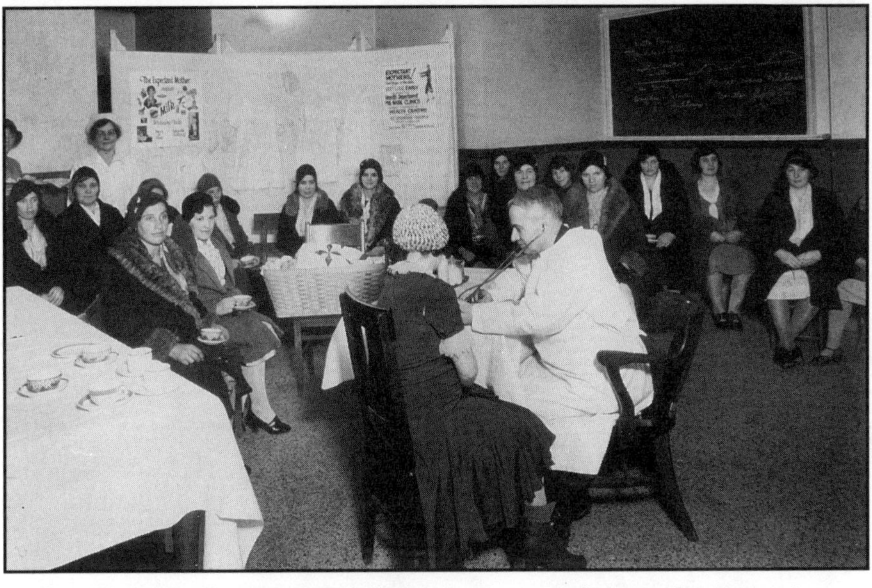

By the mid-1940s, the Department had started prenatal classes for women in conjunction with local charitable groups.

was an appropriate health education activity, there was little unanimity about who should provide the training. In cities like Edmonton, this type of service was provided solely by the Victorian Order of Nurses, from 1940 to 1966, when it became a health department responsibility.[37]

In Toronto, the Department's nurses were heavily involved in teaching prenatal courses and publicizing this new service, especially to first-time mothers. The nursing and nutrition staff who prepared the course material submitted it to the Departments of Obstetrics, Pediatrics and Psychology at the University of Toronto for approval. This reliance on medical expertise was a long-standing attribute of Departmental policy but also mirrored increasing public respect for the success of medical science. In addition, surveys of the women who participated in the classes were done in 1949–50 and 1950–51 to determine consumer reaction. Most women found the experience very positive and appreciated the chance to share their concerns with health professionals and other pregnant women. They felt that they had learned "the truth instead of old wives' tales," and that the information on labour and handling the baby made motherhood enjoyable rather than frightening. And many of them urged the staff to consider creating fathers' classes or to integrate the classes and hold them in the evening.

In 1952, the program was broadened to include expectant fathers. They were given separate classes on successive evenings by an obstetrician, a public health nurse and a nutritionist. Their sessions stressed the role which the husband should play in supporting his wife through her pregnancy and in caring for the baby after it came home. This innovation received national publicity through a 1953 article in *Health* which informed prospective fathers that "every baby needs to have the loving tender care of his father as

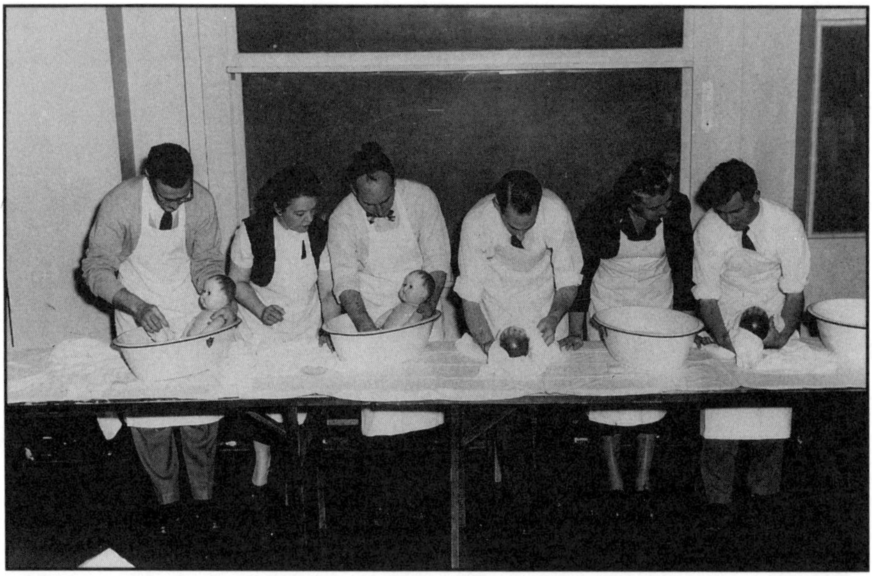

By the late 1950s, some Toronto men were learning how to bathe a baby as part of the the Department's prenatal course for first-time fathers.

well as his mother. If he is to be a pal on fishing trips later, he should be a pal in diaper days."[38] There was no mention of the fathers participating in the birth of their children, because a survey of Toronto hospitals in 1958 revealed that few of them were prepared to admit husbands to the delivery room beyond the first stages of labour. Nonetheless, the value of men's participation was recognized in 1957 when joint evening classes were introduced, and by the 1970s they were entering the delivery room as coaches and participants. This trend was apparent in Britain, Canada, and the United States, where the consumer rights movement greatly affected birth practices in the 1960s and 1970s.

New Needs, New Clients: Redefining the Prenatal Program

In contrast to the maternal welfare service of the 1930s, the prenatal classes attracted a middle class clientele. As early as 1950, Connie Gray, the Assistant Director of Public Health Nursing, was expressing concern that working class women were not attending the sessions. She recommended a more diversified approach, and stressed that a program like this must be modified to suit its consumers. In particular, the Department had to respond to the demand for the courses among working women. By 1957, 50% of the women enroled in evening classes were full-time workers. Two decades later, most prenatal classes were offered in the evenings because this trend continued.

From the 1950s to the present, the city's ethnic mix has altered as well. In 1978, the Health Planning Steering Committee's report noted that only 25% of Toronto women attended the city's classes, and recommended a sustained attempt to reach the remaining 75% who, it suspected, were not attending for financial or cultural reasons.[39] Indeed, research by a staff nurse and an associate professor of nursing at the University of Toronto, highlighted the different perceptions of the importance of prenatal classes and "scientific" medical care for Canadian, Portuguese, East Indian, and Caribbean women. Although Canadian-born women attended the prenatal classes enthusiastically, immigrant women thought group learning was a "strange idea" and preferred to seek advice from family and friends. In the early 1980s, the Department tried to overcome these cultural barriers by offering prenatal classes which incorporated their cultural values to Vietnamese, Chinese, and West Indian women through agencies such as the Immigrant Women's Centre.[40]

Other new client groups appeared as well. As society's moral code changed, pregnant teenagers opted to complete their pregnancies and to care for their own babies. Few of them had much knowledge of basic nutrition principles, and many failed to seek prenatal care prior to giving birth. During the 1960s and 1970s, the Department's nutrition consultant, and one of its assistant directors of public health nursing, participated in joint studies of aspects of the prenatal program with researchers from the University of Toronto's School of Hygiene and Faculty of Nursing. The first project, a nutrition study, demonstrated that a sample group of reasonably

To attract clients, the Healthiest Babies Possible program developed a logo which symbolized its activities.

educated, employed women, did not conform to the Canada Food Guide's daily milk, fruit, vegetable and bread consumption requirements during their pregnancies. These findings suggested that the subjects of the second study — pregnant teenagers — needed more guidance on managing their diets and their pregnancies, than was available in the prenatal course and the Department's current system of home visits.[41]

These two studies convinced the Department to set up a new prenatal outreach program called Healthiest Babies Possible (HBP) in 1979. In contrast to the prenatal classes, which like the child health centres, had been established to serve the entire community, the new program had a clear target group: high risk pregnant women. The development of the Healthiest Babies Possible programme also illustrated changing trends in public health administration. This client-specific program with built-in evaluation mechanisms, was designed and implemented by the Department's nursing and nutrition staff, not external medical experts. Using community resources like local libraries and social agencies, the HBP team was attempting to assist these women to create their own support networks and to take control of their lives. Independence through health education was the project's objective. The staff involved in the project saw themselves as facilitators and partners, not detached, objective experts.

Using television, radio, magazines, and newspapers to publicize their activities, the nurse and the nutritionist who made up the HBP team worked on 308 cases in 1979, 340 in 1980, 324 in 1981, and 348 in 1982. Through carefully maintained statistics, they were able to demonstrate that this service had lowered the number of low birth weight babies from 11% to 7% of newborns in the high risk group. In 1982, HBP was integrated into the core programs offered by the Health Department, and a High Risk Pregnancy Registration programme was set up to assess women and offer them access to appropriate resources. By focusing on individuals who most needed assistance, the staff were ensuring that Toronto maintained its enviable record of no cases of maternal mortality.

Patients or Partners?: Changing Attitudes to Pregnancy, 1960–83

Pregnancy and childbirth became a focal point of preventive activity during the early decades of the twentieth century. At that time, environmental problems were dealt with to eliminate some of the major causes of maternal and infant mortality. As we have seen, the Health Department's contributions to this process included the pasteurization of milk, improvements in the water supply, and control of communicable diseases. But what of mainstream medicine? During the 1920s and 1930s, a shift from home births to hospital births began. Similar trends occurred in Britain and the United States. In 1937, 40% of British children were born in hospitals; this increased to 91.4% by 1972.[42] Americans adapted even faster, as 55% gave birth in hospital in 1940, and 88% in 1950.[43] By 1946, 96% of Toronto's 19,000 births took place in hospitals. But how did this affect mortality? Until the adoption of sulpha drugs and penicillin to limit puerperal sepsis, and blood transfusions to assist women who were hemorrhaging, hospitals were not especially safe for women.[44]

Toronto's doctors quite correctly blamed some of the maternal mortality on septic or criminal abortions. Members of the Ontario and Saskatchewan Health Departments raised the issue during the 1934 Canadian Public Health Association Meeting in Montreal, and it was still seen as a significant factor in Toronto in 1947, in spite of the use of antibiotics to treat patients.[45] In 1960, the *Globe & Mail* described Toronto as the safest place to have a baby in Ontario, because no women had died from the four leading causes of maternal mortality found elsewhere in the province: toxemia, hemorrhage, infection and anaesthesia. The paper did note, that of the ten maternal deaths classified as preventable, five were the result of botched abortions.[46] Until the Canadian Criminal Code was amended in 1969, abortion was illegal, and the attack on maternal mortality remained incomplete.

By the 1960s and 1970s, some middle class women in Canada, the United States and Britain were beginning to question the necessity for medical intervention in childbirth. For women involved in the second wave of feminism, medical dominance of delivery represented the "medicalization" of a natural experience.[47] Although most Toronto women continued to consult obstetricians and to have their babies in hospitals, this consumers' rights movement affected the Health Department in several ways. In 1979, as a member of the Hospital Council of Metropolitan Toronto and University Training Hospitals Association Joint Committee on High Risk Pregnancy, Doreen Hamilton, the Department's Parent and Child Health Consultant, prepared a minority report which stunned the medical participants. Instead of supporting the committee's recommendation for the construction of a six million dollar neonatal intensive care unit, Hamilton advocated a one million dollar educational campaign which stressed alternate approaches. These included:

government-sponsored prenatal classes, genetic counselling, legalization of midwives, studies of present obstetrical practices, studies on the possibility of out-of-hospital childbearing centres and the education of family physicians and obstetricians regarding nutrition, lifestyle factors, prenatal classes and midwifery skills.[46]

Hamilton's suggestions were supported by the local board of health which was strongly committed to "demedicalizing" childbirth. The board was unsympathetic to the health officer's dilemma in dealing with his medical colleagues and their support for the majority report, with its high tech equipment and emphasis on medical intervention. This conflict reflected the continuing split between preventive and curative medicine, and the growing competition between medical and non-medical personnel within the Department for future funds and public support.

Further proof that the previous deference to medical expertise was over, was evident in the Department's creation of its own Task Force on High Risk Pregnancy in 1980. This team criticized both the 1979 study, and an Ontario Government Task Force report on the same subject in 1980 because neither had indicated a role for public health. In one sense, both the medical reports

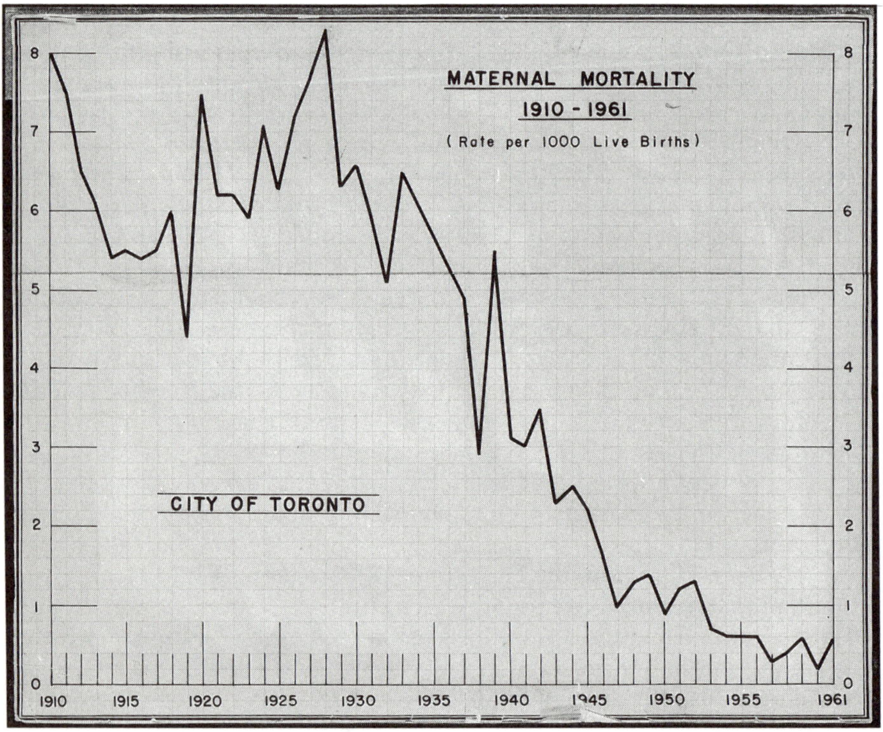

This graph shows the steady decline of maternal mortality in Toronto starting in 1942-3.

represented the ultimate expression of curative dominance in obstetrics; in another sense, they demonstrated rising public expectations about medicine's ability to save premature babies.

For the new generation of public health activists, official neglect of health promotion and health education activities in this critical area indicated that the federal government's working document, *A New Perspective on Health for Canadians,* and all the behavioural science research done during the preceding decade, were being ignored by the medical establishment. Pressure to change the Department's prenatal classes to reflect this new knowledge came from younger nurses who had studied health promotion techniques, and from board members who believed in the community action model of social development. Together these people revised the Department's prenatal course and introduced preconception classes. Both stressed the health risks which maternal behaviour, such as smoking, drinking or drug use, posed for the baby, and gave women the information that they needed to make informed choices about their actions before and during pregnancy.[49] The Health Department's efforts to combat maternal mortality provide a case study of the transition from treatment to education to health promotion.

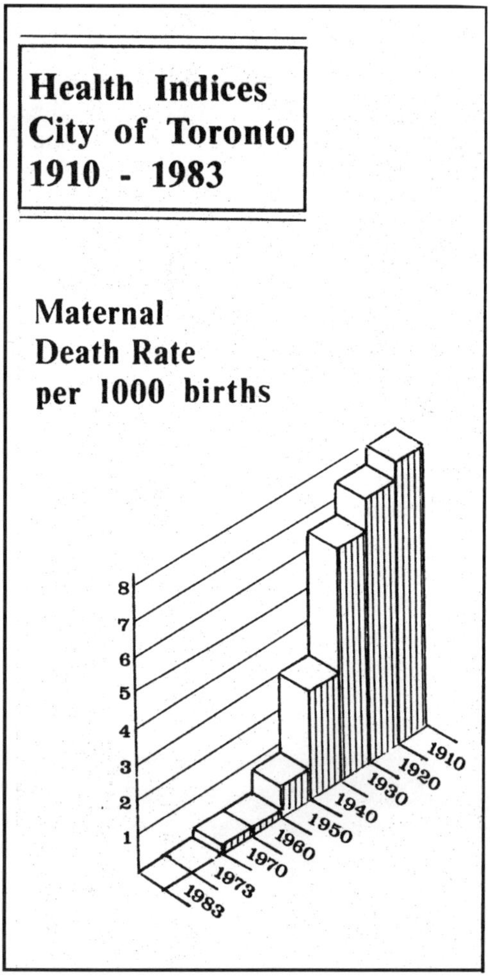

By 1983, maternal mortality was no longer a leading cause of death for the city's women.

Conclusion

The Health Department's continuing efforts to control and combat infant and maternal mortality illustrate how the international model was adapted to local circumstances. The evolution of these services and programs also demonstrated the continuing importance of voluntary groups and social activism. From the prewar supporters of well baby clinics, to the Local Council of Women during the 1930s and the women's groups of the 1960s, the Department has had both vocal supporters and caring critics.

These external influences were paralleled by changes in nursing education and practice. As the reform interests of the pioneers were displaced by the scientific objectivity of their successors, the Department's efforts in these two field were also undercut by the financial exigencies of the Depression. In the 1950s, the baby boom and the arrival of large numbers of immigrants meant that the medical and nursing staff had a new clientele to educate and little time to query the relevance of their activities.

But the rapid decline in the demand for their services at the child health centres, and the increasing difficulty of finding women at home during the afternoon visits in the 1960s, led the senior nursing administrators to begin the process of redefining health education work. The women's movement, and the criticism of hierarchical authority which it fostered, contributed to the development of new approaches. In nursing schools, courses in trans-cultural methods, health promotion and community activism replaced traditional health education training. All of these developments fostered change and renewal as the Department moved from health education to health promotion in this field.

Chapter Nine

"Keeping the Well Child Well": School Health Programs

For early twentieth century reformers, "keeping the well child well" was part of a broader effort to transform the educational system from its nineteenth century focus on rote learning, to its modern emphasis on developing well-rounded individuals. Both public health reformers and educational reformers believed that healthy children were happy students, and that doctors, nurses and teachers shared a common goal in teaching students good health habits. Such efforts paid further dividends because the children of today would be the parents of tomorrow, and training them in basic hygiene principles was expected to produce healthier future generations. In many respects, the alliance between health and education reformers was founded on the conservative humanitarianism of both groups. They wanted to improve but not drastically alter the social structure, and therefore targeted children as the most easily educated segment of society.

In 1917, Toronto's Health Department took over the Board of Education's school medical inspection system, which had uncovered large numbers of children with medical problems. Although regular examinations and daily assessments of students suspected of having communicable diseases remained the foundation of the staff's efforts, the Health Department was committed to a modern health education program. American advertising techniques were in vogue during the 1920s and health leaders adapted them to "sell" their message to children. Skits, pageants, songs, posters, and puppet shows, were used by public health nurses and teachers to teach children basic health habits.

Among the city's school population, there were children who suffered from significant physical or mental disabilities. Special classes were created for these students, and the Department's staff provided liaison between the schools, the parents, and other helping agencies. By the 1940s, Toronto's Department had a well-established program of maternal and child health services which revolved around the city's school children. In its assessment of city public health services, the Phair Committee criticized what it saw as the excessive emphasis on a small proportion of the population. This comment foreshadowed the changes that were to occur during the post-war years.

During the 1950s and 1960s, enrollment in Toronto's schools increased dramatically as the baby boom children passed through the system. For some of the doctors on staff, this was an excellent opportunity to conduct research projects in conjunction with their colleagues at the University of Toronto. For the nurses, the arrival of large numbers of immigrant children raised anew the question of the Department's responsibility in helping the newcomers adapt. In contrast to the situation at the beginning of the century, however, expertise and government agencies were under attack by community activists.

Education was especially vulnerable to the criticism that it was an instrument of social control wielded by the economic élite, and in the late 1960s, reformers won seats on the Toronto Board of Education. With their emphasis on community participation and equality for all, regardless of race, gender or social status, these men and women remodelled the city's education system. The Health Department was affected by this activity because the education reformers highlighted nutrition deficiencies, and the long-term health consequences of poverty, as factors which prevented inner city children from learning as much as their middle class counterparts. Since the reformers no longer believed that the Department's traditional programs were capable of meeting these needs, they pushed for targeted educational activities, consistent evaluation procedures and health advocacy. Their criticisms contributed to the growing pressure to reform the Department and its programs. In 1976, a Health Planning Steering Committee was appointed, and it embarked on the challenging task of forecasting future needs and redefining the Department's structure to meet them.

Promoting School Children's Health

"If a boy or girl is not impressed with the value of public health when he or she leaves school, there is something wrong with our method of instruction."[1] When Charles Hastings made these remarks at the beginning of his address to the World Federation of Education Associations in 1927, he was indicating that school medical inspection had been transformed into health education by his medical and nursing staff and their supporters in the schools. The change completed a long process of evolution, from the environmental concerns which Canniff had stressed in the 1880s through to Charles Sheard's anxiety about schools as a medium for spreading communicable diseases. Boston introduced school medical inspection to North America in 1894, and New York appointed medical inspectors in 1897, and pioneered the use of school nurses in 1902. Both the Hamilton and Montreal school boards established inspection systems in 1907, and that year Toronto's progressive reformers began their campaign for this extension of state medicine. Sheard's response was revealing because he told the local board of health that school medical inspection was "a pure fad" proposed principally by women, who were trying to get "easy billets for their friends, with good pay and little work."[2] In fact, the Local Council of Women and their medical supporters, who included Hastings, MacMurchy and Charles Hodgetts, the Secretary of the Provincial Board of Health, represented an élite group of social reformers who wanted to modernize the city's health and education services. Unable to convince the board of health to establish the program, the reformers turned to the Board of Education, and on April 24, 1910, medical inspection began.

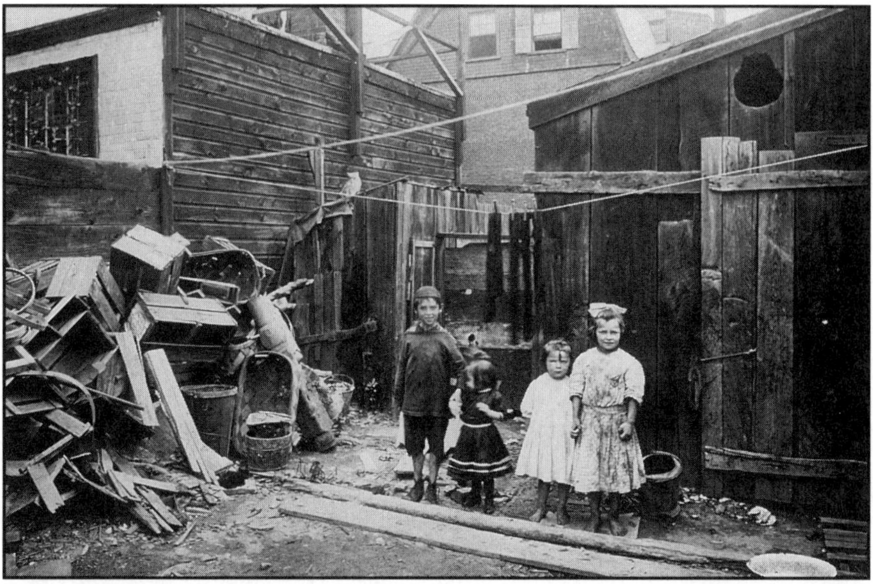

Slum children like these were the initial focus of the Board of Education's school medical inspection program.

Initially the activity was confined to downtown schools which most needed the nurses' services. Lead by Lina L. Rogers, the Canadian born pioneer of school nursing in New York City, the new system quickly identified large numbers of children with health problems. In February 1911, a Chief Medical Inspector was appointed to supervise the growing number of school doctors and to assist Rogers in organizing her ever-expanding nursing service. By 1912, the Board of Education was providing medical inspection in eighty schools for 45,000 pupils. Twenty-five nurses and eighteen medical inspectors provided routine inspection after every vacation period, individual medical inspections of those entering and leaving school, and daily inspections of specific cases. Legally, the staff was required to examine children absent more than two days and to report cases of contagious disease to the Health Department. The nurses, in particular, were very effective at discovering cases of tuberculosis and diphtheria.

As it was practiced in Toronto, school medical inspection had three objectives: control of communicable diseases, detection and correction of defects and abnormalities, and health education. When the Board of Education medical and nursing staff began their work, they concentrated on the first two goals because the need was most pressing. Children suffering from measles or mumps were a source of contagion for their classmates and had to be excluded from school. Pupils who had poor eyesight, hearing problems, physical deformities, or infected tonsils and adenoids, were not able to perform at peak efficiency in the classroom. But the most common problem uncovered was bad teeth and infected mouths. In 1911, a Dental Service was begun to teach the children proper procedures for caring for their teeth once the decayed teeth and abscesses had been treated.

Medical inspection alone did not guarantee the correction of physical or dental problems. Like their counterparts in the Health Department, the Board of Education nurses made home visits to persuade the parents to look after the child's health. The school nurses found that poverty and lack of family doctors often prevented any action being taken. They also called on charitable groups to supply assistance to needy families, and the Board of Education itself provided glasses for children who needed them.[3]

In effect, the Board of Education was duplicating the work of the Health Department. The depression from 1913 to 1915, and the outbreak of World War I produced calls for unification in 1916. Mayor Church, members of the Board of Control, Charles Hastings and even John Ross Robertson, the philanthropist whose offer to fund a demonstration project had spurred the Board of Education into action in 1910, joined the fight to transfer medical inspection to the Health Department. For the politicians, the city's deteriorating financial status was sufficient justification for the change. Medical inspection cost ratepayers $25,000-30,000 annually. By adding the Board of Education's medical, dental and nursing staff to the Health Department and integrating them into its generalized system, the money would be more wisely spent and the mill rate would not rise.[4] Rampant inflation during the war made this an attractive argument.

From the medical officer's perspective, the takeover was necessary to complete the chain of centrally directed preventive services his Department offered. Hastings argued that the transfer would eliminate the possibility of more than one nurse visiting a family and that it would provide a more efficient level of service. Not surprisingly the Board of Education objected to the loss of control. Although Rogers had retired when she married Dr. W.E. Struthers, the Board of Education's Chief Medical Inspector in 1913, she was a vehement opponent of unification. Her American experience led her to fear that political influence would affect appointments, and that medical staff would change the focus from health education to discovering and treating defects.[5] Others shared her concerns, and with the assistance of various committees of the Ontario legislature, some education trustees tried to stonewall the proposal. In spite of an effort by the Provincial Board of Health to mediate the situation, the Mayor and council decided to include a referendum question about the transfer on the election ballot for 1917. When the votes were counted, 22,815 ratepayers had voted in favour of the transfer while 6,400 opposed it.[6]

Even after such a resounding defeat, the Board of Education did not concede gracefully. According to Robertson's *Telegram*, a smear campaign was begun alleging that Catholic nurses would attend Protestant children, although the medical officer had clearly stated that Protestant doctors and nurses would serve the public schools while Catholic nurses would look after the separate schools.[7] With the support of Toronto members in the provincial parliament, the necessary legislation was quickly passed in 1917.

Toronto's traumatic experience with the politics of amalgamation was repeated in other Canadian cities. Financial pressure during the Depression led Oshawa, Kitchener, and Hamilton, to unite their health and education staff, but in Edmonton the campaign failed in 1933. Further efforts by the medical officer in 1947 suffered a similar fate, but provincial government funding, which was offered only to amalgamated services, finally compelled unification in 1952.[8]

Developing the Department's System

Through the spring and summer of 1917, Hastings and Dyke worked to ensure a smooth transition from inspection by the Board of Education to examination by the Health Department. In many respects, there were few problems since both groups shared a similar professional background and ideology. Not all of the Board of Education staff opted to join the Health Department. Some joined the Canadian Army Medical Corps while others went to the provincial government. For the doctors and dentists, Hastings created a new division, School Medical and Dental Services. By 1919, these two disciplines had separated, and they would remain related but distinct until decentralization in the 1980s. The nurses were assigned to district work, with the exception of senior staff who supervised school medical services from within the renamed Division of Public Health Nursing.[9]

From September 1917 onward, school medical inspection became a dominant feature of Health Department work. Each doctor was assigned a series of schools within a specific district, and was expected to do annual physical examinations of new and departing students as well as to diagnose cases of contagious disease. By 1920, the department had expanded from five to eight districts, and the district medical officers were now also responsible for home visits to children sick with communicable diseases, meetings with mothers to discuss treatment for scabies (a contagious disease caused by the itch mite) and pediculosis (lice), workmen's compensation care for civic employees, and staff health reports for various departments.[10]

During the 1920s, district medical officers were encouraged to complete the University of Toronto Diploma in Public Health, because their field positions were a springboard for advancement to senior administrative positions within the civic, provincial, and federal health bureaucracies, and charitable organizations. Men like Grant Fleming, John Phair, Clarence Hincks, Frederick Burke, Gordon Jackson, and Leon Pequegnat, all started their careers as district medical officers with Toronto's Health Department. Like their colleagues, they carried out complete physical examinations of all children in Grades 1 and 7, and for students with mental or physical disabilities in other grades. In contrast to the limited inspection which the Board of Education had conducted, the Health Department sent consent forms home to parents and encouraged them to attend their child's examination. During the 1920s, 70% of Grade 1 students' parents were present, while nearly 50% came for medical consultation about older children. The interviews were an opportunity to discuss the child's development, in comparison to the height and weight tables which the Department's medical staff had developed in 1923 using American models. Parents with underweight

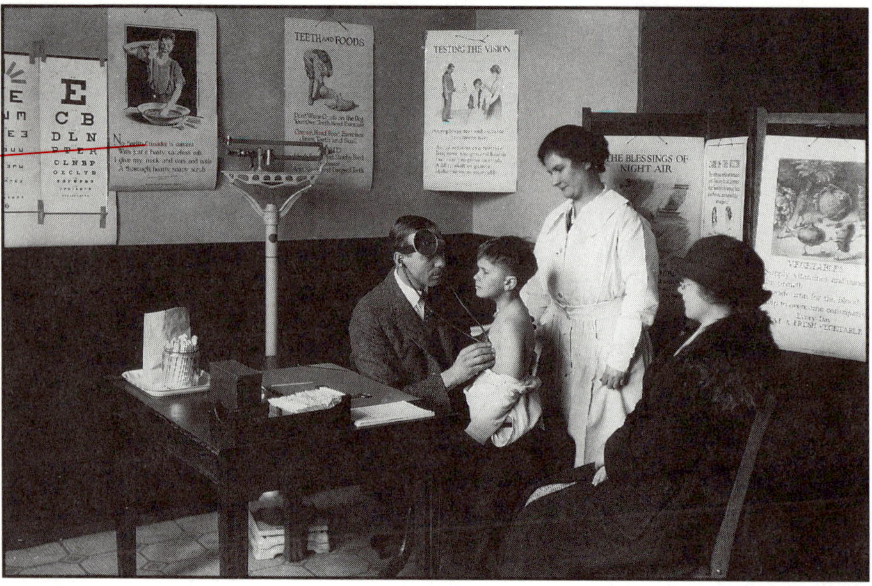

In addition to examining this child in his mother's presence, Health Department staff assumed that the posters pictured here would also contribute to developing healthy habits.

children were advised to follow the nutrition guidelines found in the Department's Health Rules brochure, while others were reminded of basic personal hygiene principles through the posters which lined the examination room.[11]

School medical inspection aroused opposition from Toronto's doctors. To overcome fears that patients would switch to the Department's medical staff or consultants, a policy of prohibiting private practice for full-time staff was instituted. As well, the Director of Medical Services hired local practitioners on a part-time basis in an effort to counteract complaints. Each doctor also received a form letter indicating that the child had been examined and that specific problems were evident. In 1928, 65% of these problems were corrected, but financial difficulties during the Depression lowered this to 58% by 1932. Pressure mounted for the Department to take over the treatment of children, but the medical officer resisted because of lack of funds and fear of further antagonizing the medical community.[12] Hastings and Jackson used every opportunity to defuse misconceptions about the Department's role by addressing the Academy of Medicine, Home and School Clubs, and voluntary groups. Their medical staff also gave speeches to local organizations and published papers describing their work in professional journals.

The duties of the public health nurses were redefined after unification. Each morning the district nurses visited two of Toronto's 87 public and 26 separate schools. There they inspected re-admissions, responded to teachers' requests for exclusion of possible cases of infectious disease, arranged physical examinations, and followed up any students with defects or abnormalities. These activities provided the nurses with another link to the families in their districts, and completed the Department's chain of contact with the public from the prenatal period through to adulthood.

The nurses also gave brief health talks to the classes that they visited. For Dyke and Rogers, health education rather than discovery and treatment of physical problems lay at the heart of school medical inspection, because like progressive education reformers, these women believed that children were more malleable than adults. The Board of Education nurses had introduced concepts of personal cleanliness through inspecting hands, fingernails, necks, and scalps; they also conducted teeth brushing and nose blowing drills. After amalgamation, health lessons were made more sophisticated through storytelling, songs, pageants, posters, and classroom competitions — innovations that were derived from American public health advertising campaigns.[13] Both the Junior Red Cross and the Girl's Health League carried on the education which Rogers had introduced through Little Mother's Classes. But Dyke was concerned that these activities might undermine a child's confidence in his or her parents by threatening deeply held values, particularly if the child came from an immigrant family.[14]

As progressives, she and her nurses believed that knowledge would change health behaviour, but as realists, they all recognized that it was a

HEIGHT and WEIGHT TABLES for TORONTO CHILDREN

If a child's weight is below the average for his age and height, it is generally an indication that he has some physical defect or that his health habits are faulty.

Up to the present time tables compiled in other countries, and therefore based upon children who may be presumed to vary in build from Toronto children, have been used as a standard. It has been the experience of those using the tables that the weights given were somewhat high.

During the winter of 1922, a height and weight survey of 60,000 school children was made in Toronto. From this survey were compiled the tables appearing on this page.

These tables represent the *average* weight for height and age. Measurements were taken in school clothes and without boots. The age was taken to the nearest year.

HEIGHT and WEIGHT TABLE for BOYS

Hgt. In.	5 Yrs.	6 Yrs.	7 Yrs.	8 Yrs.	9 Yrs.	10 Yrs.	11 Yrs.	12 Yrs.	13 Yrs.	14 Yrs.	15 Yrs.	16 Yrs.
39	35	..	..	..	..	..	..	..	..	..	..	..
40	36	37	..	..	..	..	..	..	..	..	..	..
41	38	39	40	..	..	..	..	..	..	..	..	..
42	40	40	41	43	..	..	..	..	..	..	..	..
43	42	42	43	44	..	..	..	..	..	..	..	..
44	44	44	44	45	47	..	..	..	..	..	..	..
45	46	46	47	48	49	..	..	..	..	..	..	..
46	47	48	48	49	50	..	..	..	..	..	..	..
47	..	50	50	51	51	52	..	..	..	..	..	..
48	..	52	52	53	54	54	56	..	..	..	..	..
49	..	54	55	55	56	56	58	60	..	..	..	..
50	..	56	57	57	58	59	60	62	..	..	..	..
51	..	..	59	60	61	62	63	64	..	..	..	..
52	..	..	62	63	63	64	65	66	67	..	..	..
53	..	..	64	65	66	67	68	69	70	72	..	..
54	..	..	..	68	69	70	71	72	73	74	..	..
55	..	..	..	70	71	73	74	75	76	77	..	..
56	..	..	..	..	74	76	77	77	78	79	81	..
57	..	..	..	..	78	79	80	81	82	83	84	..
58	..	..	..	..	..	82	83	84	85	86	87	88
59	..	..	..	..	..	83	87	88	89	90	92	93
60	..	..	..	..	..	85	90	93	94	95	96	97
61	..	..	..	..	..	89	93	95	98	99	100	102
62	..	..	..	..	..	..	97	100	101	103	104	105
63	..	..	..	..	..	..	102	104	106	108	109	110
64	..	..	..	..	..	..	107	108	113	114	115	116
65	..	..	..	..	..	..	..	113	118	119	120	121
66	..	..	..	..	..	..	..	..	123	124	125	126
67	..	..	..	..	..	..	..	..	127	128	129	130
68	..	..	..	..	..	..	..	..	132	133	134	135
69	..	..	..	..	..	..	..	..	135	136	137	138
70	..	..	..	..	..	..	..	..	..	141	142	143
71	..	..	..	..	..	..	..	..	..	..	145	147
72	..	..	..	..	..	..	..	..	..	..	149	153

HEIGHT and WEIGHT TABLE for GIRLS

Hgt. In.	5 Yrs.	6 Yrs.	7 Yrs.	8 Yrs.	9 Yrs.	10 Yrs.	11 Yrs.	12 Yrs.	13 Yrs.	14 Yrs.	15 Yrs.	16 Yrs.
39	34	35	..	..	..	..	..	..	..	..	..	..
40	35	37	37	..	..	..	..	..	..	..	..	..
41	37	38	39	..	..	..	..	..	..	..	..	..
42	39	40	10	41	..	..	..	..	..	..	..	..
43	41	42	42	42	..	..	..	..	..	..	..	..
44	43	44	44	44	..	..	..	..	..	..	..	..
45	45	46	46	46	47	..	..	..	..	..	..	..
46	47	47	47	48	49	..	..	..	..	..	..	..
47	..	49	49	50	50	51	..	..	..	..	..	..
48	..	51	52	52	52	53	54	..	..	..	..	..
49	..	53	54	54	55	55	56	..	..	..	..	..
50	..	..	57	57	58	58	59	60	..	..	..	..
51	..	..	59	59	60	60	61	62	..	..	..	..
52	..	..	61	62	63	63	64	65	..	..	..	..
53	..	..	..	65	66	67	67	68	69	..	..	..
54	..	..	..	67	69	69	70	71	72	..	..	..
55	..	..	..	..	73	73	74	74	75	77	..	..
56	..	..	..	..	76	76	77	77	79	79	..	..
57	..	..	..	..	..	78	80	80	83	85	88	..
58	..	..	..	..	..	86	84	85	86	90	91	95
59	..	..	..	..	..	89	89	90	92	94	97	100
60	..	..	..	..	..	..	91	92	96	98	101	102
61	..	..	..	..	..	..	94	95	100	102	106	107
62	..	..	..	..	..	..	100	101	102	105	108	110
63	..	..	..	..	..	..	105	107	107	110	110	113
64	..	..	..	..	..	..	..	110	112	112	118	119
65	..	..	..	..	..	..	..	115	116	118	120	123
66	..	..	..	..	..	..	..	..	119	122	123	126
67	..	..	..	..	..	..	..	..	123	126	126	128
68	..	..	..	..	..	..	..	..	126	128	130	132
69	..	..	..	..	..	..	..	..	..	131	133	135
70	..	..	..	..	..	..	..	..	..	134	136	138

DEPARTMENT OF PUBLIC HEALTH
CITY HALL, TORONTO

Health Rules For School Children

Healthy living means proper food, long hours of sleep, and plenty of fresh air. Obey the following simple rules, and eat the kind of meals described, if you want to be strong and well.

RULES FOR EATING

Eat no solid food between meals.

Eat slowly and chew your food well. Do not wash it down with water or milk.

Drink water between meals, but not at bedtime.

Drink at least one pint of milk every day.

Wash your hands before you eat.

Food should be warm and well-cooked, served on clean dishes and at a clean table.

Flies must be kept away from food. Flies carry germs.

Milk should be kept cold and on ice if possible.

Dinner for children should be at noon.

SLEEP

Go to bed early enough at night so that you do not have to be wakened in the morning. MAXIMUM SLEEP MEANS MAXIMUM HEALTH.

Young children should be asleep by 7 or 7.30 ; older children not later than 8.30 p.m. The child of six needs 12 to 13 hours of sleep if well and more if he is run down. The child of fourteen needs 10 to 11 hours of sleep.

FRESH AIR

Fresh air is necessary for health. When going to school you can get only two or three hours outdoors, but you can get ten to twelve hours of fresh air while asleep.

Keep your bedroom window open during sleeping hours.

No. 3960. May, 1923.

Health Department staff distributed this pamphlet to teachers, students and parents.

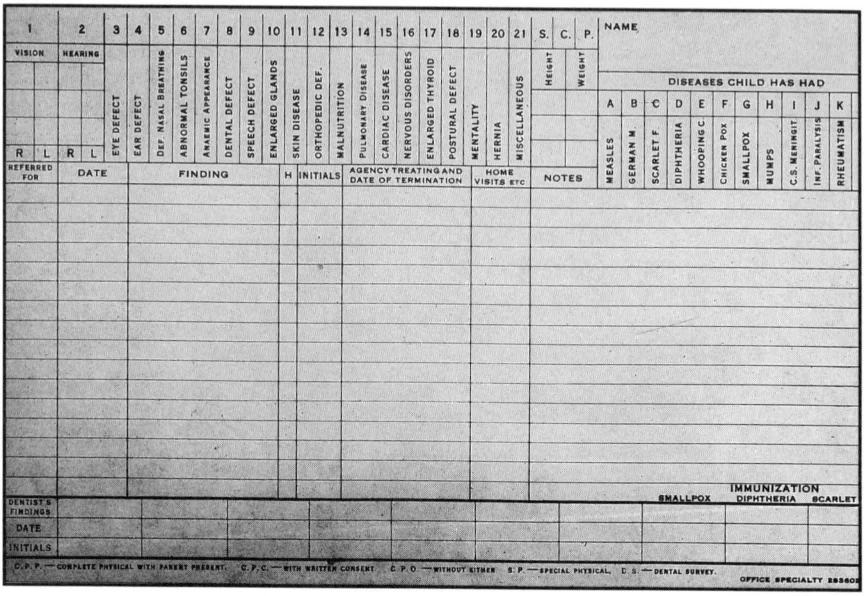

1 VISION R L
2 HEARING R L
3 EYE DEFECT
4 EAR DEFECT
5 DEF. NASAL BREATHING
6 ABNORMAL TONSILS
7 ANAEMIC APPEARANCE
8 DENTAL DEFECT
9 SPEECH DEFECT
10 ENLARGED GLANDS
11 SKIN DISEASE
12 ORTHOPEDIC DEF.
13 MALNUTRITION
14 PULMONARY DISEASE
15 CARDIAC DISEASE
16 NERVOUS DISORDERS
17 ENLARGED THYROID
18 POSTURAL DEFECT
19 MENTALITY
20 HERNIA
21 MISCELLANEOUS
S. C. P. HEIGHT WEIGHT
NAME
DISEASES CHILD HAS HAD
A MEASLES B GERMAN M. C SCARLET F. D DIPHTHERIA E WHOOPING C. F CHICKEN POX G SMALLPOX H MUMPS I C.S. MENINGIT. J INF. PARALYSIS K RHEUMATISM
REFERRED FOR | DATE | FINDING | H | INITIALS | AGENCY TREATING AND DATE OF TERMINATION | HOME VISITS ETC | NOTES
IMMUNIZATION: SMALLPOX DIPHTHERIA SCARLET
DENTIST'S FINDINGS
DATE
INITIALS
C. P. P. — COMPLETE PHYSICAL WITH PARENT PRESENT. C. P. C. — WITH WRITTEN CONSENT C. P. O. — WITHOUT EITHER S. P. — SPECIAL PHYSICAL. D. S. — DENTAL SURVEY.
OFFICE SPECIALTY 28360

Toronto's school doctors and nurses completed this form for each school child.

lengthy process that required tact and determination. In 1928, Annie Dove, the Superintendent of the Runnymede District office, organized exhibits and demonstrations of infant care, school medical inspection, and Red Cross home nursing, as part of a fund raising effort in one of the local schools. Pupils who had completed the Department's nine week Health League course for older girls, showed visitors how to give babies their baths, while younger students demonstrated proper teeth brushing techniques. Several nurses and a dental officer were also present to answer questions and discuss the content of the displays. Dove's efforts attracted the attention of other Home and School Clubs and represented a forceful attempt at raising community awareness of the Department and its message.[15]

By the early 1930s, the faith of the progressive reformers in their persuasive abilities was waning. Widespread public acceptance of the Department's role still raised questions among public health nursing leaders about the effectiveness of didactic methods. As behavioural psychology permeated the curriculum, the nurses reassessed their emphasis on health education as an appeal to students to put "class honour and Canada's need for healthy men and women" ahead of their own interests. Instead, they argued that active practice of health habits such as "washing hands, drinking water, playing out of doors and living in well ventilated rooms," through teaching aimed at the "child's intellectual level" would serve to create life-long patterns by fulfilling his specific needs.[16] During the Depression, making these changes proved difficult, and the provincial Department of Education, in conjunction with the Ontario Health Department, developed its own health teaching manuals for teachers.

The nurses and the teachers shared a common goal but some tension arose concerning who should teach the children. Many of the Department's nurses had done teacher training prior to nursing, but in 1932, Esther Beith pointed out that the nursing curriculum should be expanded to include teaching techniques if public health nurses were to make a significant contribution. Although some effort to incorporate this material was made during the 1920s and 1930s, school nurses visited classrooms only on invitation from the teacher and devoted most of their effort to routine inspection and home follow-up.

Creating Special Classes

During school medical inspections, the nurses and doctors uncovered children with sight problems, hearing defects, mental retardation, and behavioural problems. To deal with these disabilities, special classes were created by the Board of Education. In 1912, two Forest Schools were opened in Victoria and High Parks, for children "who bear the earmarks of incipient disease and whose poverty precludes any hope of summer vacation away from the dirt and degradation of their homes."[17] They were intended to be a scientific experiment to test the current medical hypothesis, that rest, improved nutrition and health education, would turn dull, listless, underachievers into healthy, energetic students. Since nearly 70% of the students were immigrants, these schools had another mission: assimilation.[18] Amalgamation split control of the forest schools between the Board of Education and the Health Department, but they shared a common goal which was to restore the children to regular classes.

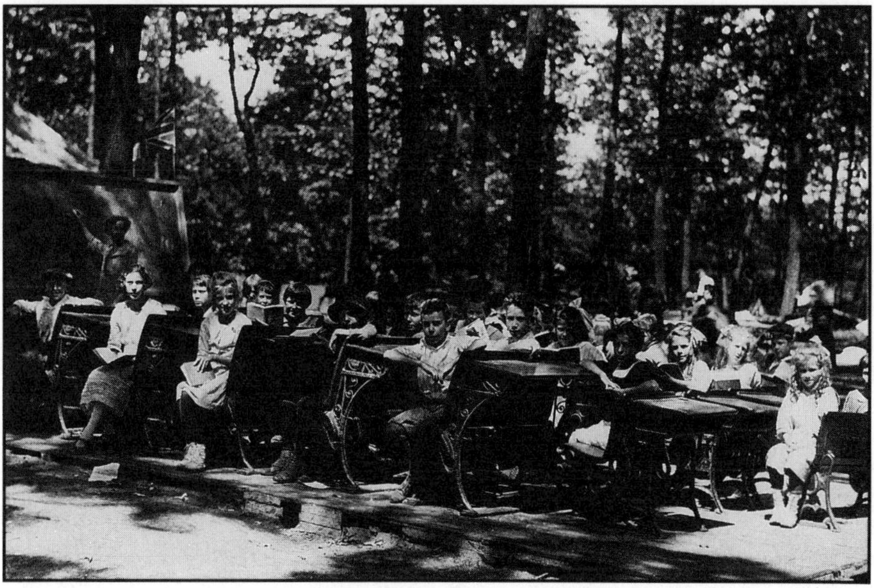

The High Park Forest School in July 1922.

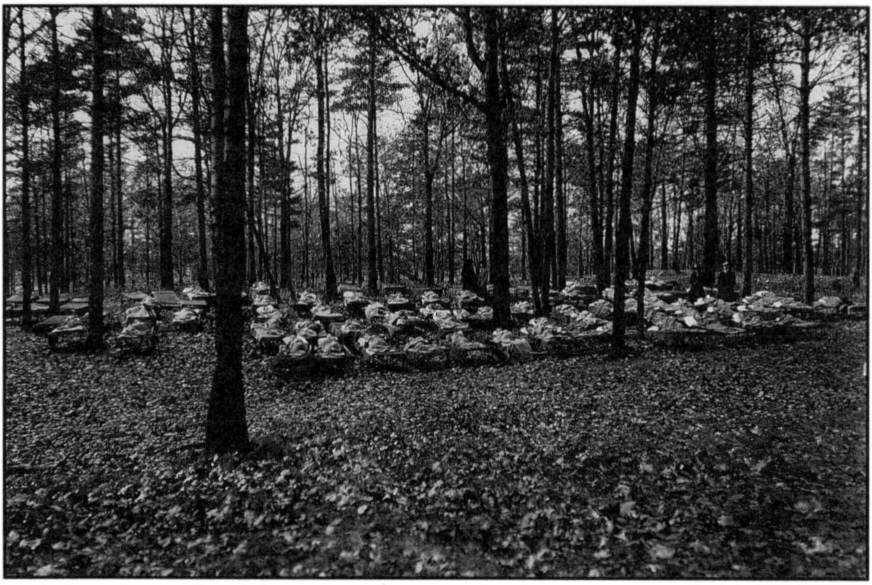

The Forest Schools opened in May and closed in October. Daily rest periods were thought to help the children regain their health.

With the decline of immigration during the 1920s, the Forest and Open Air schools in Toronto became less interested in acculturation, and more concerned with weight gain and improvements in the child's mental and emotional state. This paralleled the Health Department's work with children suffering from vision and hearing problems or mental retardation. With the Board of Education's assistance, sight saving and lip reading classes were created early in the 1920s to ensure that these students received appropriate training. The Department's doctors and nurses, aided by the teacher, not only discovered these children, but also referred them to consultants and counselled their parents on the best way to make them healthy citizens.[19]

Mentally retarded children received similar service. In 1917, Clarence Hincks, the Department's psychiatric consultant, began using the Binet-Simon intelligence test on selected school children. He and his staff from the Department found many more retarded students than the Board of Education could accommodate. By the end of 1921, Toronto had 21 special auxiliary and industrial classes. Each one had 16 students compared to regular classes of 45. As Hastings noted: "This of course is not preventive work. It is making the best of irreparable conditions."[20] Still, according to teachers and principals, all students benefited from this change because "normal" ones were able to receive all their teacher's attention while the "subnormal" were no longer frustrated by their inability to keep up.[21] This rationale was repeated by the city's health officer as he justified hiring Dr. Eric Clarke on a full-time basis, and created a new Division of Mental Hygiene in 1925.

By 1928, attention had shifted to normal children and their behaviour problems, according to the Supervisor of Mental Hygiene Nursing, Emma Clarke. In several articles published in the *Canadian Nurse,* Clarke outlined the trials and tribulations of this new nursing education field. Lack of psychiatrists meant that many assessment duties became the nurse's responsibility. She also had the task of interviewing the teacher, the parents, and the child to prepare a report for the consulting doctor, and later, to visit the home and classroom to interpret his findings to the individuals involved.[22]

Like many of her medical colleagues in this specialty, Clarke blamed poor parenting for much of the disruptive and manipulative behaviour that children displayed. This viewpoint was presented to Toronto parents through American trained staff like Clarke, and through the advice literature which was provided by the National Association for Mental Hygiene. In 1932, the first of several parent education groups was established to enable worried mothers to evaluate their parenting skills using the latest research and educational material. These groups were not successful, partly because of lack of funds and partly because they appealed to women who were already fairly knowledgeable.[23]

During the 1930s, the Department created two Child Guidance Clinics with the Board of Education, for pupils who engaged in "temper tantrums, bed wetting, self abuse, laziness, irritability, fears, imagined illness and truancy."[24] Like Vancouver's Provincial Child Guidance Clinic, which opened in 1931, Toronto's clinic diagnosed children's behavioural problems and then referred them to private physicians, if they could afford it, or sent them to the outpatient clinic at the Hospital for Sick Children. A survey by the Big Brother's Association in 1929, blamed rising juvenile delinquency rates on "dull normal" students and recommended the construction of vocational schools to train these children. During the Depression, however, the Board

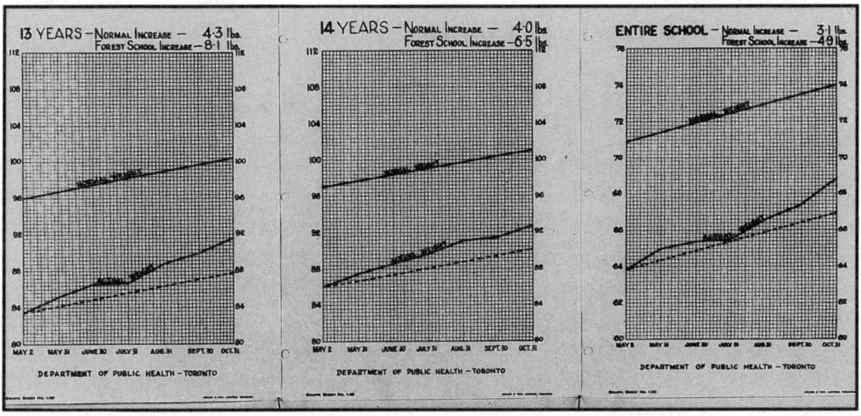

The Health Department published these charts in 1927 to demonstrate the weight gains which the nourishing meals provided at the Forest Schools produced among underweight children.

of Education simply continued to increase the number of auxiliary classes and to convert three existing schools for this purpose.[25] After 1945, new schools were built, and the Department's medical and nursing staff continued to provide the community links which assisted these students in adjusting to the work world.

In 1941, the Mental Hygiene Director enlisted, and the Department had to accept a part-time replacement for him. Since younger members of the nursing staff also joined the armed forces, the Department was understrength and using retired staff to fill gaps when the Phair Committee conducted its survey in 1942. As a former Director of Medical Services, Phair was particularly interested in Toronto's system of school medical inspection. He and his colleagues presented a strong critique of the Department for allocating 50% of its budget, and 50% of staff time, to 20% of the population. He was sarcastic about the "teaching" which the public health nurses provided, but did admit that their other duties limited the development of health education. The Forest Schools were singled out for condemnation because they only served 500 students, and Phair could not see that they contributed to enhancing pupils' health.[26] Only the Mental Hygiene Division escaped, although the Committee observed that it lacked qualified personnel because salaries were too low.

In response to these comments, Jackson agreed to seek the local board of health's support for alterations in the school medical inspection program. The medical officer indicated that the provincial capital would willingly participate in an experiment to test more targeted inspection work. He agreed to the closing of the Victoria Park forest school, but urged the Board of Education to create special "health classes" for malnourished and chronically fatigued children. To improve the nurses' mastery of education techniques, promising younger staff were encouraged to return to the University of Toronto to complete Bachelor of Arts degrees, and many did in 1948 and 1949. In spite of this upgrading, there was no resolution of the long-standing split between teachers and public health nurses on the subject of who should be in charge of health education in the classroom.

Medical Research or Community Action?

After Jackson's death in 1951, his successor, Leon Pequegnat, took advantage of the national health grants system to provide funds for research into myopia, hearing problems, ineducable children,[27] and specific topics, like colour-vision defects, cardiac defects, and scoliosis. Each of these projects was directed by a medical specialist, and represented the Department's continuing effort to interact with the mainstream of the profession. Nursing staff were used to organize the clinics, conduct the initial test, and provide information about children who needed follow-up examinations. During the 1950s, the number of students available for clinical trials increased markedly. Between 1951 and 1957, 14,000 children entered the city's educational system, and in the latter year, the Department's nurses were visiting 123 elementary schools with 89,252 pupils, and 16 secondary schools and

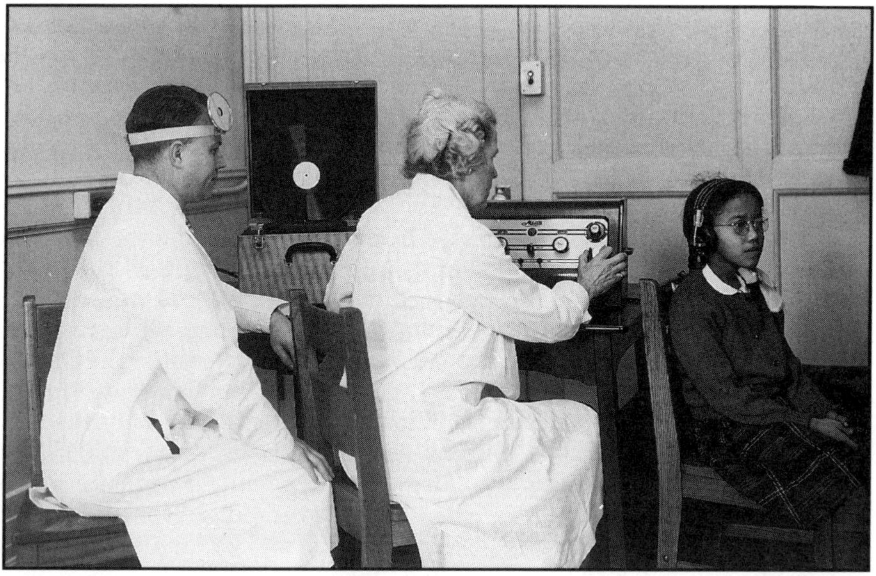

If an initial hearing test indicated problems, Toronto children were assessed by the Department's audiologist and his technician.

three handicraft schools, with an enrolment of 18,855 students.

Although the research projects conducted during the 1950s and 1960s provided new data for medical experts, the nurses began to question the use of their time for secondary prevention. By the early 1970s, many of the doctors involved in this clinical research work had died or retired, and pressure mounted to rethink the role of therapeutic and screening activities for the school population. As well, the growing interest in health promotion and behaviour modification led younger nurses to query the public perception of their role as "emergency" medical caregivers, and to express discontent at the limited contact that they had with students as health educators.

External forces also contributed to the demand for change. During the late 1960s, community activists won trustee positions on the Board of Education. From this vantage point, they launched an attack on the middle class WASP ethos that dominated Toronto schools despite a continuing influx of immigrants and refugees. Multiculturalism became a hot issue. So did poverty.[28] In 1971, the Board of Education expressed interest in a joint survey with the Health Department and the Hospital for Sick Children, to evaluate the health of students living in the Niagara Street district in the downtown core.[29] By 1976, multiculturalism and poverty had become an explosive combination for the Board of Education when charges of racism and discrimination against black students, in particular, were made public.

In this heady atmosphere of conflict and confrontation, the Health Department joined the Board of Education in setting up the School and Community Organization to Revitalize Education program. The SCORE project was designed to identify children with learning disabilities in low income areas of the city. Health Department staff participated in the early identification program and the nutrition and growth charting portions of the project. With its built-in evaluation mechanisms and limited lifespan of three years, SCORE provided a sharp contrast to the traditional single item focus of the school inspection and screening services,[30] and served as a pilot project to demonstrate the effectiveness of comprehensive, coordinated community-based programs.

This new approach was welcomed by many nurses who were seeking to escape from the public perception of their role in the schools as "Band Aid givers." It was less pleasing to the doctors who still wanted to use school children and clinic clients as experimental subjects in preventive research. With declining enrollments and more use of family doctors after the Ontario Health Insurance Plan came into effect, the nurses began to argue in favour of eliminating medical inspection, and instead concentrating on health education through personal and group counselling sessions. As a result, in 1980 the school nurses formed teams to carry out the assessment work during the fall, and then prepared and presented health education lessons to the students in the winter and spring. For kindergarten and Grade 1 students, the nurses presented "Clean Clappers" to demonstrate the importance of hand washing, while material on fitness, the "choose not to smoke" program, and information on family life were presented to Grades five and six.[31] In addition to enhancing the nurses' satisfaction with their jobs, focused work has the added benefit of serving the people who most need it. After decentralization, the Department established a Task Force on School Health. Its purpose was to define the approach which staff would use to achieve optimum health for school children in the twenty-first century, drawing on the experience and expertise of the past and the present.

School Dental Services

> My Hilda was awake an' bawlin' all last night with a toothache. It's them school dentists what does it. He filled her tooth about a month ago, and it looks like tin he's put in, if you ask me.[32]

This contemptuous statement appeared in Hugh Garner's novel *Cabbagetown* as two of the female characters reflected on the effect that their poverty had on the treatment that they and their families received from public agencies. They were sceptical of the competence of the doctors and dentists who worked for the Health Department, and like many of their contemporaries, thought that only individuals in private practice were true professionals. Such views were a sad commentary on the service and oral hygiene education, which the Department's overburdened dental staff tried to provide during the dirty thirties.

Dental inspection in Toronto originated with the Board of Education, but in 1913 the Health Department opened an extraction clinic to serve the needy.[33] Unification of the health and education dental staff did not bring immediate efforts to prevent tooth decay because the demand for treatment was so great. In 1922, the three dentists who carried out the dental surveys examined 65,742 students and found 33,179 with various problems. Although the dentists gave short talks and distributed literature while their assistants completed the necessary paperwork for each class, no additional staff were available to reinforce this effort. Not surprisingly, the Dental Division's work was focused on treatment. In 1922, the Health Department had 28 dental clinics in the city's schools, and the full and part-time dentists who worked there gave 32,285 treatments, which included 18,120 extractions and 21,509 fillings.[34]

The Department was ambivalent about providing this service, and the colour coded cards which children took home to their parents strongly urged them to take the students to the family dentist. Like the school medical inspectors, Toronto's dentists did not wish to infringe on their colleagues' practices, but from 1920 until the 1950s pediatric dentists were in short supply and most dentists in private practice preferred to treat adults. To encourage student dentists to consider careers in pediatric practice, the dental staff supported the creation of children's clinics in the University of Toronto Faculty of Dentistry and in the Hospital for Sick Children. The Department also opened an Orthodontia Clinic in 1932 and a Preventive Orthodontia Clinic in 1950, both to serve children and to train specialists. The latter clinics offered advice and very limited treatment because they lacked staff and funds.[35]

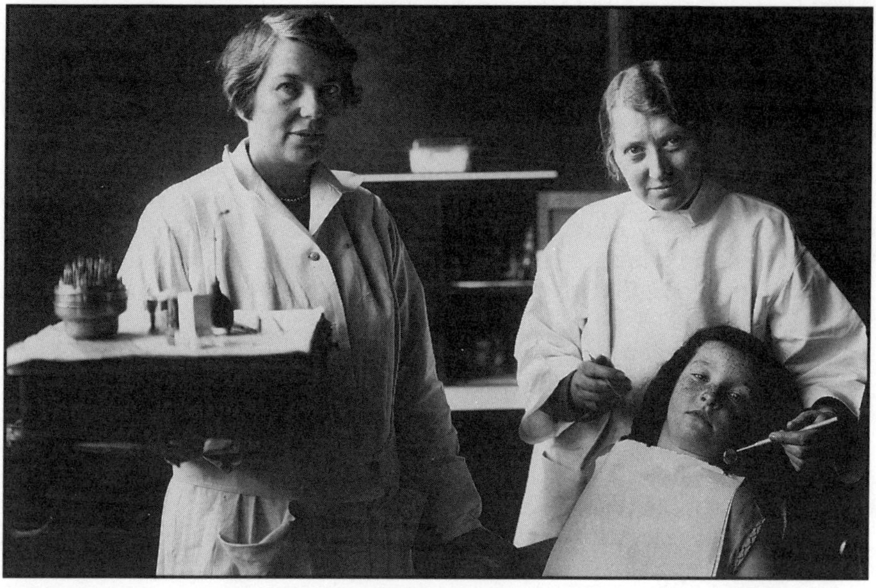

The dentist and her assistant pictured at the Kimberley School Dental Clinic in September 1930 provided dental care for that district.

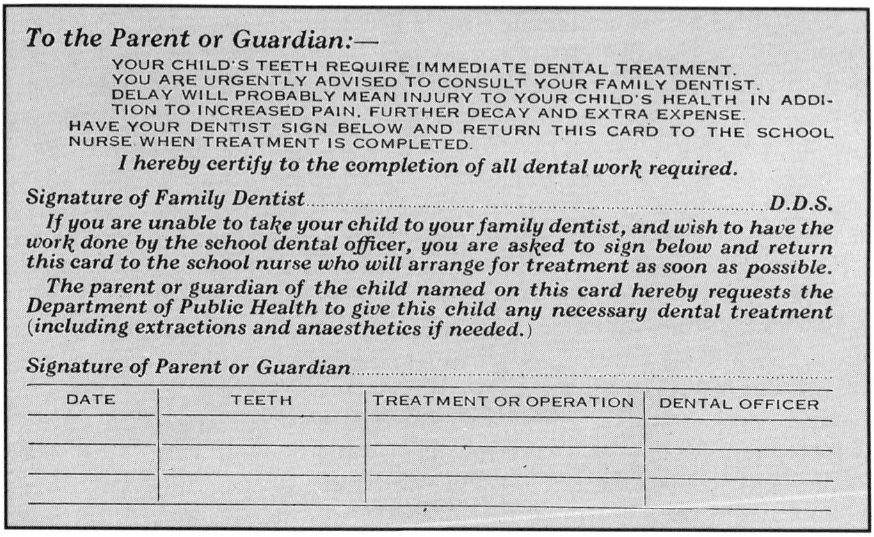

To the Parent or Guardian:—

YOUR CHILD'S TEETH REQUIRE IMMEDIATE DENTAL TREATMENT.
YOU ARE URGENTLY ADVISED TO CONSULT YOUR FAMILY DENTIST.
DELAY WILL PROBABLY MEAN INJURY TO YOUR CHILD'S HEALTH IN ADDITION TO INCREASED PAIN, FURTHER DECAY AND EXTRA EXPENSE.
HAVE YOUR DENTIST SIGN BELOW AND RETURN THIS CARD TO THE SCHOOL NURSE WHEN TREATMENT IS COMPLETED.

I hereby certify to the completion of all dental work required.

Signature of Family Dentist .... *D.D.S.*

If you are unable to take your child to your family dentist, and wish to have the work done by the school dental officer, you are asked to sign below and return this card to the school nurse who will arrange for treatment as soon as possible.

The parent or guardian of the child named on this card hereby requests the Department of Public Health to give this child any necessary dental treatment (including extractions and anaesthetics if needed.)

Signature of Parent or Guardian ....

DATE	TEETH	TREATMENT OR OPERATION	DENTAL OFFICER

The Dental Division encouraged parents to use family dentists to treat the problems which the dental survey teams uncovered.

In 1931, the Department purchased a film projector and the dental survey teams started to show "Bobby's Bad Molar" during their inspections because "There is no better means to impress the minds of young children."[36] Such efforts were vital because one consequence of the Depression was cavity-causing diet deficiencies among school children. To encourage preventive work, Dr. Edmund Guest, who was chairman of the Board of Education and the Oral Hygiene Committee of Toronto's Academy of Dentistry, arranged for the latter group to confer an Honour Certificate on classes with 100% dental health when the dental inspectors arrived. This replaced the Honour Roll which had been introduced in 1915. By 1934, seventy classes had qualified for certificates even though the Depression was making it increasingly difficult for parents to pay for dental care. In 1935 Alderman F.J. Conboy, the former director of Dental Services for the Ontario Health Department, asked for a report on the use of school dental clinics. Jackson was able to assure him that as in the past, the demand was so great in low income areas that no clinics were offered in affluent districts, such as South Parkdale, Rosedale, Moore Park or Oriole Parkway. And he noted that all possible means were used to send children to private dentists.[37]

During the Second World War, Dental Division staff went overseas and finding replacements was very difficult. In spite of this, the service was extended to high school students in 1942. New movies approved by the Academy of Dentistry and the Ontario Dental Association were used for education purposes, and by 1942, 200 classes had won Honour Certificates. These publicity measures did not impress the Phair Committee, which criticized the Department for putting undue pressure on struggling parents and for failing to meet its treatment objectives. In his response to these criticisms, Jackson commented: "Almost paradoxically it seems we must urge more parents to go to their own dentist but we must not embarrass them about it." He also observed that the Department's quota for client service was 40% of children with defects, but that the Depression had increased this to 60% of those surveyed — much too large a group for the limited resources available. To prove his contention that the dental health of Toronto's children had improved greatly since the introduction of dental inspection, the medical officer noted that in 1943 Toronto children had an average of 2 cavities, while the children of war workers who had come from parts of the province without dental services often had 7–10 cavities. Likewise, the number of children with abscessed teeth and other types of mouth infections was 1% in Toronto and as high as 50% elsewhere.[38] Nonetheless, he looked forward to the end of the war when new staff could be hired and new programs introduced.

Service or Prevention?: The Dental Dilemma

During the 1950s, the Dental Division participated in several research studies funded by national health grants. For pre-school children in the Riverdale district, dental hygienists joined the public health nurses at the child health centres and for kindergarten preregistration, to examine the children's teeth and offer topical applications of fluoride to those without cavities. Keeping track of the children in this experiment was difficult, because many moved to other districts when their immigrant parents earned enough to buy a home. Linguistic barriers also caused problems, and the Division's education material was translated into seven languages to accom-

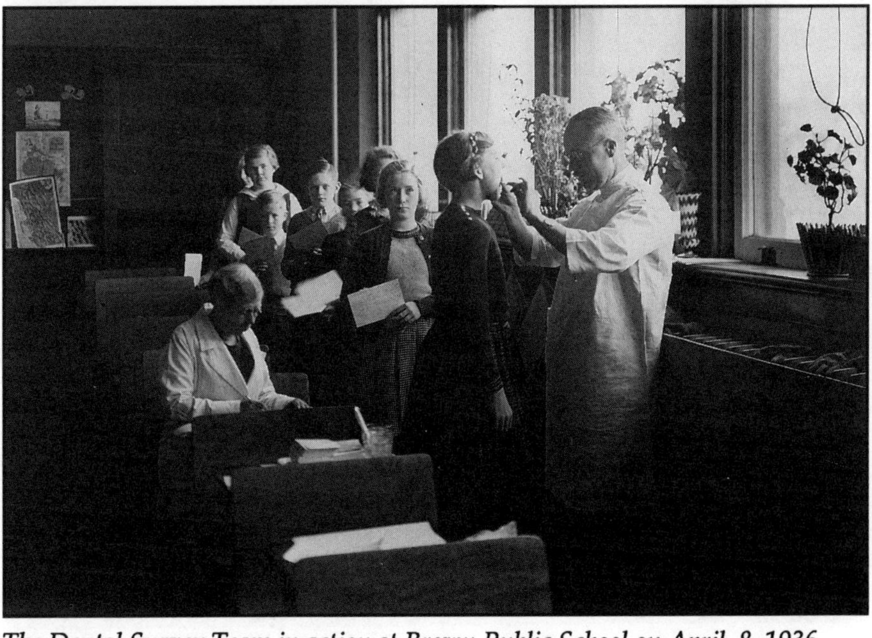

The Dental Survey Team in action at Brown Public School on April 8, 1936.

modate the newcomers. By 1960, the project was considered so successful that it was implemented in all the other districts in spite of on-going shortages of qualified hygienists.[39]

Other research activities reflected the continuing close ties with the Faculty of Medicine and the Ontario Health Department. The University of Toronto's Division of Preventive Dentistry analyzed samples from two Grade five classes involved in a nutrition and salivary lactobacillus experiment, in addition to participating in the Riverdale project. The Ontario government used random samples of Toronto school children's dental records as part of the epidemiological material it required to create a uniform statistical system for the province. The Dental Director, Dr. F.H. Compton, noted that this capped a decade of experimentation in Ontario as local governments tried to determine the optimal dental care system. To ensure

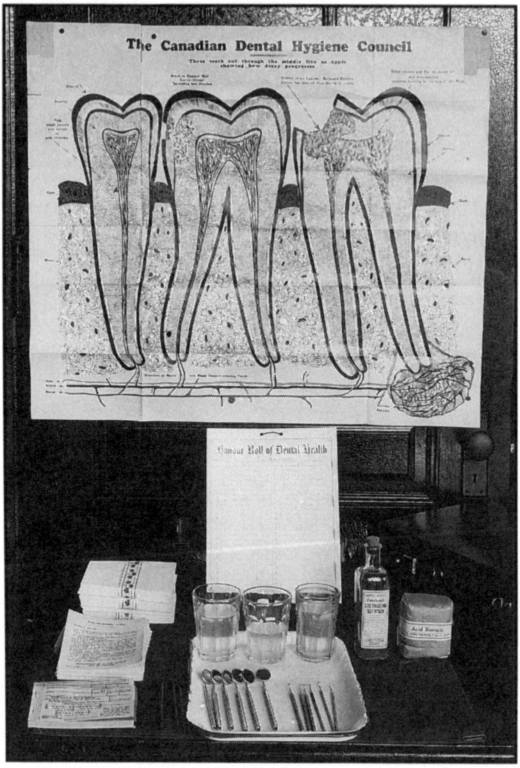

The Dental Survey team discussed the causes of tooth decay and presented the Dental Health Honour Roll to classes which had 100% cavity-free students during the team's annual visit.

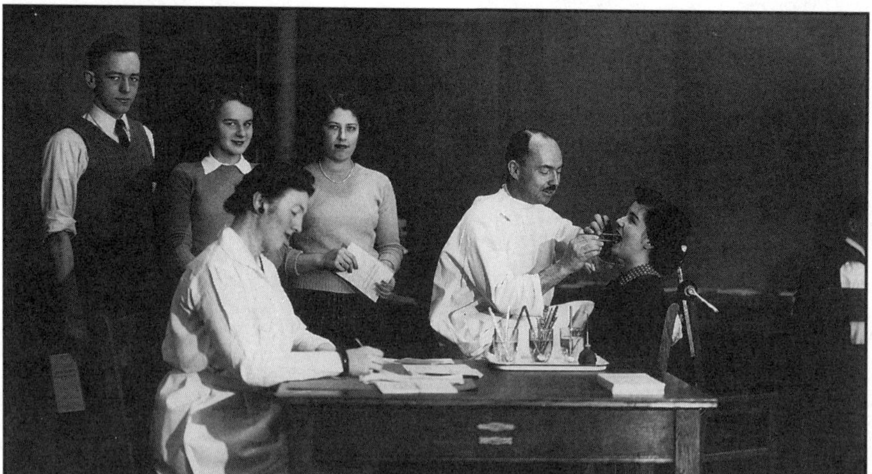

The Dental Survey Team in a Toronto high school, November, 1942.

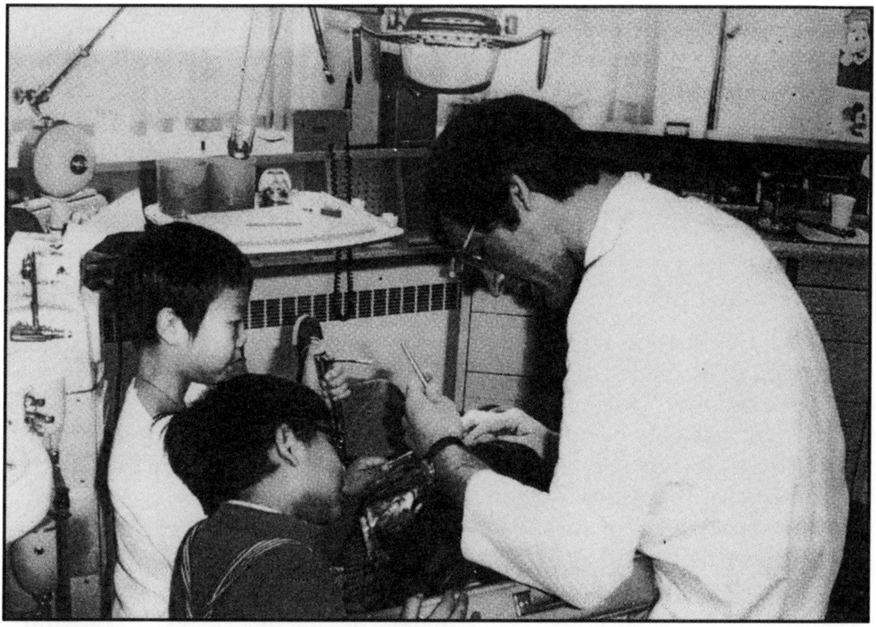

Through the 1970s, the Department's dentists continued to provide clinical treatment, especially to immigrant children.

that Toronto remained abreast of the latest developments and planned for the future, Compton assisted the Academy of Dentistry, the Public and Separate School Boards of Education, Home and School groups, and the Metropolitan Social Planning Council in organizing a Dental Workshop Conference. The gathering's principal recommendation was the creation of a Council on Dental Health whose function was to coordinate local efforts.[40]

Throughout the decade, Compton spearheaded the fight for fluoridation. Victory was finally achieved in 1963. Although this benefited children born in Toronto, the dentists quickly realized that immigrant students, particularly those from the Far East, still had numerous cavities and other dental problems. During the 1970s, the dental survey hygienists began to express concern that the 15 to 45 minutes that they spent talking with each class annually, was not effective. Like their predecessors, they wanted more support from parents and teachers.

Both the dentists and the hygienists agreed with the members of the Health Planning Steering Committee that a provincial dental plan should be implemented. Indeed, demand for their services had declined in North Toronto during the decade because so many families had private dental insurance. In less affluent districts, the province paid for welfare recipients' dental needs. Many people who were not covered still wanted their children to use city services, and as a result, the dentists' workload did not decrease. But did the Health Department have a responsibility to these people? Was this service an essential component for the future? In *Public Health in the 1980's*, the authors carefully defined the amount of service that they thought was a legitimate city responsibility and argued that advocacy of a provincial program, nutrition research and preventive education should be the focus of future work. With decentralization, many dental staff retired or left the Department. Those who remained reorganized their work, and in 1987, the 40 clinics were consolidated into 8 centrally located and easily accessible facilities. That year the Ontario government finally extended dental care coverage to the province's children.[41]

Meet Mr Vitamin: Modern Nutrition

Modern nutrition science began just before World War I when researchers started to discover the role that vitamins and minerals played in growth and development. During the war, Hastings acted as Toronto's Food Controller. He took this opportunity to educate citizens about the dangers of malnutrition in workers and children, and about the threat that wasting food posed for the Allies. Although the public health nurses discussed diet and the importance of milk with individual mothers during their home visits and at the well baby clinics, Hastings wanted more practical training, so he arranged to have domestic arts teachers from Central Technical School give cooking demonstrations at one of the child health centres. In the August 1919 *Health Bulletin,* he pointed out that malnutrition in New York City's children had increased from 5 to 19% between 1914 and 1918. He recommended a similar survey of Toronto students, called for a nutritional clinic at the Hospital for Sick Children, and urged "let us eat more intelligently."[42]

When 1,400 of the 20,000 Toronto children surveyed in 1920 were described as malnourished, the medical officer and his supporters organized a milk drinking campaign. The publicity which this generated led the Home and School Council to sponsor milk supplements in downtown schools. The Health Department's nurses assisted with the project because only children without other health problems, such as bad teeth or infected tonsils, were eligible to participate. The Department's medical staff gave the children weekly talks on the importance of fresh air, proper diet, exercise, and sufficient sleep, weighed them, and when they had reached their normal weight, presented them with a certificate indicating their achievement. School health classes and the Junior Red Cross skits, pageants, and songs, reinforced the nutrition message, as American researchers proved the benefits of cod liver oil, orange juice and vitamin supplements during the decade.[43]

Nutrition Education: Toronto's First Nutrition Consultant

The Depression and World War II brought nutrition concerns to the forefront. In 1933, Toronto's council set up a committee to study the nutritional adequacy of relief diets. Continuing public complaints after the committee's report led the Health Department to accept student dieticians for field work, and to send them into the city's homes with the public health nurses. During the 1930s, public health nutrition became a research field at the School of Hygiene. Led by Dr. E.W. McHenry, staff and students cooperated with community organizations such as the Visiting Homemakers Association, to evaluate the diets of low and middle income Torontonians. Publication of their findings worried many citizens, including Elsie Hickey, the Director of Public Health Nursing. In 1940, she informed Jackson that a nutritionist was needed if Toronto was to maintain its leadership in the public health field, because "we must admit that other health departments have gone further than we, as practically all well organized departments have nutritionists on their staffs." Further pressure came from Alan Brown and the Local Council of Women. All of these factors contributed to the appointment of Toronto's first nutritionist in June 1942.[44] During the war, the Canadian government rationed food, but unlike the British government, did not arrange milk and vitamin supplements for pregnant women and young children.[45]

By the late 1940s, the nutritionist had been integrated into the Department's home visits and health education activities. She advised the public health nurses, and if necessary, went with them to offer personal consultation to clients, particularly in lower income districts like Moss Park, Riverdale and University. She also prepared the menus in the Forest Schools and health classes, served as liaison between the dietician at the Riverdale Isolation Hospital and the Health Department, and provided practical experience for student dieticians interested in community nutrition. Although there was a fairly rapid turnover in the position, each woman gave guest lectures to Home and School Associations, created public displays, and participated in educational activities. In 1949, nutritionists at various institutions united to form the Toronto Nutrition Council, and the Ontario Health Department's Interdepartmental Nutrition Committee.[46] These bodies were

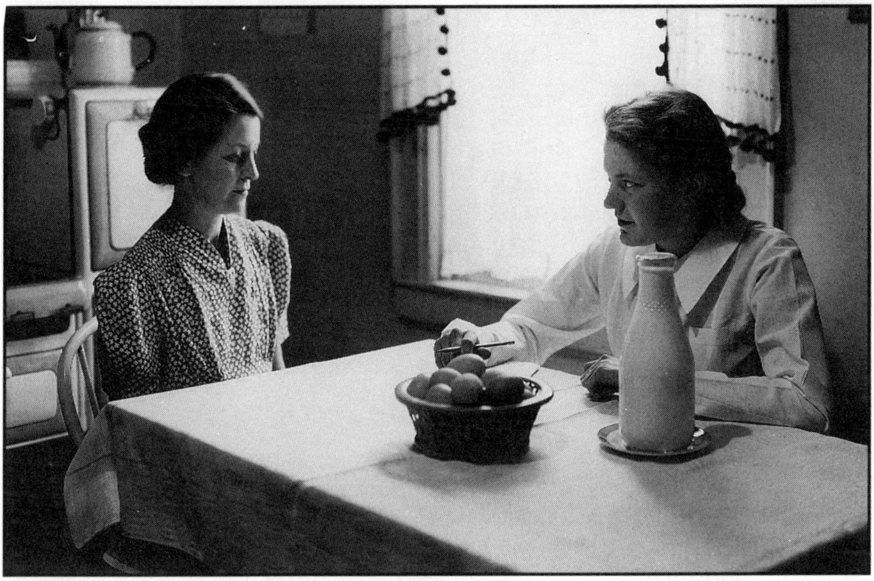

Nutrition counselling at home in the 1940s.

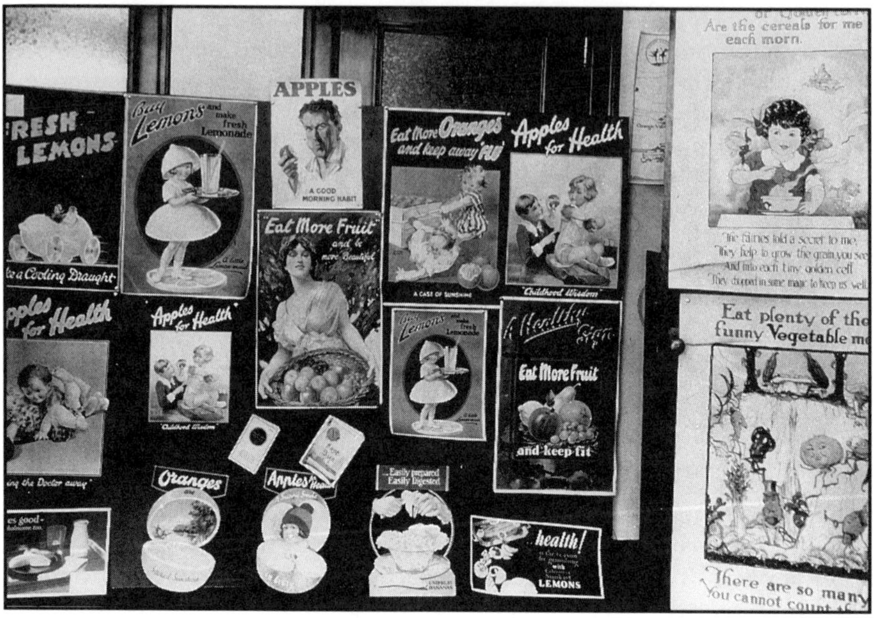

Through the 1930s and 1940s, poster campaigns were designed to "sell" nutrition concepts to homemakers and their children.

a forum for discussing professional concerns, establishing camaraderie, organizing nutrition research projects, and combating misinformation in newspapers, magazines and other media.

Much of the nutritionist's work entailed remaining up-to-date, to enable her to offer the public and her colleagues the most accurate information on food and its value. As Ruth Moyles, Toronto's second nutritionist observed, the purpose of nutrition education was behaviour modification. To achieve this successfully, the "ignorance, carelessness, disinterest, food whims and modern-day over-indulgence" of consumers had to be overcome. How was this to be accomplished? In 1949 McHenry reflected on his years of study in an article called "Confusion and Stupidity in Nutrition Education." Among his suggestions for a more dynamic approach to the problem were advertising, the inclusion of nutrition education in teacher training courses, and unification of the efforts of nutritionists so that the public received consistent information. He was concerned that Canada's Food Rules sounded too draconian and recommended simplicity and repetition focused on children because:

> Nutrition education not only has to overcome inertia; it has to compete with high-pressure advertising with regard to some foods at least...It is almost impossible to drive any distance without seeing an attractive bill-board [sic] urging people to drink a brand of pop. How many bill-boards about milk have you seen?[47]

In Toronto Moyles' successor, Janet Wardlaw, implemented some of McHenry's suggestions. In "Food Facts and Fallacies," she stressed the importance of expert advice and warned her readers to beware of food faddists. She also demonstrated that while Canada's Food Rules were the foundation of scientific study in nutrition matters, consumers merely had to recognize food groups and balance their use to create acceptable diets.[48]

In addition, she assisted the public health nurses with nutrition activities in Toronto's schools. To educate children, Toronto's teachers were encouraged to hold poster contests, to do food intake surveys, and to have students conduct food identification projects. The most effective teaching tool proved to be feeding experiments using white rats. In 1957, twenty-three pairs of the rodents were distributed among schools in each health district, and specific classes were responsible for feeding one animal a balanced diet and the other a junk food diet. The effect of these two regimens on the growth and longevity of each rat gave the students a graphic illustration of the dangers of excessive sugar consumption.[49]

In addition to educating children, the nutritionist also participated in a survey of the foods used by immigrants. In 1957–8, the members of the Toronto Nutrition Committee analyzed the results of their survey and created a booklet called *Food Habits of New Canadians*; it was intended to enable nutritionists and public health nurses help the newcomers choose less expensive Canadian substitutes for expensive imported foods. Through the 1960s and 1970s, this information was updated as new groups arrived and the Department's nutrition pamphlets were translated into many languages. The difficulty of assisting immigrant parents was illustrated early in one nutritionist's career, when she had a case in which a young diabetic was sent home from the Hospital for Sick Children with diet sheets that used

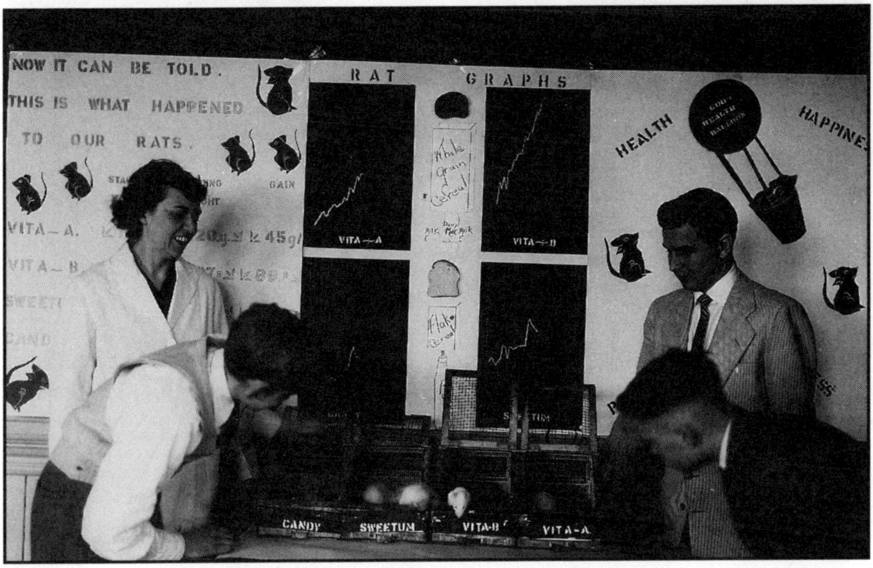

School nurses and teachers supervised the rat feeding experiment undertaken in 1957.

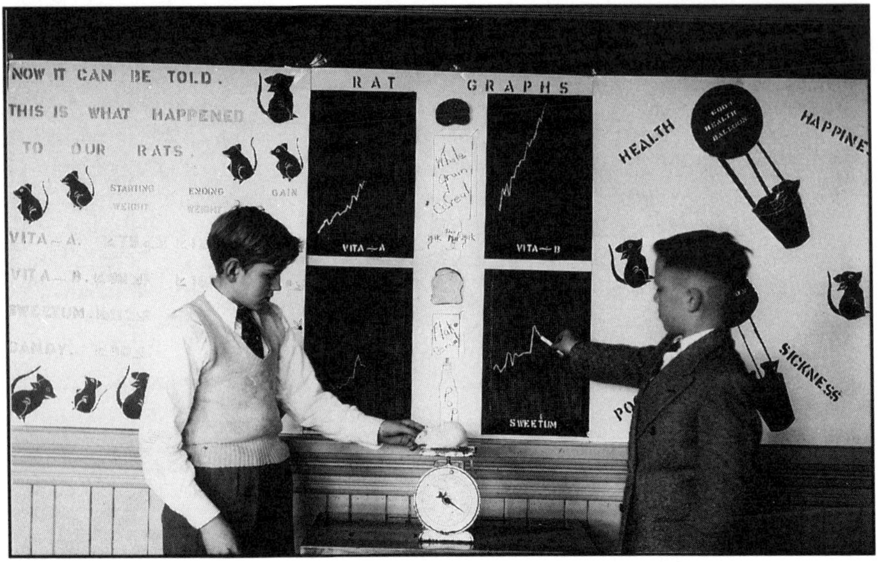

Weighing the rats showed the difference in growth patterns as a result of different diets.

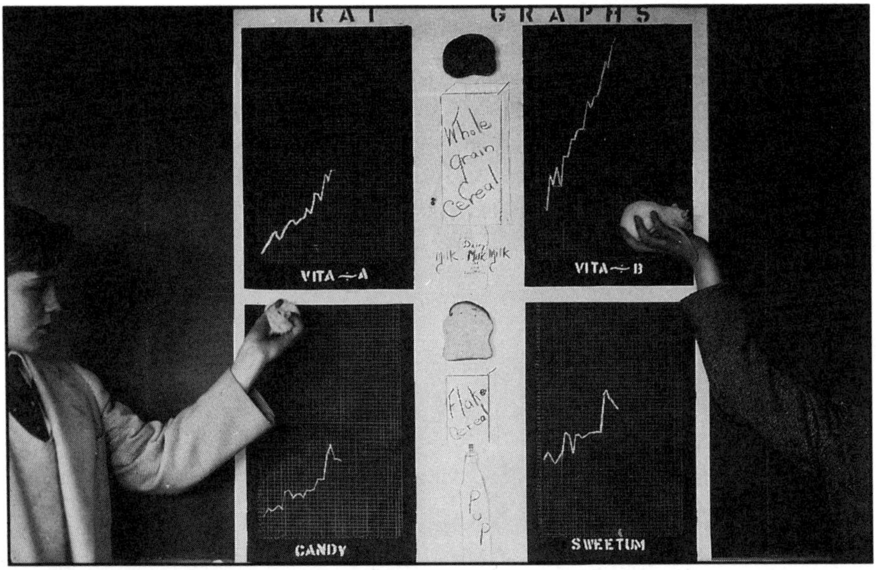

Graphs comparing the two rats reinforced the lessons about healthful food choices which the experiment had been designed to foster.

Canadian foods for her meals. The little girl's parents were unable to follow these directions and she was re-admitted to the hospital. With the assistance of the district nurse, nutritionist Linda Latchford visited the family, counselled the parents, and then sent the meal plans away for translation. But the child still continued to have diabetic crises. After six months of effort, the district nurse finally discovered that the parents could not read, so she and Latchford drew pictures of the items and amounts of food that the child could eat.[50]

Through the 1960s, Toronto nutritionists, like the Department's medical and nursing staff, contributed to a variety of surveys and research projects. They included a Vitamin C use survey with the Hospital for Sick Children, a breakfast survey at Charles G. Fraser school, a nutrition survey of Grade nine girls, a study of infants' iron levels, and the prenatal diet survey already noted.[51] But during the decade, each nutritionist had to respond as well to public queries such as "How much strontium 90 is contained in Toronto milk?" or "Will peanut butter on my porridge harm me?"

By the mid–1970s, Toronto's nutritionists had been pursuing traditional public health education tactics for three decades, yet the constant introduction of new foods and the amount of public misinformation about them did not seem to be diminishing. Moreover, deaths from the diseases of both poverty and affluence dominated the post-1945 mortality statistics. Dieting, physical fitness, and concern about food additives became central to the lives of many Britons, Americans, and Canadians, as they tried to prevent heart attacks, cancer and other lifestyle diseases, and to stay slim.[52] Gradually, researchers demonstrated that childhood eating habits, in part, determined an individual's susceptibility to chronic disease. As a result, both *A New Perspective on Health for Canadians* in 1974, and *Public Health in the 1980's*, questioned food producers and advertisers who exploited children by "selling" valueless snacks. In Toronto, the city's nutritionist urged the board of health to support targeted programs like Healthiest Babies Possible, and to assist parents' groups who wanted to educate their children about lifestyle diseases caused by junk food.[53] Advocacy now joined education as the focus of the nutritionists' efforts.

Conclusion

The changing pattern of the services and programs which the Health Department staff have provided in the city's schools mirrors both changes in the larger society and developments in public health training and practice. When the Department took over school medical inspection, many health problems were still common among Toronto children. Combining service and education, the city's doctors, dentists, nurses, and ultimately, its dental hygienists and nutritionists, created community-wide programs which were intended to establish basic health standards and knowledge. Their efforts were supported by the health classes which the Board of Education included in the curriculum, and by the activities of voluntary organizations such as the Junior Red Cross.

During the 1950s, the staff's workload increased with the arrival of the baby boom and immigrant children in the city's classrooms. By the beginning of the following decade, the consensus which had dominated society since the 1910s collapsed, as critics emerged to point out the social inequalities and racism, which they argued, persisted in spite of the education system. The members of the Health Department were swept along in the tide of change, as their long-established approach to school health programs was criticized as obsolete and ineffective. External pressure for reform co-incided with internal conflict between the medical research model and health promotion. Together these forces coalesced to develop targeted health education programs for students, and to redefine the services and health promotion activities which the staff would perform.

Chapter Ten

Administration or Advocacy?: STD and Family Planning

In 1898, a muck-raking journalist, C.S. Clark, published *Of Toronto the Good, A Social Study: The Queen City of Canada As It Is*. In several brief chapters, he outlined the moral laxity he found hidden under a veneer of Victorian prudery, and informed his readers that prostitution was widespread, venereal disease was rampant, and condoms, and other unnamed birth control devices were available to those who knew where to look.[1] On the eve of the new century, these revelations helped to focus public attention on two neglected health concerns: venereal disease and family limitation. But were these medical or moral problems? What role should Toronto's Health Department play in dealing with them?

For "social purity" reformers and concerned clergymen, venereal diseases and birth control practices were an affront to Christian society. For many of the city's doctors, the human cost of these diseases and the maternal mortality which resulted from excessive childbearing demanded action, in spite of the social stigma attached to sexually transmitted diseases (STD) and the legal prohibitions against the discussion and sale of contraceptives. The social and political implications of dealing with these issues meant that public officials approached them with caution unless, like Charles Hastings, they believed that these "lamentably neglected" aspects of modern life caused too much preventable sickness and death. For Ontario's municipal health officers, World War I was the catalyst which added control of venereal diseases to their statutory duties. They would not become involved in family planning matters until the 1960s.

The First World War not only broke down significant social taboos about the discussion of human sexuality, but also demonstrated the effectiveness of central government involvement in the nation's economy. In the aftermath of the conflict, the Borden government finally created a National Health Department, and one of its primary goals was controlling and preventing VD. Like the rest of the provinces, Ontario passed legislation which created clinics and made local health authorities responsible for ensuring that disease victims were identified, provided with treatment, and offered the opportunity to name their contacts. The combination of federal funding and provincial legislation led to the development of Toronto's approach to these diseases. Instead of the leadership role which the Health Department had created in its sanitation, communicable disease control, and health education efforts, it was assigned a co-ordinating function. This remained the foundation for staff activities throughout the twentieth century.

All levels of government agreed that educating the public to prevent the spread of these diseases was an essential component of the attack against them. None of them, however, wanted to lead the crusade, and in 1919, the Canadian National Council to Control Venereal Disease was created in Toronto, with funds from federal and provincial authorities and interested citizens. Led by Dr. Gordon Bates, the CNCCVD capitalized on public concern by creating a national network of information centres. But public interest was fickle. In the rush to return to normalcy, wartime fears about the impact of VD faded, and not until World War II would another strong educational effort occur. Indeed, during the 1920s, the federal government gradually eliminated its funding for VD education and the treatment clinics. In the following decade, the province cut back its spending in response to the Depression. In spite of this, Toronto's Health Department continued to fulfil its statutory duties, and surveys carried out by voluntary organizations indicated that the incidence of the disease was declining.

World War II brought renewed interest from the federal and provincial authorities and a new therapeutic measure in the form of penicillin. When the Phair Committee assessed Toronto's Health Department in 1942, however, it argued that the city probably had one of the highest incidence rates in the nation. To overcome this, it proposed closer links between the city and the province and encouraged the Health League of Canada, a successor to the CNCCVD, to mount further educational campaigns aimed at both doctors and the public. In the aftermath of the war, these initiatives seemed somewhat redundant as penicillin and the sulpha drugs cured the venereal diseases quickly. But were these scourges truly vanquished? By the early 1960s, penicillin-resistant strains of VD were appearing — just as society was loosening moral strictures and the "sexual revolution" was beginning. As the Department's statistics demonstrated that syphilis and gonorrhea rates were increasing, health authorities began to question the effectiveness of their disease control and health education methods. By the 1970s, behaviour modification through health promotion was attracting attention at both the federal and municipal levels. Through a variety of targeted advertising and educational campaigns, the new health activists tried to modernize the staff's approach to their work and to educate the public.

In contrast to government support for VD education, treatment, and control work, any reference to birth control was illegal until 1969. Although Canadian women had begun to control their fertility as the nation urbanized during the nineteenth century, doctors and health agencies were prohibited from discussing contraceptive techniques by the 1892 amendments to the Criminal Code. During the 1930s, lay philanthropists broke the public silence on this matter, but local health departments did not follow suit until effective measures were available in the 1960s. The rise of the women's movement, and the establishment of the Planned Parenthood Association in 1961, provided the community pressure which led the Health Department to sponsor birth control counselling through a clinic at Toronto General Hospital in 1965. A decade later, family planning was respectable, except in the eyes of recent immigrants, and, with provincial funding, Toronto created an innovative, multidisciplinary, Division of Family Planning Services. It combined contemporary program creation procedures with modern advertising techniques to help citizens make informed choices on preventing unwanted pregnancies.

From 1918 to the present, Toronto's Health Department has worked to fulfil its statutory duties with regard to sexually transmitted diseases, and to respond to public demands for birth control information. In so doing, it has moved from a focus on administration to a commitment to advocacy.

Lifting the Veil of Secrecy: STD

On July 1, 1918, Ontario's Venereal Disease Prevention Act went into effect after five years of intensive campaigning by outspoken lay, medical, and military reformers. In 1913, Toronto's Local Council of Women asked the city council to set up a commission to investigate the "white slave trade." In so doing, these women were imitating the vice commissions which many American cities created between 1910 and 1916. These research projects were intended to establish the extent of prostitution in each city, and the need for education and legislation to combat the perceived consequences of illicit sex — gonorrhea and syphilis.

"NEW CONDITIONS HAVE TAUGHT NEW DUTIES"

Evidence of Advances in Public Health Administration

The Forty-Second Annual Meeting of the American Public Health Association. recently held at Jacksonville, might well be termed an "epoch-making convention." Never before has such evidence of advanced thought in Public Health administration been evinced. The true issues in the field of preventive medicine were more definitely defined, consequent upon a more accurate knowledge of the real sources of disease and the means by which they are transmitted from one to another.

It was made clear that much work was now being done by Departments of Health that had only an indirect bearing on the prevention of disease and should, therefore, not be charged up to Public Health Service, and that many of the vital problems had been neglected, as, for instance, Industrial Hygiene and Industrial Diseases.

It was shown that this is part of a community hygiene, and that the dangers from improper heating and ventilation and the trade dusts were in themselves prejudicial to health, and not an infrequent cause of the development in transmission of disease, and that in addition to this there were the dangers resulting from the trades themselves—as lead poisoning, mercurial poisoning, etc.—and yet these have been lamentably neglected. However, the Association took sufficient cognizance of this to arrange for a special section in Industrial Hygiene for subsequent meetings.

This action on the part of the Association was well timed from the economic standpoint alone, inasmuch as Sir Thomas Oliver has pointed out that the aggregate cost of illness due to occupations alone in the United States amounts to $772,892,860, and this is for the most part preventable.

The problem of venereal diseases also received due consideration. and was referred to as another lamentably neglected branch of preventive medicine. Those who are competent to judge are of the opinion that these diseases constitute probably the most important of all factors in the degeneration and depopulation of the world. As has been expressed, we are paying the penalty of centuries of an ignorant, ill-considered false modesty in terms of morbidity and mortality that probably surpass the amount of all other communicable influences combined.

The ravages of Cancer were also considered, and in connection therewith the duties of Departments of Health to institute an educational campaign by which they may convince the public that this disease can be robbed of its terrors by early diagnosis and early treatment.

The curses of the Drug Habit and the Patent Medicine faker constituted the subject of an interesting and instructive discussion. Startling facts were revealed by those who took part in the discussions. It was shown that there are at least four million (4,000,000) victims of Morphine, Opium and Cocaine in the United States, or four out of every 100.

The people of the United States and Canada spend over $110,000,000 on patent medicine every year. The people of Toronto spend over

*Charles Hastings publicized contemporary issues such as the health costs of venereal disease in the **Health Bulletin**.*

When Toronto's commission reported in 1915, a new factor had been added to the equation. Canadian troops at home and in Europe were suffering high rates of infection from both venereal diseases. By 1917, military authorities had created "blue light" centres for Canadian servicemen, and public health physicians, women's groups, and politicians, were starting to worry about the return of infected veterans. As a result, in August that year, concerned Toronto activists set up a committee to investigate solutions to this problem. This group, in turn, persuaded the Hearst government to create a commission to examine the impending crisis. Dr. C.K. Clarke, Superintendent of the Toronto General Hospital, had already informed the federal Commission on Conservation that serological tests conducted on public ward patients revealed a venereal disease infection rate of 12–13%. These were the first reliable Canadian statistics, but they were incorrectly extrapolated to Ontario's population as a whole, to justify demands for government intervention.[2]

But what could the government do? Like their European counterparts, Toronto's doctors knew that syphilis and gonorrhea caused pain, sterility, congenital birth defects, and paralytic dementia (general paresis). Could these diseases be prevented, controlled or treated like other communicable diseases? Or did their mode of transmission mean that they would remain stigmatized? In 1906, August Wassermann had developed the complement fixation test which helped doctors diagnose syphilis. Four years later, Paul Ehrlich announced the discovery of salvarsan, an arsenic derivative which killed the syphilis bacteria. These advances and better diagnostic techniques for gonorrhea provided the foundation for control and treatment.[3]

The problem, however, lay in public attitudes to these diseases. For some, discussing sex-related topics was unacceptable. For others, gonorrhea and syphilis represented the "wages of sin." To counter such Victorian morality, social purity crusaders argued that women and children suffered unnecessarily as a result of infection. These arguments, however, had a limited effect until the First World War, when the demand for fighting forces and war workers compelled all levels of government to recognize the high price that the nation was paying, for what Hastings informed readers of the December *Health Bulletin*, was "centuries of an ignorant and ill-considered false modesty in terms of morbidity and mortality" from venereal diseases.

As a result, Toronto's medical officer and his colleagues, such as Gordon Bates, argued that Ontario should adopt Western Australia's tough venereal disease legislation, which gave medical officers summary powers to compel testing and treatment, while conducting an educational campaign to lift the veil of secrecy surrounding these diseases. Ontario's 1918 act fulfilled their demands, because the regulations which defined its operation empowered the medical officer to oversee individuals, general practitioners, and hospital clinics.[4]

The federal government, too, had debated controlling the spread of these diseases after the troops came home. In 1919, in response to the threat of venereal disease, and after the influenza epidemic of 1918–19 demonstrated the inadequacy of provincial disease control procedures, the Borden government created a National Department of Health. With very limited appropriations, the new department identified venereal disease as a health threat worthy of government funding and publicity. From 1919 until 1924, federal authorities provided per capita grants to each province to support venereal disease clinics and preventive education activities.[5]

Controlling VD: The Initial Campaign

For cities like Toronto, the combination of federal funding and provincial legislation led to the creation of venereal disease clinics because curing the disease limited the potential spread of infection. To co-ordinate the services provided at the Toronto General, Western, St. Michael's, Wellesley, and East General hospitals, and the Hospital for Sick Children, the Health Department appointed a supervisor of venereal disease nursing who introduced this new task to the Hospital Social Service nurses. This Division had been created in 1914–15 to assist tuberculosis victims and public ward patients who were being sent home. The Hospital Social Service nurses were assigned this new duty because of their close links with hospital staff, and their experience in arranging social, as well as medical services.

Francis Brown, who was the first supervisor of venereal disease nursing, outlined Toronto's system in speeches and articles. She stressed the importance of the initial interview and the nurses' role in creating a 'good atmosphere' in the clinics because patients had to come weekly for treatment which was "long and tedious and frequently painful." When patients ceased to attend, the Department's nurses had to track them down and persuade them to resume treatment. They also had to try to elicit a list of contacts in order to control the spread of the disease. The case-finding aspect of the nurses' work was difficult because some clients ignored their legal obligations and gave false names and addresses. Others had only the slightest knowledge of the person from whom they had contracted the disease, and all were frightened of the loss of confidentiality.[6]

Much of the VD control work focused on prostitutes arraigned in district court because of the somewhat misguided assumption that these women were the focal point for infection. The Venereal Disease supervisor spent a portion of her working day in court persuading, or requiring, prostitutes to take Wassermann tests. She also visited women in the Don Jail and at the Jail Farm for the same purpose. Although the Department could compel people charged with prostitution-related offenses to undergo tests while in jail, prior to trial, persuasion rather than coercion remained the preferred approach.[7] Toronto's approach was regarded with approval by provincial authorities, who recommended that recently appointed VD nurses from other Ontario communities spend three weeks to a month in the capital observing the system in operation.[8]

By the 1930s, serological examinations constituted 40% of the Department's laboratory work and were the foundation for all the staff's efforts to combat syphilis. In the United States, blood tests slowly became mandatory for marriage licenses and hospital patients, especially pregnant women.[9] During the 1920s, however, American attempts to deal with prostitution foundered on public opposition to infringement of civil liberties, and the lack of medical support for state or municipal clinics.[10] In Toronto, few fears about imposing on civil rights were expressed until the 1960s. Instead, the staff viewed their links to the courts as a way of finding defaulting clinic patients and controlling the spread of the diseases.

Like many of her Canadian and American contemporaries, Brown believed that education was the key to preventing venereal diseases. She objected to the pessimistic view that human nature would never change and argued against the double standard of sexual morality. Her views were echoed by the Women's Christian Temperance Union which had supported the purity campaign prior to 1914. Although most commentators argued that parents should provide the child's introduction to the subject, many realized that social taboos and lack of knowledge prevented them from doing so. As early as 1914, Dr. W.E. Struthers, the Board of Education's former Chief Medical Inspector, was arguing in favour of sex education in Toronto schools; his views were echoed by Dr. J.G. FitzGerald of the University of Toronto in 1926, in his well-known textbook, *An Introduction to the Practice of Preventive Medicine.* Such suggestions were far in advance of public opinion. Nevertheless, voluntary groups like the Canadian Girls in Training gingerly started to provide some information to young women during the interwar years.[11]

Public Education: Success and Frustration

The most prominent educational organization was the Toronto-based Canadian National Council for Combating Venereal Disease. The Council took a dynamic approach to publicity and showed the American anti-venereal disease film, *The End of the Road,* throughout the province. In the early 1920s, it also organized speeches by leading medical authorities and international activists like Mrs. Emmeline Pankhurst, and set up poster displays and exhibits at the CNE. As a member of the Toronto branch of the Canadian Social Hygiene Council, the new name for the CNCCVD, Brown participated in the development of educational programs and publicity materials. An exhibit at the St. Charles Hotel in 1923, opened by Toronto's mayor, Hastings, and J.W.S. McCullough, Ontario's Chief Medical Officer, attracted 13,000 spectators during its time on display.[12] With the support of the Ontario Health Department, the exhibit then toured the province. These educational efforts were based on modern advertising techniques but the displays and presentations were segregated by sex to ensure that propriety was maintained. The moral stigma co-existed uneasily with experts' assumption that providing information would assure changes in behaviour.

In 1924, the Social Hygiene Council appointed two regional organizers to reanimate quiescent branches and develop new groups in the rest of the country. Leon Pequegnat worked as the Eastern organizer during 1925, and learned first hand about the difficulties of maintaining public interest in this topic as memories of wartime concern faded. He joined Toronto's Health

Department in 1926, and strongly supported the city's annual grants to the Canadian Social Hygiene Council between 1928 and 1939, after federal and provincial venereal disease control funds were slashed. Although a renewed educational campaign by the Council in the early 1930s produced more literature, and another internationally recognized film, *Damaged Goods*, it failed to overcome the social stigma of the disease.[13] As a result, municipal health authorities devoted most of their attention to controlling the disease and providing service to stricken individuals.

Administering Provincial Legislation

According to the Venereal Disease Prevention Act, individuals who suspected that they were infected could seek diagnosis and treatment from private practitioners. Indeed, the Health Department's nurses and medical staff encouraged people to go to their family doctors for treatment, but many were deterred by the cost and the potential embarrassment. In spite of the secrecy provisions of the legislation and its 1922 amendment, many victims feared discovery and preferred to seek treatment from non-medical sources and patent medicines. Those who did seek medical help were sometimes treated as "moral lepers" since most doctors shared society's moral code. Moreover, few general practitioners had the specialized knowledge or skill to carry out the complex and expensive, 18 to 24 month treatment for the disease.[14] During the 1930s then, more patients turned to public clinics for service because they were free and anonymous.

In 1935, Pequegnat described the problems facing health departments in administering the venereal disease legislation for the Social Hygiene Section of the Canadian Public Health Association. As he reminded his audience, "Immorality does not of necessity imply the presence of venereal disease" [sic] and therefore, the staff hired to carry out the provisions had to have compassion and tact. He strongly urged his colleagues to consider the Toronto approach, which stressed courtesy letters and home visits, rather than coercion to achieve treatment, because "We will all agree that results are desired rather than penalties."[15] In effect, the deputy health officer was arguing in favour of regarding the venereal diseases like any other communicable disease for the purpose of reporting and care. By adopting this neutral stance toward the problem, he was trying to eliminate the moral stigma.

He concluded his remarks by calling for further provincial funding, since the federal grants had stopped in the mid–1920s and the province had limited its support during the 1930s. Through the Depression, Toronto's Health Department faced annual budget cuts. Since surveys by the Canadian Social Hygiene Council indicated that the incidence of VD was declining in the city, the Department began to downplay its control work. By 1939, the medical director, the nurse supervisor, and the stenographer all worked on a part-time basis while the Division clerk was the lone full-time employee. Would this be sufficient to deal with a wartime situation?

In October 1940, Pequegnat addressed the Academy of Medicine about the recent amendments to provincial legislation because venereal disease rates were beginning to rise and wartime conditions were expected to compound the problem. Without notification from general practitioners, neither the city nor the province could mount an effective campaign to control the spread of the disease. Under the 1918 act, doctors were required to notify local health departments of positive test results and the amount of treatment which they provided. If patients stopped coming before treatment was completed, general practitioners were supposed to report this to the health department. And they were also expected to try to uncover the names of contacts. As Brown had noted in 1924, few doctors felt that they could ask such intimate questions, and according to Pequegnat the situation had not greatly improved by 1940. That year, the law was changed to require that practitioners report to the Ontario Health Department and that they send regular reports on the patient's progress to the provincial Department. Pequegnat was critical of doctors who complained about filling out two sets of forms and remarked: "Occasionally one still has to contend with misunderstanding of respective function, encroachment, wrong attitudes, and with inadequacies born of lack of precision (in examination and reporting)."[16]

In 1943, Gordon Bates conducted the fourth survey of venereal disease incidence in Toronto carried out by the Health League of Canada, the successor to the CSHC. In it, he asked physicians to indicate how many of their patients had been drinking when they contracted their infection. This moralistic question was intended to elicit information about the social milieu in which the diseases were spread. As well, Bates included a query about the number of patients who had told the doctor the names of their contacts. Of the 352 doctors who were treating VD victims, 97 asked their patients for information, 5 asked 15–75% of their patients, 203 never asked these questions, and 47 did not reply. Was this reticence a result of the belief in the confidentiality of the physician-patient relationship? Did it reflect fear that the Health Department staff lacked the skills to do contact tracing discreetly? Or was it simply the doctors' way of expressing their discontent with the extension of state medicine into another area of their practice? In the United States, public health administrators faced similar opposition from their medical colleagues in the interwar period until the Surgeon-General, Thomas Parran, launched a national campaign in 1936–7 with the support of President Roosevelt.[17]

Renewed Concern: VD in World War II

In addition to changing its reporting requirements, the Ontario Health Department responded to the outbreak of World War II by re-establishing its Division of Venereal Disease Control. To direct public health nursing efforts, the province "borrowed" Pearl Stiver, the Toronto Health Department's VD nursing supervisor, for the duration of the hostilities. The federal government also recreated its VD program in 1943, in part, because of concern that the civilian population was at risk. The Health League's survey that year provided further cause for alarm because the number of positive Wassermann tests at Toronto General was up and the hospital reported 168 new cases in 1943, as opposed to 41 in 1937, when the previous survey was done. Moreover, general practitioners were treating 26% of the syphilis victims and 46% of the gonorrhea cases, while the public clinics cared for the remainder. A year earlier Toronto had reported 1,801 cases of syphilis and 1,218 cases of gonorrhea to the province.

This rapid rise continued and on October 11, 1944, the medical officer, G.P. Jackson, reported to the local board of health that VD cases had increased by 51% since 1938 for a total of 18,000 cases. He also told the members that prostitution was not the main cause of this high rate but that for inhabitants under the age of 30, "street pick-ups" in dance halls, restaurants, hotel corridors, and "to some extent beverage rooms" were the source of much of the infection. Jackson was using these statistics to reinforce the Phair Committee's recommendation for a more comprehensive and effective approach to VD control.

For Mayor Conboy, these revelations prompted an immediate request to city council for an appropriation of $10,000 to combat the diseases, and to the Health League for a renewed educational campaign. Late in 1944, Pequegnat was appointed as the Director of the Division, but the demands of other duties and the lack of municipal funding hampered efforts to implement the provincial Health Department's suggestions. In the fall of 1945, Dr. A.L. McKay, the provincial government's VD expert, became the director of Toronto's VD Control Division after he was demobilized from the navy.[18] In contrast to its limited efforts during the 1930s, the province maintained its interest in controlling venereal disease after 1945 and established close links with Toronto's staff.

In addition to the director, ten new public health nurses were hired in 1944–45 as epidemiologists to do contact tracing.[19] To maintain confidentiality, people suspected of having these diseases were invited to Room 314 in the City Hall to discuss their health status with one of the nurses. Since the Department had to deliver notices requiring testing directly to the individual, VD staff spent much of their time prowling around the less salubrious parts of Toronto at various hours of the day and night. Occasionally this lead to some awkward confrontations and eye-opening experiences. As one of the nurses who joined in the 1940s recalled:

> It was an old apartment on Bloor Street and I had to go down a dark hall to a rather dark door. When the door was answered, a man and woman came...and were very loath to answer whether the person I asked for was there or not. However, as I say, we did develop some skills in establishing our credibility without being too threatening and without admitting why we wanted to see this person. So, I finally did get into the most amazing room that I, as a little, naive public health nurse had ever seen with satin drapes

> and satin covers on the bed and overstuffed furniture in a rather small room. And the girl was not English-speaking, so when I talked to her, I felt I had to raise my voice. In the midst of telling her that she needed to have an examination because she had been in contact with a VD, she was getting very excited. The door opened, and in rushed this man and woman waving a slipper or something, raising their hands and telling me to get out and get out fast. I didn't need to be told, I was out of there so fast. That had a happy conclusion, I quickly gave her my card and told her to go to a doctor for her health's sake and within a week I had a report from a doctor saying she had gone.[20]

Prostitutes of either gender were very susceptible to sexually transmitted diseases and therefore received close attention from the Department's staff. Dealing with Toronto's homosexual community often proved difficult for the VD nurses because of the stigma attached to both aspects of the problem. Male inspectors, and after 1960, male public health nurses, were sent to investigate cases which were deemed too difficult or dangerous for female staff. As a former VD inspector remarked, calming upset clients was a challenge to which he responded by telling them that: "It is no shame to get an STD, but it certainly is a shame to pass it on."[21]

Solving the Problem: Education or Antibiotics?

Once the war was over, education was again expected to play a role, and in 1945 various women's groups, the Health League, and the Welfare Council of Toronto were asked for their opinions about a film which Pequegnat wished to use.[22] In 1948, the provincial and city health departments assisted the YMCA with an exhibit on "the causes, means of spread and the results of prompt treatment." Toronto's Laboratory staff provided microscopes and samples of syphilis and gonorrhea for interested visitors while other staff gave evening lectures. This demonstration attracted 4,000 young men and women during the week.[23] Measuring the effectiveness of such publicity was difficult because the faith in a direct correlation between knowledge and individual behaviour that had been the bed-rock of educational campaigns in the 1920s no longer existed.

Indeed, many experts hoped that widespread use of penicillin by the civilian population, once adequate supplies were available, would cure existing cases and gradually limit the need for education. In 1954, Toronto united its venereal and communicable disease control divisions because most experts agreed that the need for separate campaigns was over. Now monitoring was sufficient. In the United States, federal and state funding for anti-venereal disease efforts had declined markedly during the 1950s, and concern about the cost/benefit ratio in the 1960s and 1970s further undermined control efforts, by demonstrating that mass blood testing was expensive and turned up limited numbers of new cases.[24] For a decade, it seemed that antibiotics had cured an age-old scourge and that the stigma of venereal diseases would be lifted.

By the end of the 1950s, the incidence of sexually transmitted diseases was increasing and penicillin resistant strains of the diseases were appearing in Toronto and other North American cities. In 1961, a *Globe & Mail* reporter questioned the health officer, Dr. A.R.J. Boyd, about the rise in VD cases and the possibility of resistant strains of these diseases. Boyd was reluctant to comment on the clinical aspects of the problem because Toronto no longer conducted its own serological tests, and the city's hospitals and general practitioners provided treatment. Moreover, Toronto's director of communicable disease control was not dismayed by these statistics, noting that the Department now had its nurses doing contact interviewing for family physicians, and had introduced an American innovation — cluster testing — as a means of uncovering hidden cases. To ensure that staff carried out this approach effectively, the director proposed sending some of them to American cities where it was practiced, and requested approval to attend a World Forum on Venereal Disease in Washington.[25] All of these activities were intended to enable the Department to fulfil its statutory duties and continue to co-ordinate existing services.

External factors altered this arrangement. The "sexual revolution" of the 1960s produced an outpouring of concern about increases in venereal infections, especially among teenagers and young adults.[26] Yorkville acquired a reputation for swinging sex, and parents of runaway young girls worried that their children would be infected while experimenting with an alternate

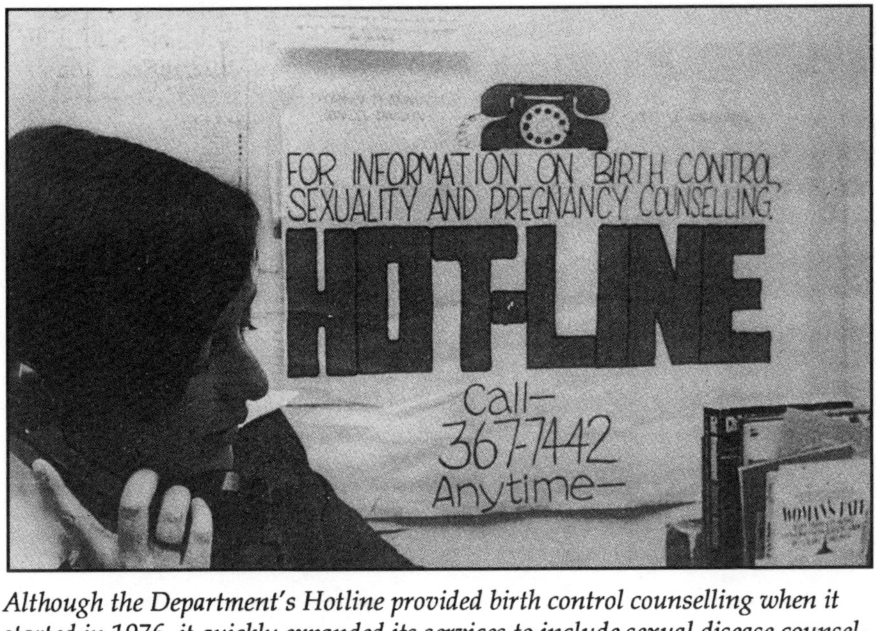

Although the Department's Hotline provided birth control counselling when it started in 1976, it quickly expanded its services to include sexual disease counselling.

lifestyle.[27] In response to rising disease rates, counter-culture activists created their own health care facilities by opening the Rochdale Free Clinic in 1969, and replacing it with the Hassle Free Clinic in 1973.[28] Neither of these were run by the Department, although nursing staff were assigned to do contact tracing for the Hassle Free Clinic. Public health nurses and inspectors who had to deal with the hippies, found their confrontational attitude a challenge to the Department's reliance on persuasion and education in controlling venereal diseases.[29] Nevertheless, the Health Department supported city funding for these non-governmental clinics and lobbied the municipal and provincial governments on their behalf.

Health Promotion: The Contemporary Approach

By 1965, venereal diseases topped the federal government's list of ten leading notifiable health threats. During the 1970s, federal and provincial authorities stated that gonorrhea had reached epidemic levels across Canada. Evidently, traditional educational and treatment efforts had failed, so a new generation of activists turned to behaviour modification through health promotion. In the 1974 working document, *A New Perspective on Health for Canadians,* the authors commented on the continuing stigma which affected attempts to control and prevent sexually transmitted diseases, yet also labelled these diseases a "self-imposed risk" to health, because they believed that "promiscuity and carelessness" were responsible for Canadians' high rate of infection.

To develop a more sophisticated attack on these problems, the federal government offered funding for advertising campaigns and experiments in behaviour modification techniques. In 1976, the Department's Venereal Disease Action Committee recommended combining VD work with the new family planning division, and creating a joint educational campaign using available media contacts. In spite of these efforts, the stigma remained. Community groups consulted during the re-evaluation of the Department's

REPORTED CASES OF SYPHILIS AND GONORRHEA FOR TORONTO AND PROVINCE OF ONTARIO RESIDENTS, 1976 - 1980

Year	Number of Cases: City of Toronto Residents		Number of Cases: Province of Ontario Residents		City Cases as Percentage of Provincial Total	
	Syphilis	Gonorrhoea	Syphilis	Gonorrhoea	Syphilis	Gonorrhoea
1976	926	4,192	2,129	16,612	43.5	25.2
1977	685	3,751	1,772	16,188	38.7	23.2
1978	563	3,963	1,577	15,859	35.7	25.0
1979	658	3,822	1,653	16,658	39.8	22.9
1980	743	3,996	1,759	16,055	42.2	24.9

This chart illustrates the large number of cases of sexually transmitted diseases which Toronto's Health Department supervised in comparison to the rest of the province.

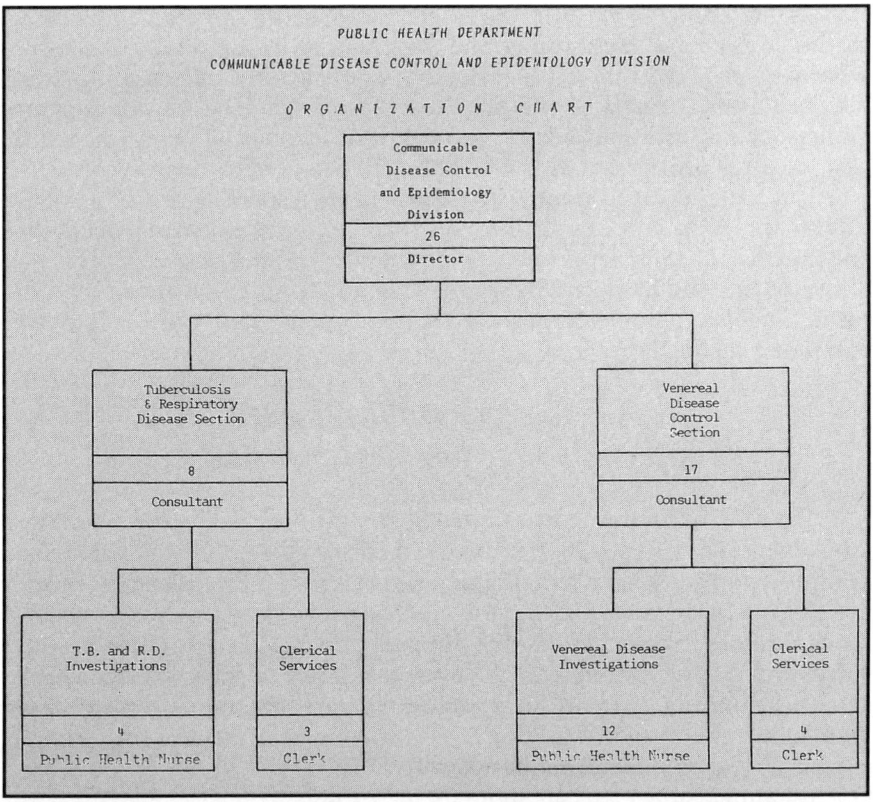

Most of the staff in the Communicable Disease Control and Epidemiology Division devoted their efforts to VD control.

role suggested more education programs, screening clinics, and in-depth counselling in city clinics, because dealing with the disease "demands a reassessment of living habits" by the sufferer. Two years later, the Department's Health Planning Steering Committee used *Public Health in the 1980's* to propose Toronto's next strategy: identifying high-risk groups and devoting educational efforts and screening programs to their needs. In 1976, the Department set up a telephone hotline which provided birth control information; sexual disease counselling was added in 1980 and over 23,000 callers were given advice on these concerns.

Still, well-established contact tracing activities continued because Toronto had the highest reported incidence of sexually-transmitted diseases in Ontario, even though it only contained 7% of the population.[30] In 1981, Toronto police raided bath-houses patronized by the city's homosexual community. Since the inmates were charged with keeping a common bawdy house or being found-ins, an enterprising *Toronto Sun* reporter wondered if they would be treated like other people charged with these offenses. When a senior staff member was asked this question without being told the circumstances, he replied in the affirmative. His response was greeted with outrage by the homosexual community and members of the local board of health, who were shocked that the Department's policies still reflected the draconian provisions of early twentieth century legislation. The episode triggered an inquiry into the compulsory provisions of provincial laws and led the new medical officer, Dr. A.S. Macpherson, to set up a review committee whose mandate was to change Toronto's approach to this procedure.[31] The combination of public opposition, new theories about individual behaviour, and the role of health departments in promoting healthy lifestyles, prompted reassessment and change. The stigma attached to sexually transmitted diseases, however, remains since society has not yet decided whether they are a moral or a medical problem.

Are You An Askable Parent?: Family Planning Controversies

"Says Birth Control Solves Grave Economic Problem." This headline in the *Toronto Star* on April 28, 1927, marked Hastings' second attempt to rouse Torontonians' interest in "intelligent birth control." Like his earlier effort in the August 1924 *Health Bulletin,* the medical officer's arguments focused on the high costs that society paid to support "unlimited reproduction of the sub-normal type." But in 1927, he also stated that he supported American anarchist Emma Goldman's contention that preventing conception was a women's rights issue, and that access to this information was vital for working women, since middle class fertility rates had already declined. Once again Hastings was an anomaly in Toronto. When the *Star*'s reporter asked various ministers to comment on Goldman's address, they indicated "that it was a subject quite outside the bounds of propriety." The president of the OMA, also refused to discuss the matter, and Gordon Bates, the director of the Canadian Social Hygeine Council, stated: "The subject is a very controversial one, one that we (the CSHC) are keeping clear of."[32]

Why did the medical and religious establishment display such strong opposition? Like venereal disease, contraception aroused deep fears about personal morality. Many commentators justified their opposition on the grounds that the declining birth rate would produce "race suicide" among Anglo-Saxon Protestants, while others felt that easily available contraceptives would encourage promiscuity. Still others, justified their position by pointing out that selling contraceptives or providing birth control advice had been made illegal in 1892 through the amendment of the Criminal Code. But for the leaders of the British and American birth control movements, Marie Stopes and Margaret Sanger, most of the opposition centred on male objections to female sexuality and reproductive choice. In Canada, socialist groups in British Columbia argued the feminist position, but they lacked the resources to mount a successful educational campaign, and no municipal department could offer such service because of the legal prohibition.[33] Private philanthropists stepped in to fill the gap.

The economic crisis of the 1930s made birth control respectable. A Kitchener rubber manufacturer, A.R. Kaufman, established the Parents Information Bureau to send nurses to visit poor families who wrote asking for information and cheap supplies of condoms and spermicidal jellies. In 1931–2 a retired Toronto minister, A.H. Tyrer, attempted to set up a birth control clinic modelled on Stopes's Constructive Birth Control Clinic, but he was unable to obtain support from the local board of health and turned to Kaufman for assistance instead. Women's groups in Hamilton opened a birth control clinic in 1932, and Kaufman used this as a model for the clinics that he supported in Toronto and Winnipeg between 1933 and 1938. Although Toronto's clinic served 9,000 clients in five years, Kaufman concluded that it was not as efficient as his corps of nurses, who visited 11,000 working class Torontonians in their homes during the same period. He also believed that the board of health and welfare groups should provide this information, but when the city's Board of Control refused to take over running the clinic, Kaufman passed it on to Toronto's League for Race Betterment. The Board of Control's action reflected the continuing stigma associated with family planning, in spite of Kaufman's victory during the 1937 Palmer case, in which one of his nurses successfully fought a charge under Section 207c of the Criminal Code.[34]

Changing Attitudes and Changing Policies

For Toronto's public health nurses, birth control was not an issue until the 1950s. Staff who joined the Department in the 1940s do not recall women asking for advice, and admit that they would have been unable to provide it because they knew so little themselves. Although there does not appear to have been an official policy preventing discussion of family planning and abortion, the nurses began to agitate against contemporary social restrictions during the 1950s, when more information became available and the School of Hygiene began evening seminars on the topic for health professionals. The staff in the lower income districts like Moss Park were particularly keen to help their clients limit the size of their families, but legal and social conventions restricted their activities.[35]

In fact, the last successful prosecution for the sale of contraceptives took place in Toronto in 1960. This led two British immigrants, George and Barbara Cadbury, to spearhead the formation of the Planned Parenthood Association of Toronto in 1961.[36] Their goal was to obtain public support for amending the Criminal Code to bring Canada into conformity with countries like Great Britain, which had created publicly sponsored birth control clinics in the 1930s. Their timing was excellent. During the 1960s, a second wave of women's groups emerged to challenge patriarchal structures and to demand freedom — including access to the oral contraceptive and the intrauterine device, to ensure reproductive choice.

For the city, family planning became an issue when the Welfare Department discovered that it had been paying for welfare recipients' oral contraceptives. An outcry by women's groups and doctors when the Welfare Department stopped paying for these supplies showed how widespread public support for the pill was in 1964. Pressure mounted for the Health Department to use existing services to dispense birth control information. From January to March 1965, Dr. Boyd was strongly condemned for his refusal to allow the nurses to discuss the topic with women during home visits, at the child health centres, and after they gave birth in hospitals.[37] In fact, the Department was circulating an internal memorandum to the effect that such advice should be given under congenial conditions, while taking the woman's religious and moral convictions into consideration.[38] This careful approach illustrated the senior administrators' view that the Department's duty was to publicize, but not provide, this type of medical service because hospital clinics already existed.

Birth Control: A Medical Service or a Community Program?

In an article in the *Canadian Public Health Journal,* the deputy health officer presented several arguments in favour of hospital-based family planning clinics. Pointing out that public health doctors were administrators rather than clinicians, Dr. Moss stressed that hospitals had the staff and the facilities to carry out complete physical examinations, while health departments could provide publicity, clients, and follow-up services. The legal implications were also discussed, as was the potential for such work to lead to better understanding of contraception and its impact on family life.[39] With the firm support of the local board of health, the Department entered into an agreement with the Toronto General Hospital, which established the first of many clinics where citizens could seek advice and treatment.

In 1969, the Trudeau government finally amended Canada's Criminal Code to permit birth control education and the sale of contraceptives. This change was a response to vociferous women's groups, and to nation-wide civil disobedience by hospitals and health departments. Edmonton's local board and Health Department staff started to provide information in December 1966, but were not able to open their first clinic until 1969. The services proved so popular that more funding was requested from the federal and provincial governments, but none was made available and the city opened more of its own clinics in the 1970s.[40]

Between 1965 and 1970, Toronto's nurses, who had raised the topic during an interview, reported that more and more women were already practicing some form of family limitation. Most were receiving assistance from their family doctors or the hospital clinics. Only new Canadians seemed less willing to discuss such matters, and they expressed disapproval that the subject was taught in the city's schools.[41] In 1970, the Nursing Division even set up a birth control information booth at the CNE. The cost factor and some public opposition meant that this type of publicity was not repeated until 1979.

If the 1960s witnessed public acceptance of birth control as a legitimate subject of discussion, the 1970s saw the issue become a focal point for old and new feminist groups. In 1971, the Association of Women Electors asked the local board to expand birth control services through a network of neighbourhood clinics. This request triggered press criticism of the Department for lack of effort.[42] Both the medical officer and his deputy counter-attacked quite sharply. Moss argued that the Department's 183 nurses were "mobile information centres" who offered advice to women in the child health centres and their homes. He also noted that the Ontario Health Insurance Plan (OHIP) insured family planning services and stressed the role of the general practitioner in this area. Boyd stated that public health nurses and interpreters visited non-English-speaking women in their homes to provide advice.[43] Since the senior administrators clearly could not foresee expanding community services, local women's groups opened the Bay Centre for Birth Control in 1973, and Centro Donne, later the Immigrant Women's Centre, in 1975. These centres were created because of feminists' concern about male, medical dominance of reproductive health issues; they offered teenagers, young adults, and new Canadians, an alternative to hospital clinics and moralistic private practitioners.

Modern Health Education: Networking and Community Development

In 1975, the Ontario Ministry of Health offered health departments and health units throughout the province full funding to create family planning divisions. For the reform-oriented members of Toronto's local board of health, this was an excellent opportunity to realign the Department's birth control efforts toward education, and to build a network of community-based facilities to "demedicalize" fertility control. In contrast to the medical focus of the other divisions, the Family Planning Services Division was multidisciplinary from its inception. Community workers with social work degrees were hired to apply the current community development model, by creating programs which suited each district. All activities were carefully monitored to see if they fit the new division's "management by objectives approach to planning and promotion." In other words, this division was intended to be a prototype for public health in the 1980s and beyond — interdisciplinary and community-oriented with built-in evaluation procedures.

The Family Planning Services Division challenged the *status quo* within Toronto's Health Department in two ways. On the one hand, it ended the medical emphasis on an arm's length relationship to significant social issues. On the other hand, it introduced current concepts in health promotion through activities such as the annual birth control week, which it sponsored each February. Using slogans such as "sex education: it's everybody's business" and "are you an askable parent?," the family planning staff tried to arouse public and professional interest. To reassure parents that it was not

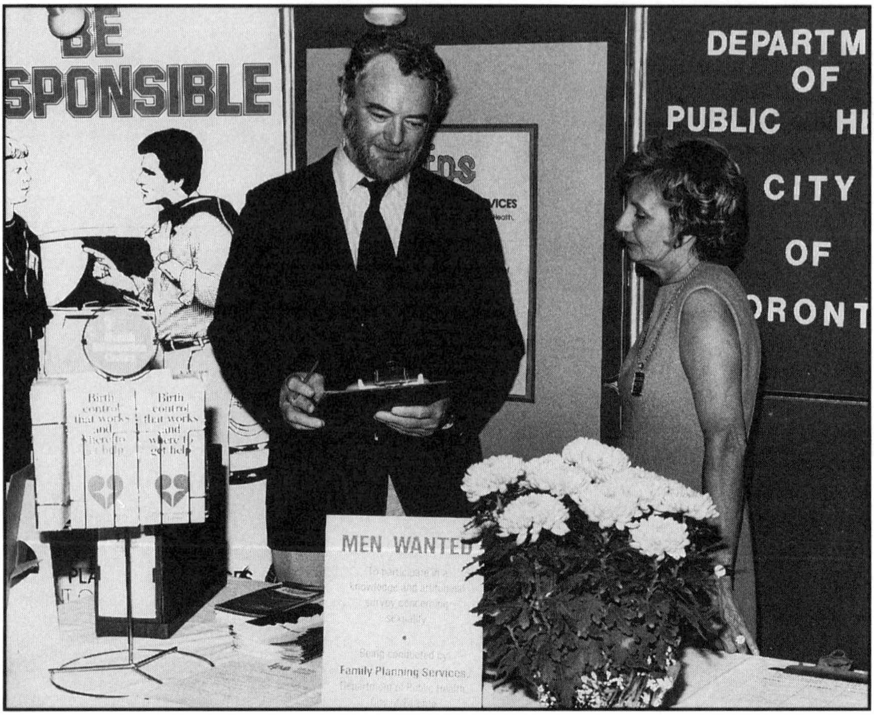

Dr. A.S. Macpherson examining material prepared for the 1981 Birth Control Week campaign, "Be Responsible." Young males were the target group that year.

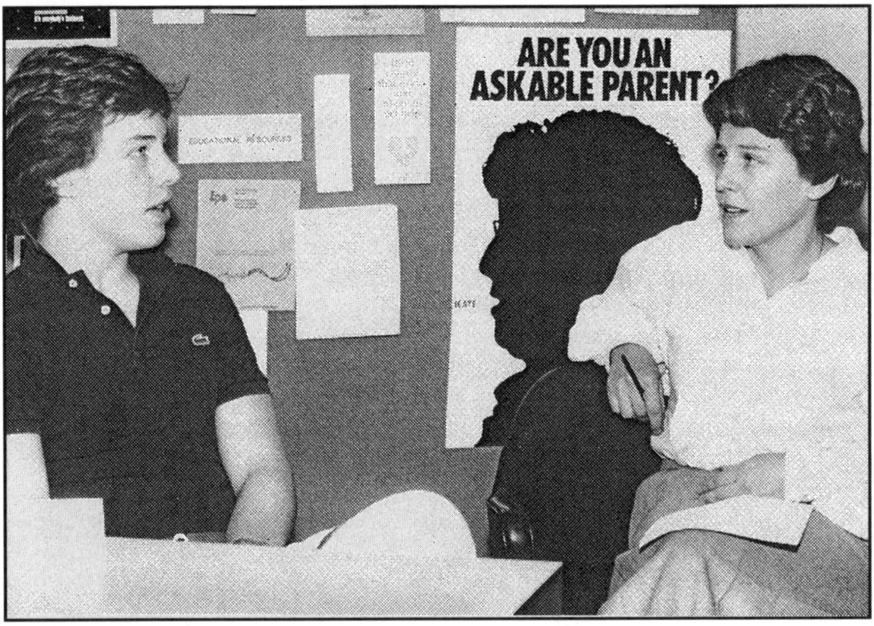

A Health Department member counsels her son.

endorsing teen sex, the division carried out a series of surveys of current practices and knowledge, including one of young men's understanding of birth control methods and their responsibilities. In 1984, free condoms were distributed through various clinics to publicize preventive methods for males. Outraged parents and educators condemned the Department for this action because they did not see it as an appropriate publicity gimmick like the key chains, book marks, and coffee mugs given out in other years. The condom controversy illustrated the limits of public tolerance and prompted a reassessment of birth control week as a publicity measure.[44]

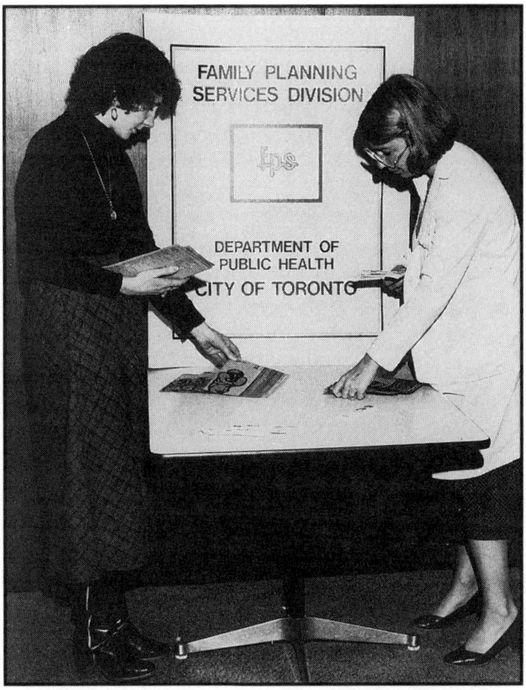

Members of the Family Planning Services Division preparing for an education session in 1980.

Community development required a more subtle form of activity. Each of the eight community workers was expected to assess her district and to develop projects which were appropriate to the citizens' needs. In 1980, for example, the Hillcrest community worker co-ordinated local groups to provide a six week after-school program for teenagers in the Pelham Park Ontario Housing Unit. Called "About Life, About Love", the program, which examined health and healthy relationships, was well received. That same year, the Moss Park worker organized a seven part program on life cycle issues for the Toronto Dominion Bank's employees. These sessions were held twice weekly at lunch hours and attracted over 100 people. And in Riverdale where teen pregnancies were a significant problem, the community worker encouraged local groups to start lobbying the board of health and city politicians for a birth control clinic in the district. The underlying purpose of all this activity was to enable individuals to participate actively in their own health concerns.

Such focused efforts were the basis for making family planning one of the core programs which the Department offered. Indeed, Toronto's expertise in this field was recognized by the Ministry of Health, which used the Family Planning Division staff to organize local and provincial training sessions and professional networks. In addition to its community efforts, the division also worked closely with the Board of Education in developing educational material, suitable first for high school students, and later for public school students. All of these activities demonstrate public acceptance of birth control as a legitimate responsibility for local health agencies. Problems such as teenage pregnancies and the use of abortion as a method of birth control, however, remain to challenge health activists.

Conclusion

Human sexuality and its consequences have always aroused great social tension. So too, have attempts to deal with sexually transmitted diseases and family limitation methods. For Toronto's Health Department, the social purity campaign prior to 1914 highlighted a new area of endeavour, but federal funding and provincial legislation were required before the staff could move into such a potentially controversial area. From 1918 onward, the Department's efforts centred on controlling the disease, and ensuring that case-finding and contact-tracing were done to prevent it from spreading. Community health education, which had become the dominant feature of the nurses' work with women and children, was generally left to voluntary groups, most notably the Canadian Social Hygiene Council and its successor, the Health League of Canada. Dividing responsibilities among local and provincial health departments, and non-governmental organizations, was done in the interests of efficiency and in order to prevent public disapproval from being directed at city staff.

One unforeseen result of this division of duties, however, was the routinization of reform activity. This process was intensified by the use of penicillin and sulpha drugs to treat venereal diseases. Not until these diseases began to spread rapidly among the general population during the 1960s, did local health authorities question the approach which they had been following since the 1920s. By the 1970s, widespread opposition to all forms of authority had compelled the staff to modify their reliance on legal means to achieve their goals, and turned their attention to health promotion. This change coincided with the election of a new generation of community reformers and their appointment to the local board of health. Together these people redefined the Department's educational programs to focus on the problems of the 1980s — genital herpes and AIDS — as well as informing citizens about syphilis and gonorrhea.

The Department's involvement in family planning contrasted sharply with its activities in controlling and preventing venereal diseases. Since providing such information was a criminal offence until 1969, senior administrators from the 1930s to the 1960s did not encourage staff to discuss this matter with clients, until it became socially and politically acceptable to do so. Initially, the Department linked its efforts with those of hospital-based clinics because the medical officer and his deputy believed that birth control information had to be provided by clinicians. This perspective alienated women's groups and led them to create free-standing clinics. During the late 1970s, health promotion activities developed after the Family Planning

Services Division was created to modernize the Department's approach to this contemporary concern.

The evolution of the Department's activities in these two areas illustrates the interplay of federal and provincial funding and policy, the impact of national crises, such as the World Wars and the Depression, and the influence of voluntary groups and philanthropists. It also demonstrates how medical science and health education programs failed to develop a clear cut solution to age old human concerns.

Chapter Eleven

Limits to Prevention: Adult Health Problems

Between 1920 and the present, health workers throughout North America learned that:

> Unfortunately, the causal relationships between behaviour and health are not nearly as clear-cut as they are between 'germs' and disease. Today's illnesses and injuries and the disabilities to which they give rise are the result of numerous interacting factors. This means that prevention is a far more complex undertaking than we may at one time have imagined.[1]

Adult health problems, such as mental illness, alcoholism and drug addiction, showed the limits of existing health education techniques, and the difficulty of separating treatment and prevention. Indeed, the Health Department's efforts in these areas did not fall under provincial health legislation, but rather devolved on the staff as a result of the interest of reformers, like Charles Hastings, in such stigmatized behaviour. Hastings, in turn, derived his concern from the international public health and prohibition movements, which launched an all out attack on drug and alcohol abuse prior to the First World War.

During the hostilities, the large number of troops who succumbed to "shell shock" surprised army officials and assisted in legitimating psychiatry as a medical specialty. Once the war was over, psychiatrists' services were welcomed by people who believed that environmental influences, especially interpersonal relationships, moulded individuals and contributed to their mental health or illness. For local health departments, employing psychologists and psychiatrists was an attempt to enhance the services that they provided, by helping individuals to avoid mental breakdowns. Integrating such activities into the existing structure, however, was difficult because of limited funding during the interwar years, and because there were few experts available and willing to work for a public agency. As a result, much of the work was done by public health nurses, and not surprisingly, focused on children. The rising suicide rate during the Depression and increased committals, however, suggested that Toronto's adults also needed expert advice and guidance.

After the Second World War, psychiatry gained even more prominence because it was linked to drug treatment for various forms of mental illness. As a result, the provincial health department introduced a policy of deinstitutionalization, which had a marked effect on district public health work.

Since many of the recently released patients also had drug and alcohol problems, dealing with them was very time consuming and somewhat frustrating. In contrast to other Ontario cities, Toronto created a corps of mental health nurses to alleviate some of the stress on its staff, but they were quickly overwhelmed by the demand for their services during the 1960s and 1970s. In 1974, the federal government's working document, *A New Perspective on Health for Canadians,* noted that mental illness and mental retardation were still stigmatized in Canadian society, and that they had become leading causes of hospitalization among adults. Moreover, suicide was the fourth leading cause of death among Canadian men and women. What could be done to prevent such suffering and tragedy?

By the 1970s, the advisory and co-ordinating role which the city's mental health directors had developed since the 1950s, did not satisfy the members of the local board of health, former psychiatric patients, and community activists. These people proposed redefining the city's efforts in terms of health advocacy and health promotion. When the city's two largest newspapers ran exposés of the appalling living conditions which former patients endured in 1981, the local board, community agencies, and the mayor, set up a series of task forces to examine social inequality and housing problems. The reports which these projects produced, pinpointed a lack of provincial planning and funding as the culprit. But within the Department, a conflict between traditional public service and primary prevention was brewing. Would advocacy be an effective alternative to the treatment and referral activities which had been the focus of the Mental Health Division's programs? Only time would render a verdict.

Erasing the Stigma: Adult Mental Health

Shame, fear, and loathing have been the dominant attitudes towards people suffering from mental illness during the nineteenth and twentieth centuries. As Ontario's system of mental hospitals slowly evolved, institutionalization for long-term care became the favoured method of dealing with these individuals. In 1918, however, an important step toward public acceptance of mental illness as an illness was taken when Dr. Clarence Hincks established the National Committee for Mental Hygiene. This organization and its successor, the Canadian Mental Health Association, worked to educate Canadians about conditions in mental institutions, to erase the stigma associated with the various mental illnesses, and ultimately, to help former patients rejoin society.[2] With its headquarters in Toronto, the Mental Hygiene Committee developed close links with the Health Department, and provided assistance to the public health nurses who dealt with adult patients.

Prior to the 1950s, however, the Department's work with adults was fairly limited. During the interwar years, individuals suffering from mental problems were assessed by district medical officers and a medical colleague, since two signatures were required for committal to the Ontario Hospital at 999 Queen Street, or to the Toronto Psychiatric Hospital, which had been opened in 1926. The workload increased during the Depression when "the strain of unemployment and financial worries" led to "an increased number of admissions to mental hospitals."[3] In 1931, Toronto recorded 111 suicides, the highest number in its history to that point. In spite of such clear evidence of the need for adult mental health counselling, the Division of Mental Hygiene stressed children's behavioural problems and mental health needs.

This focus reflected the prevailing understanding of Freudian psychology, and suggested some of the limitations of the preventive model. What environmental factors contributed to mental illness? Did all adult psychoses and neuroses originate in childhood as Freud suggested? Or were they a result of the stress of urban life or adult crises? In contrast to its techniques for controlling communicable diseases, or its general health education strategies, Toronto's Department lacked a coherent approach to this problem.

During the Second World War, the Director of Mental Hygiene enlisted, and only a part-time substitute was available because most of Canada's small cadre of psychiatrists served with the armed forces. From 1941–46, Dr. E. P. Lewis, the Director of Mental Hygiene, also served as the part-time Director of the Toronto Psychiatric Hospital. He used both positions to provide clinical material for students from the University of Toronto's Faculty of Medicine. Under Lewis, who became full-time in 1946, the Department developed an emergency treatment and referral service for adults who were suffering from a variety of psychoses and neuroses. This occurred because of growing public and professional acceptance of short-term hospitalization as an effective method of dealing with illness episodes. As a result of his interest in clinical services for adults and children, the Mental Hygiene Division's budget had increased from $18,871 in 1940 to $50,465 in 1950. In view of this shift in emphasis, Jackson began to question both the Division's stress on treatment and its expenditures.[4]

Redefining Mental Health Services

By the 1950s, the work of Freud and his disciples had thoroughly penetrated popular consciousness, and many Americans and Canadians believed that psychiatrists held the key to the mysteries of mental illness.[5] Dr. Lewis's death in December 1949 raised the issue of the Health Department's future role in mental health work. For Jackson, this was an opportunity to rationalize the Division's work, and to change its focus from treatment to assessment and referral. Not only was the latter approach more in keeping with modern public health administrative practices, but it would also enable Jackson to trim the Division's budget and apply the savings to other programs. The medical officer's strong views on the matter ultimately caused a sixteen month controversy which pitted him against his usual allies and the press.

Why had this occurred? In 1950, Jackson argued that a well-trained district medical officer with a diploma in public health could effectively direct the work of the new Division of Mental Health, because he was sceptical about the public's faith in psychiatry which he characterized as a specialty of "doubtful or unproved value." As the chief executive of the Department, the medical officer had also been perturbed that Lewis had run his division as an autonomous unit whose efforts had been devoted almost solely to children. Jackson recommended integrating the activities of this division with those of other staff, by stressing preventive work, in-service training, and assisting district medical officers and nurses with "acute and serious situations in the home." This proposal and the medical officer's justification for it angered Home and School groups, the Toronto Board of Education, and the Women Electors' Association because these organizations believed that only a fully trained psychiatrist could deal with children's mental problems. Not surprisingly, these groups were supported by the Canadian Mental Health Association. Jackson's call for a "broader vision" of preventive mental health work was drowned in a chorus of criticism led by these interest groups, the *Toronto Star* and the *Globe & Mail*.

The controversy raged throughout the fall of 1950 and spilled into January 1951. That month, the Council bowed to public pressure and voted 13 to 8 to reject the compromise which the medical officer, the Board of Control, the local board of health, and the mayor had worked out. Jackson had stood firmly against the tide of public opinion because of the data he had collected from American cities like New York, Milwaukee, Los Angeles, Kansas City, and Detroit — none of which used psychiatrists to direct their mental health work. He also knew that Ontario faced a shortage of trained specialists in this field, and during the job search which he conducted, learned that Toronto's salary and pension benefits did not match those of other levels of government. After this political humiliation, he was relieved when the Board of Education created its own Child Adjustment Centre, and hired its own psychiatrist in June 1951. As a result, some of the Health Department's child psychologists and school nurses moved to the new centre, and the Health Department was now free to reorganize its mental health services.[6]

In April 1951, Dr. Clarence Robinson, who held degrees in psychiatry and public health, became the city's Mental Health Director. He intended to focus on adults and prevention, but almost inevitably, he and his successor provided clinical treatment to emergency cases who were unable to afford medical care or lacked access to it. But as the city was reorganizing during the 1950s, significant external changes began to modify the Health Department's activities. As a result of the Ontario Health Survey's revelations about the shortage of psychiatric clinics in the province, the Ontario government offered national health grant funding to general hospitals for the construction of psychiatric units. In 1949, the Wellesley Hospital opened a 32 bed unit and other Toronto hospitals quickly followed. By providing short-term care, these clinics contributed to the belief that mental illness could be cured through modern medical intervention.

In fact, research into the causes of mental illnesses, and drugs to treat them, had demonstrated that some forms of disease were caused by chemical imbalances which could be corrected through administering specific drugs. The introduction of psychotropic drugs, such as tranquillisers and anti-depressants, enabled clinics and general practitioners to treat and discharge patients rather than committing them. The treatment model strengthened the bond with curative medicine and its institutions. It also called into question the long held view that the environment contributed to mental health problems.[7] Without that foundation for preventive action, the Health Department had to redefine its role.

In 1954, the province amended the Mental Health Act. The new legislation included a clause which permitted the Minister of Health to negotiate with local boards and medical officers regarding the establishment and co-ordination of mental health facilities. Since the province expected interested municipalities to pay one-third of the cost of such facilities, few local health departments accepted the suggestion.[8] In Toronto, the Ontario Hospital had begun to use neuroleptic drugs and to send patients home as quickly as possible. As a result, some districts were swamped by former patients who needed assistance adjusting to their medication, and to their return to the community. The amount of work that assisting these people entailed for the Department's doctors and nurses, limited any interest that they had in taking over existing hospitals or clinics.

Specialization: Developing Mental Health Nursing

By 1958, the Department's senior medical and nursing staff were searching for a more effective way to provide service to the growing numbers of former psychiatric patients. London's Ontario Hospital provided a model, because a decade earlier it had introduced an outreach program in which staff nurses did community follow-up work with former patients. In Toronto, continuing staff shortages had prevented the city's Ontario Hospital from undertaking such a program, and the institution's administrators were pleased when the Health Department proposed a pilot study of such a service. Beginning in the Runnymede, Parkdale, and Hillcrest districts, the project provided pre-admission and post-discharge information about specific patients to the staff at 999 Queen Street. The perceived success of these efforts led the Directors of Mental Health and Public Health Nursing to conclude that they needed a new staff member: the mental health nurse.

Beginning in 1959–60, experienced district nurses were sent to the University of Toronto for a one year training course which focused on mental health issues, and public health administration and supervision.[9] As soon as staff were available, each mental health nurse was assigned to a district office, where she offered immediate support during mental health crises. The nurses continued to do follow-up work for discharged patients and helped with early case-finding, leading to diagnosis and referral. By 1965, Toronto was one of the few cities in Canada with its own corps of mental health nurses; this attracted visitors from across the country for observation and discussion.[10]

In addition to former patients, the mental health nurses also had to adapt to new client groups, including successive waves of immigrants who flooded into the city after 1945. During the 1950s, the Division continued to

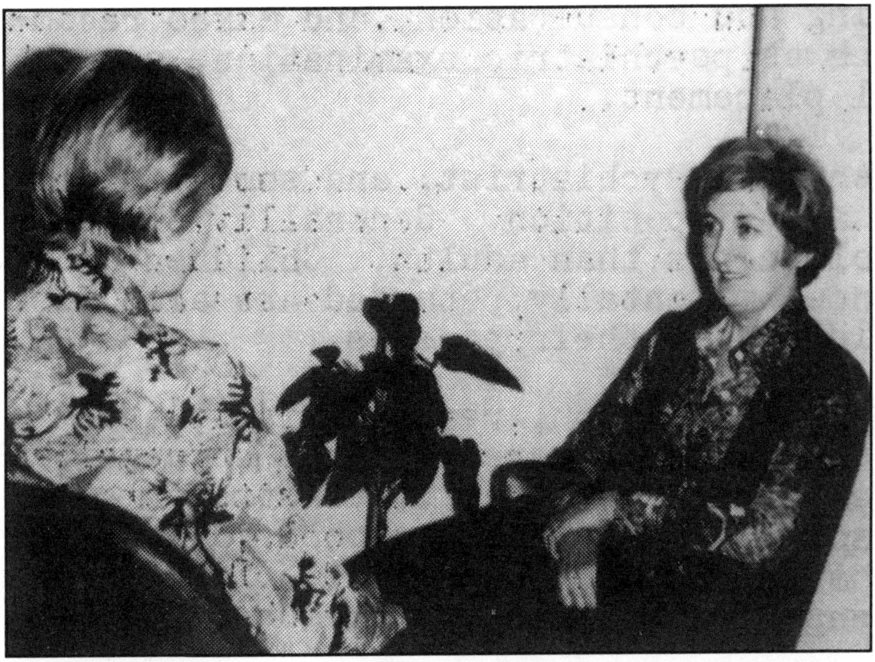

This reproduction from the Annual Statement shows that mental health nurses also visited clients in their homes.

offer psychological testing and assessment for the Separate School Board, and Robinson reported sympathetically on the strains which adjusting to a new culture imposed on immigrant children. Adults from other countries also experienced mental problems. Displaced persons, Holocaust survivors, and refugees, all faced language barriers, the stress of urban life, and the pressure of assimilation. Like native-born Canadians, the stigma associated with mental illness often meant that families closed ranks around the victim and refused to seek help until the situation drastically deteriorated.[11] In spite of Robinson's argument that "mental illness is a sickness to be treated, cured, and not one of which to be ashamed," many immigrant families refused to use psychiatrists because their cultural beliefs prohibited such external intervention. Nevertheless, Toronto Western Hospital opened a comprehensive mental health clinic staffed by district nurses in 1968, and subsequently created a transcultural psychiatric unit for emergency cases from the surrounding Portuguese community. In the late 1970s, the arrival of Vietnamese boat people revealed the psychic trauma of deprivation and torture among refugees once again. In 1980, the Mental Health Division's director served as a member of the Greater Toronto South-East Asian Task Force, which supported the creation of the Hong Fook Centre for Vietnamese and Chinese Torontonians.[12]

Seeking a Role for Prevention

But what about prevention? By the early 1960s, Robinson was discussing the difficulty of applying the three stage preventive model that was becoming the credo of public health administrators to mental health work. In his opinion:

> Unlike the groups of preventable bacterial and viral diseases, there is no sharp dividing line between prevention and treatment in the field of mental health. Most mental illnesses involve somatic, psychological and social factors.[13]

As a result, he called for more statistical data about the number of "mental health admissions; the amount of alcoholism and drug addiction...; the number of suicides; the number of divorces, separations or desertions; the number of convictions...for crimes against person and property" and several other variables.[14] The research which these topics demanded was beyond the Department's capabilities, but the call for such information indicated the broader perspective that was emerging. Indeed, in 1962, in its submission to the Hall Commission on Health Services, the Canadian Public Health Association pointed out how markedly mental health programs had changed, or were changing, as a consequence of deinstitutionalization and medical treatment in hospital clinics. As a result, they argued that "early diagnosis, early treatment and effective rehabilitation" would constitute local health authorities' contribution to improving mental health.

Early in the 1960s, the Ontario government started a "total push" program to encourage long-term patients to leave mental institutions. One unforeseen consequence of this policy was an increase in the number of suicides. In 1965, Metro Toronto's Coroner's Office reported 175 deaths by suicide, in comparison to 120 from automobile accidents. Several staff from the Mental Health Division participated on the Metropolitan Toronto Committee on Suicide Prevention and Crisis-Centred Mental Health Services to analyze this problem. They reported these statistics to the local board of health, and pointed out that approximately 1,500 people, usually young adults aged 15–44, had attempted suicide in spite of the stigma attached to it. As the committee argued, "the suicidal act should not be considered a criminal act, but rather the impulsive action of a person in despair, overwhelmed by adverse circumstances." To help lower the rate, the local board approved the request for training for the nurses to recognize symptoms, and in conjunction with community groups, to offer "a strong supportive service...to check the suicidal impulses harboured by depressed patients."[15]

During the 1960s, the province expanded its policy of deinstitutionalization, in spite of a shaky economy which made rehabilitation and integration difficult. In 1963, Clarence Robinson pointed out that "For optimum mental health, most persons require gainful employment; adequate shelter, food, sleep and recreation; recognition as a contributing member of society; and a philosophy that involves survival."[16] But did Toronto's Health Department have the staff and resources to provide effective aftercare for recently released patients? With the support of the Canadian Mental Health Association, the Salvation Army, and other religious and charitable groups, the mental health nurses tried to serve these needy clients. In 1964, the federal Department of Manpower and Immigration funded Adult Training Centres to assist young men and women in retraining to meet the needs of a changing economy. The Health Department's district nurses arranged physical examinations and discussed the results of psychological tests with the trainees. As they discovered, many of these people were unable to complete the course because of emotional problems, often triggered by family crises. In 1969, George Brown College took over the retraining program, and the Department withdrew from this attempt to deal with adult mental health needs, because the amended Mental Health Act of 1967 no longer contained a clause encouraging co-ordinated community mental health services. Indeed, the province's narrow definition of the role of local health departments in mental health, preventive education, and assessment, further limited the development of after-care services.[17]

By the late 1970s and early 1980s, Ontario's Conservative government was under constant attack by community groups for failing to provide decent housing, retraining courses, and assistance to former patients. Vocal patients' rights groups gained support from community activists and politicians because the problem was intensifying as a result of the provincial decision to close the Lakeshore Psychiatric Hospital. By 1983 nearly 7,000 patients were being released in Metro every six months.[18] Much to the dismay of nearby merchants and homeowners, many of them remained near the Queen Street Mental Health Centre, which had replaced 999 Queen

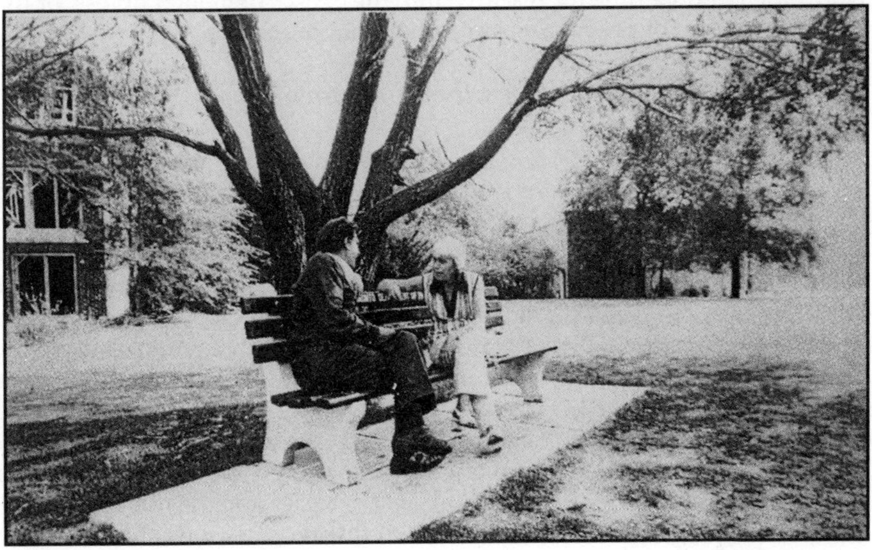

Mental health nurses offered counselling in the environment which made the client most comfortable.

The Mental Health Division has the following responsibilities:

- to provide a preventive and community mental health program, to promote mental hygiene;
- to provide prevention and intervention services to children under five years including those in day nurseries and day care centres;
- to provide nursing services to three special secondary schools and three schools for retarded children;
- to provide information, education, psychological testing and counselling, psychiatric assessment and consultation, and referral service where special treatment is indicated; also for the mentally retarded;
- to provide services through home visits by mental health nurses including after care services for patients discharged from psychiatric hospitals and clinics;
- to provide an Adult Protective Service Worker for rehabilitation of developmentally handicapped persons (the mentally retarded).

The Mental Health Division performed many functions.

Street in 1970. Through this period, Toronto's mental health staff tried to provide personal service to the increasing stream of poor, unemployed, ex-psychiatric patients. Their efforts to help people avoid the "revolving door" syndrome left little time for research into the causes of mental illness, or for the development of preventive or promotional programs.

From Service to Advocacy

The Mental Health Division's reliance on "counselling, assessment, referral and treatment" were criticized by the Health Planning Steering Committee. As a proponent of primary prevention, the committee concluded that preventing mental illness was one of the most difficult problems facing health workers. In their opinion, neither the social variables which contributed to the disease nor the physiological and chemical imbalances which triggered certain forms of it were adequately understood. In spite of agreeing that medical and social scientists were still uncovering the root causes of many forms of the disease, the Steering Committee recommended eliminating the Department's treatment and service activity. It also argued in favour of geographically limited studies of high risk groups, and the development of behaviour modification strategies for over-stressed residents. In keeping with its growing interest in advocacy, the committee also suggested that the Mental Health staff study "the inadequacies and unmet needs" of the current system, and then lobby the provincial government to fulfil its responsibilities.[19] This set the stage for conflict between the old and new views of preventive activity.

In 1981, a study team from the Health Advocacy Unit prepared a epidemiologic study of suicides in the city for the local board of health. Although the members discovered that suicide rates had not increased markedly since 1970, their data demonstrated that low income districts, such as Moss Park, Parkdale, Hillcrest and Runnymede, had higher rates than North Toronto. Since previous research had indicated that parasuicide remained a significant drain on local hospital emergency rooms and psychiatric clinics, the Advocacy Unit's researchers recommended better liaison between clinical facilities and the Department, and collecting further data on suicide attempts. In contrast to their predecessors, who relied on personal contact and group education sessions to prevent suicide, the HAU team called for primary prevention through gun control laws, restrictions of prescriptions, modifications in drug packaging, and social programs for families.[20] Since these broad-ranging suggestions were beyond the Department's jurisdiction, staff in the new health areas developed their own programs after decentralization was completed. In 1983, the Western Health Area, which included the former Parkdale and Runnymede districts, introduced weekly discussion groups on self-esteem and group dynamics for

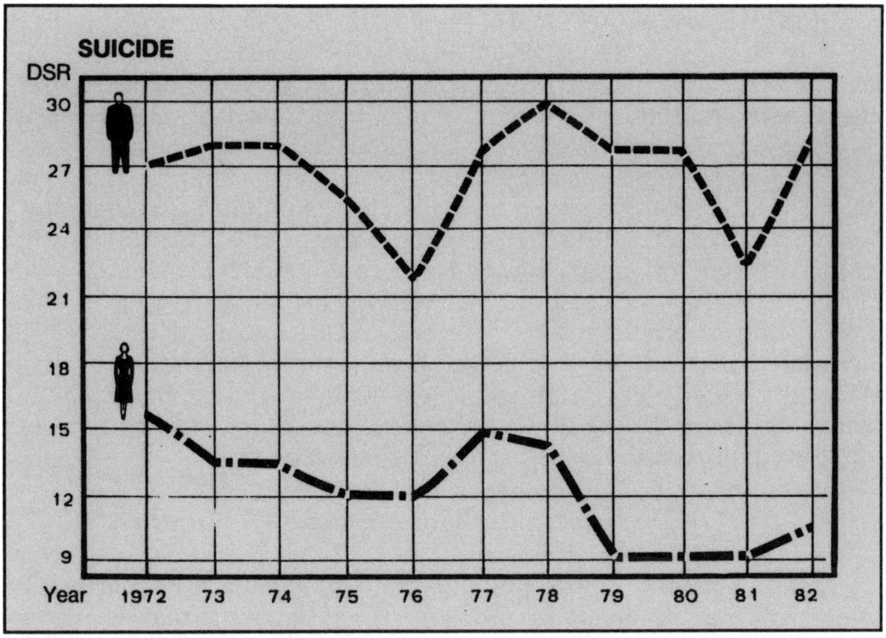

As part of their efforts to modernize the Department's epidemiological capacity, the staff statisticians evaluated the city's health status to determine the leading causes of mortality. As this retrospective table based on directly standardized rates (DSR) demonstrates, suicide was a leading cause of male mortality during the 1970s.

people recovering from mental illness. This type of primary prevention reflected contemporary theories about community service, and marked the end of the Department's reliance on treatment.

"The National Curse of Habit-Forming Drugs": Lifestyle Issues

By 1900, Toronto had earned its reputation as a bastion of Victorian morality. Clergymen and women's groups, such as the Women's Christian Temperance Union, directed the Canadian counterpart of the American crusades against alcohol and narcotics. The concerns that these groups expressed led the local board of health to discuss the dangers of patent medicines which contained opium, morphine or alcohol, but there was little that local governments could do. As a result, the National Council of Women and the WCTU pressured the Laurier government to stop the drug traffic and to control the prescription of narcotic drugs, because they argued that using drugs led to crime and prostitution. In 1908, the Canadian government passed its Narcotic Drugs Act. This was the opening round in an unending struggle to control drug use and addiction. Prior to 1914, similar arguments had little effect in ensuring the prohibition of alcohol because public sentiment did not support the measure.

In 1915, Hastings used the February *Health Bulletin* to launch his campaign against alcohol. Using arguments from both medical science and the prohibitionists, the medical officer stated that excessive drinking contributed to organic diseases, lowered resistance to pneumonia and tuberculosis, predisposed individuals to criminal behaviour, and led to mental illness and hospitalization. From his vantage point, the role of the public health administrator was to publicize this social evil and to gain public approval for its limitation. In October 1915, he was able to report to his readers that his efforts had been duplicated elsewhere in North America. To convince Torontonians of the dangers of drink, he stressed the social consequences of poverty and ill health, and cited British and Australian statistics which indicated that abstainers lived longer, healthier lives than heavy drinkers. Hastings's rhetoric was typical of the war years, and he and other prohibition advocates were pleased when the provincial and federal governments introduced the measure in 1916–17.

From Prohibition to Government Monopoly

Unfortunately, complete prohibition of the manufacture and sale of alcohol did not eliminate the problem. The progressive reformers were shocked and disillusioned when public opposition to the measure resulted in lawlessness and violence. Bootleggers and their supporters defied the police, while veterans fumed at the narrow-minded attitudes which prevented them from having a drink. By the mid–1920s, the western provinces opted for government controlled sale of liquor and beer in an effort to end the controversy. The provincial government followed their lead in 1927, when it created the Liquor Licensing Board of Ontario. To limit the political fallout from creating this government monopoly, the politicians continued to allow local option. Toronto became a patchwork of wet and dry areas as local residents voted on the matter.

The social stigma also lingered. Prior to entering a liquor store to buy their monthly allotment, Ontarians were legally obliged to purchase permits which cost $2.00. The permit had to be renewed annually until the system ended in 1961 and enabled the purchaser to buy a limited quantity only. As well, the hours of operation for taverns and pubs were restricted to discourage excessive consumption. Social convention dictated that women did not drink and the continuing influence of the prohibition movement affected many men as well.

Nevertheless, alcohol consumption rose, and by 1929, the members of the Ontario Medical Association's Mental Hygiene committee were arguing in favour of a separate institution to treat drug addicts and alcoholics. Under Ontario's Mental Health Act, these individuals could voluntarily admit themselves to the province's mental hospitals for treatment or be admitted for two weeks on a court order. Few addicts availed themselves of the

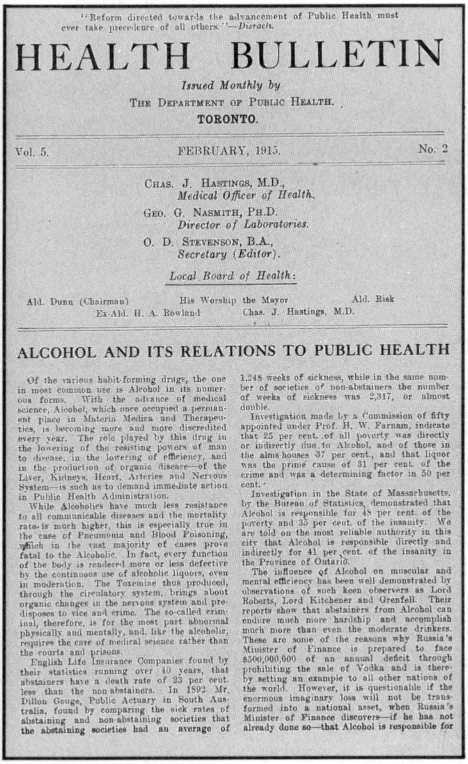

"Reform directed towards the advancement of Public Health must ever take precedence of all others."—*Disraeli.*

HEALTH BULLETIN

Issued Monthly by
THE DEPARTMENT OF PUBLIC HEALTH.
TORONTO.

Vol. 5. FEBRUARY, 1915. No. 2

CHAS. J. HASTINGS, M.D.,
Medical Officer of Health.
GEO. G. NASMITH, PH.D.
Director of Laboratories.
O. D. STEVENSON, B.A.,
Secretary (Editor).

Local Board of Health:

Ald. Dunn (Chairman) His Worship the Mayor Ald. Risk
Ex-Ald. H. A. Rowland Chas. J. Hastings, M.D.

ALCOHOL AND ITS RELATIONS TO PUBLIC HEALTH

Of the various habit-forming drugs, the one in most common use is Alcohol in its numerous forms. With the advance of medical science, Alcohol, which once occupied a permanent place in Materia Medica and Therapeutics, is becoming more and more discredited every year. The role played by this drug in the lowering of the resisting powers of man to disease, in the lowering of efficiency, and in the production of organic disease—of the Liver, Kidneys, Heart, Arteries and Nervous System—is such as to demand immediate action in Public Health Administration.

While Alcoholics have much less resistance to all communicable diseases and the mortality rate is much higher, this is especially true in the case of Pneumonia and Blood Poisoning, which in the vast majority of cases prove fatal to the Alcoholic. In fact, every function of the body is rendered more or less defective by the continuous use of alcoholic liquors, even in moderation. The Toxemiae thus produced, through the circulatory system, brings about organic changes in the nervous system and predisposes to vice and crime. The so-called criminal, therefore, is for the most part abnormal physically and mentally, and, like the alcoholic, requires the care of medical science rather than the courts and prisons.

English Life Insurance Companies found by their statistics running over 40 years, that abstainers have a death rate of 23 per cent. less than the non-abstainers. In 1892 Mr. Dillon Gouge, Public Actuary in South Australia, found by comparing the sick rates of abstaining and non-abstaining societies that the abstaining societies had an average of 1,248 weeks of sickness, while in the same number of societies of non-abstainers the number of weeks of sickness was 2,347, or almost double.

Investigation made by a Commission of fifty appointed under Prof. H. W. Farnam, indicate that 25 per cent. of all poverty was directly or indirectly due to Alcohol, and of those in the alms-houses 37 per cent., and that liquor was the prime cause of 31 per cent. of the crime and was a determining factor in 50 per cent.

Investigation in the State of Massachusetts, by the Bureau of Statistics, demonstrated that Alcohol is responsible for 48 per cent. of the poverty and 35 per cent. of the insanity. We are told on the most reliable authority in this city that Alcohol is responsible directly and indirectly for 41 per cent. of the insanity in the Province of Ontario.

The influence of Alcohol on muscular and mental efficiency has been well demonstrated by observations of such keen observers as Lord Roberts, Lord Kitchener and Grenfell. Their reports show that abstainers from Alcohol can endure much more hardship and accomplish much more than even the moderate drinkers. These are some of the reasons why Russia's Minister of Finance is prepared to face $500,000,000 of an annual deficit through prohibiting the sale of Vodka and is thereby setting an example to all other nations of the world. However, it is questionable if the enormous imaginary loss will not be transformed into a national asset, when Russia's Minister of Finance discovers—if he has not already done so—that Alcohol is responsible for

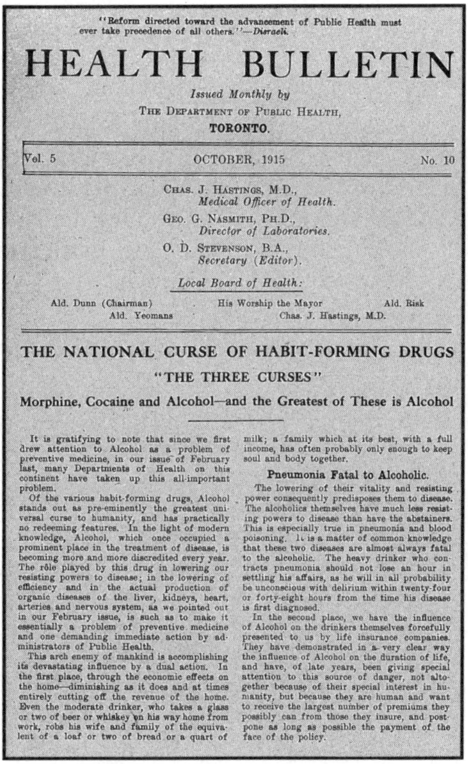

"Reform directed toward the advancement of Public Health must ever take precedence of all others."—*Disraeli.*

HEALTH BULLETIN

Issued Monthly by
THE DEPARTMENT OF PUBLIC HEALTH,
TORONTO.

Vol. 5 OCTOBER, 1915 No. 10

CHAS. J. HASTINGS, M.D.,
Medical Officer of Health.
GEO. G. NASMITH, PH.D.,
Director of Laboratories.
O. D. STEVENSON, B.A.,
Secretary (Editor).

Local Board of Health:

Ald. Dunn (Chairman) His Worship the Mayor Ald. Risk
Ald. Yeomans Chas. J. Hastings, M.D.

THE NATIONAL CURSE OF HABIT-FORMING DRUGS

"THE THREE CURSES"

Morphine, Cocaine and Alcohol—and the Greatest of These is Alcohol

It is gratifying to note that since we first drew attention to Alcohol as a problem of preventive medicine, in our issue of February last, many Departments of Health on this continent have taken up this all-important problem.

Of the various habit-forming drugs, Alcohol stands out as pre-eminently the greatest universal curse to humanity, and has practically no redeeming features. In the light of modern knowledge, Alcohol, which once occupied a prominent place in the treatment of disease, is becoming more and more discredited every year. The rôle played by this drug in lowering our resisting powers to disease; in the lowering of efficiency and in the actual production of organic diseases of the liver, kidneys, heart, arteries and nervous system, as we pointed out in our February issue, is such as to make it essentially a problem of preventive medicine and one demanding immediate action by administrators of Public Health.

This arch enemy of mankind is accomplishing its devastating influence by a dual action. In the first place, through the economic effects on the home—diminishing as it does and at times entirely cutting off the revenue of the home. Even the moderate drinker, who takes a glass or two of beer or whiskey on his way home from work, robs his wife and family of the equivalent of a loaf or two of bread or a quart of milk; a family which at its best, with a full income, has often probably only enough to keep soul and body together.

Pneumonia Fatal to Alcoholic.

The lowering of their vitality and resisting power consequently predisposes them to disease. The alcoholics themselves have much less resisting powers to disease than have the abstainers. This is especially true in pneumonia and blood poisoning. It is a matter of common knowledge that these two diseases are almost always fatal to the alcoholic. The heavy drinker who contracts pneumonia should not lose an hour in settling his affairs, as he will in all probability be unconscious with delirium within twenty-four or forty-eight hours from the time his disease is first diagnosed.

In the second place, we have the influence of Alcohol on the drinkers themselves forcefully presented to us by life insurance companies. They have demonstrated in a very clear way the influence of Alcohol on the duration of life, and have, of late years, been giving special attention to this source of danger, not altogether because of their special interest in humanity, but because they are human and want to receive the largest number of premiums they possibly can from those they insure, and postpone as long as possible the payment of the face of the policy.

Charles Hastings launched the Department's war on alcohol and other drugs in February and October 1915.

opportunity, because the wealthy could go to private hospitals while many of the poor, like Mabel Trilling in the novel *Cabbagetown*, refused to accept the stigma associated with mental facilities, failed to get treatment and died.

Growing public concern about alcohol-related illness among Canadian soldiers during World War Two led the Ontario government to create the Alcohol Research Foundation in 1949. Initially, the LLBO sponsored a treatment centre for alcoholics, but the emphasis soon shifted to research.[21] Using profits from the sale of the product, the government-sponsored researchers studied many of the physiological characteristics of the dependency, and tested the effectiveness of newly developed drugs like antabuse. Outside government agencies, Alcoholics Anonymous and other self-help groups flourished after 1950. Using a mixture of Christian rhetoric and concepts drawn from the behavioural sciences, these groups provided a non-judgmental atmosphere which enabled many people to learn to control their addictions. They also contributed to lifting the stigma of alcoholism, and to informing the public about the signs and symptoms of alcohol abuse.

With the arrival of large numbers of European immigrants after 1945, many of the restrictions on alcohol use were gradually lifted in response to the new, cosmopolitan, multicultural society that was emerging. Underpinning these changes was the rapid growth of the liquor industry. To maintain their share of the profits, large corporations spent extensive sums on advertising their products. Most of these ads portrayed alcohol use within the context of a sophisticated lifestyle. Such social manipulation was one target of the health advocates who produced *Public Health in the 1980's*. Their successors in the Health Advocacy Unit were even stronger in their condemnation of the substance which they argued was a major cause of illness, traffic accidents, and interpersonal violence. Although these activists were challenging an accepted form of relaxation, their criticisms contributed to the demand for increasing restrictions on lifestyle advertising and a gradual change in public attitudes.

Government Services: Regulation or Health Promotion?

The human cost of alcohol dependency was especially evident to the public health nurses who worked in Moss Park and other less affluent areas. But what role were they to play in combating its use during the 1960s and 1970s, as the drinking age was lowered from 21 to 18 and the regulations governing licensed premises' hours of operation were altered? As one former supervisor noted, the nurses looked the other way during the 1950s because there was so little that they could do to assist alcoholics. Two decades later, alcohol consumption had spread to elementary school children, and the Department was hard pressed to develop education programs to meet this new aspect of the problem.

In *A New Perspective on Health for Canadians*, federal researchers argued in favour of health promotion to supplement regulatory strategies, and called for further research and more efficient training programs for counsellors. They also noted that alcohol addiction was a self-imposed risk that had dire consequences for its victims. According to federal morbidity and mortality statistics, individual alcoholics were more susceptible to cirrhosis of the liver, encephalopathy, and malnutrition, than non-drinkers, and the social use of this beverage contributed to automobile accidents and obesity. Furthermore, 7% of the population purchased nearly 40% of the alcohol sold in Canada, 25% of male admissions to psychiatric facilities occurred because of alcohol use, and absent alcohol abusers cost their employers a million dollars a day in lost productivity.[22] Such a multi-faceted problem demanded a multi-pronged response.

The Ontario government had a contradictory approach to the issue. On the one hand, provincial treasurers raised tax revenue from the sale of alcoholic beverages and used the money to fund the province's economic expansion. On the other hand, the Ontario Health Department mounted a series of educational campaigns during the 1970s, using the resources of the recently renamed Addiction Research Foundation.[23] But at the same time that one section of the provincial health department was pursuing this activity, the Mental Health Branch was adding to the problem by releasing hundreds of psychiatric patients, many of whom were addicted to alcohol and drugs. For Toronto's district and mental health nurses, the needs of these clients became enmeshed in the growing critique of government activity and the demand for detoxification centres.

As an occupational therapist for the Queen Street Mental Health Centre, Anne Johnston saw the inefficiency of the system, and with the support of community groups and potential users, organized one of the first detoxification centres in the city. At the beginning of her campaign, she approached the local board of health only to be told that this was a task for the Social Services Department. When the latter informed her that it was a health matter, she became determined to make Toronto's Health Department and its provincial counterpart responsive to citizens' requests. From her perspective, achieving this objective required active participation in municipal politics, and shifting the Health Department's activities away from established programs and on to contemporary issues.[24]

As proponents of a move from controlling alcohol abuse to preventing addiction, both the federal and municipal health promoters criticized the "blame the victim" syndrome, which they argued, still existed in the public mind. In addition to condemning advertisers, the new reformers surveyed teenagers about their alcohol and drug use, mounted public campaigns against drinking and driving, and tried to develop effective educational programs to persuade adults to lower their consumption levels. The baby boom generation's stress on physical fitness and personal health coincided with these government programs, and there has been a steady decline in the amount of alcohol drunk by the majority of the population during the last ten years.

But the issue of compliance still challenges the success of health promotion activities. What factors affect an individual's decision to start or stop drinking? Peer pressure? Family circumstances? Or work-related stress? Health professionals are only now taking these factors into consideration when planning behaviour modification strategies.[25] And to further complicate the matter, the Health Department's own 1983 report, *An Unequal Society: A Challenge to Public Health,* pointed out that alcoholism was a disease of both affluence and poverty, but that the poor faced greater health risks such as "unemployment, malnutrition and 'bottoming out,'" than did their wealthier counterparts. As it did in the late nineteenth century, this complex issue continues to demand attention from public health staff, community groups and other levels of government.

Battling Drug Addiction

Since 1930, public health workers' initial optimism that drug use could be controlled or eradicated has faded. Charles Hastings sounded the alarm on this issue as well. In 1914, 1915, and 1923, he used the *Health Bulletin* to warn his fellow citizens that they wasted thousands of dollars on potentially addictive patent medicines every year. He also criticized doctors who overprescribed morphine or other addictive drugs. In 1923, he offered a short history of Canada's drug legislation, and argued that modern living, with its combination of monotony and stress, was the cause of much of the problem. He also urged people to recognize addiction as an illness and to hospitalize victims rather than jailing them. He saved his most severe criticisms for drug pushers who lured young men into addiction by providing them with "pleasure powder" or "snow" (a combination of cocaine and boracic acid) in the city's ballrooms. For pushers, he wanted jail with hard labour and the lash.[26]

In 1923, Dr. A.K. Haywood, the superintendent of Montreal General Hospital, also painted a lurid picture of the drug trade in his city. Like many of his contemporaries, he was scandalized by what he saw as the direct connection between drug use and crime. He told his audience about New York City's extensive problem, and about its unsuccessful attempt to introduce an "ambulatory or slow reduction cure" rather than the "sudden withdrawal method." The New York clinic had become a haven for drug sellers, and no cures were recorded using the former method, whereas some were accomplished through careful supervision of the latter method.[27] For Hastings and Haywood, the important question was the one asked by Professor Dixon of Britain's Royal College of Surgeons: "Can we control character, convert weakness into strength, so that temptation will disappear?"[28] Self-control and willpower were seen as the way to eliminate both alcoholism and drug addiction by the early twentieth century reformers. These beliefs conditioned the public to see drug use as a criminal activity and contributed to the marginalization of its victims.

Social Change and the Drug Problem

Toronto evidently had some narcotics problems. In 1930, Gordon Jackson told the Academy of Medicine that the city laboratory analyzed suspected narcotics samples and reported its findings to the Police Department. This service was not the beginning of a program to assist drug users because there was little public understanding or sympathy for the problem. By the end of the 1950s, Clarence Robinson was complaining about the lack of treatment facilities for drug users, but the real crisis came in the 1960s. Timothy Leary's quip about "turning on, tuning in and dropping out" justified experimental drug use for many young people. Hallucinogenic substances, marijuana, and eventually hard drugs like heroin and cocaine, caused intense public concern, as parents, politicians and the police struggled to deal with the recreational use of illegal drugs. The Department's mental health staff were called to hospital emergency wards to "talk down" kids on bad trips. They were also assigned to community groups trying to cope with the annual influx of young travellers, many of whom were heading for Rochdale College, which had acquired a reputation as Canada's equivalent to San Francisco's Haight-Ashbury district. The Rochdale Free Clinic also treated people suffering from overdoses since most drug users distrusted medical authorities.[29]

Similar developments occurred in Edmonton. In Alberta's capital, the local board of health decided to co-ordinate the activities of the 47 agencies providing service to drug users. Like their Toronto counterparts, the staff of Edmonton's Mental Health Division linked their efforts to treatment facilities by providing assessment and referral. They also assisted the city's young people in forming a youth-oriented drug crisis centre, but it disappeared in January 1972, as a result of lack of funding. And to round out its efforts, the board of health asked the city's news media to stop "glamourizing" drug use.[30]

In 1969, the Trudeau government appointed a Royal Commission on the non-medical use of drugs. Over the next four years, the LeDain Commission conducted surveys and prepared annual reports. It ultimately called for the legalization of marijuana, but the public outcry demonstrated that the stigma against drug use still existed. Toronto's Mental Health Division also contributed to the discussion by producing a report on the topic for the local board of health in 1970. Ten years later it prepared an update on marijuana use. In both instances, the researchers concluded that there was no simple solution to the problem.

The reports' authors concluded that drug use among teenagers and young adults represented a form of rebellion against parental and social values. Since the Mental Health Division's staff was so busy providing clinical service during the 1960s and 1970s, studies of the extent and severity of the problem, and the initial educational activities were undertaken by the Addiction Research Foundation and the Council on Drug Abuse, a community and business-based voluntary group. The school nurses used the educational material which these groups produced for counselling high school students, but by the late 1970s an increasing number of dropouts became high risk candidates for drug addiction as they clustered on the infamous Yonge Street strip. The formal system which the Department had in place did not reach the "street kids." Traditional strategies had to be rethought, and in the early 1980s, the Department began to hire street workers to take the preventive message to those who needed it most.

The authors of *Public Health in the 1980's* identified other groups who were suffering from drug dependency: women and the elderly. During the 1950s, valium had been developed to tranquillize mentally ill individuals, and when its use spread into the wider community, it was routinely prescribed to women diagnosed as suffering from stress. Like sleeping pills and other non-prescription drugs, valium can be addictive unless its use is carefully monitored by the patient and the physician. Seniors were even more at risk, given their deteriorating health and the unpredictable side effects of mixing various drugs. To aid these people, the Steering Committee recommended encouraging doctors to change their prescribing practices and to suggest referrals to public health nurses or other social agencies, rather than drugs, to help the elderly with their problems. The committee also called for more public education and information about the effects of drugs on seniors. And it concluded by arguing in favour of the creation of special behaviour modification groups to aid people in overcoming alcohol and substance abuse.

With its stress on advocacy, the Steering Committee was also attempting to take the Department in new directions. After the implementation of decentralization, focused efforts of this kind became possible. In 1983, the staff of the Downtown Health Area carried out community organizing with the Portuguese Inter-agency Network on alcohol and drug abuse, while the Western Health Area held sessions on the same topics in local halfway houses.[31] Health promotion, not just care or regulatory activities, had now become the focus of the Department's efforts to deal with these "hard-core" problems.

Conclusion

Since Charles Hastings staked a claim to involvement in stigmatized social issues such as mental illness, alcoholism, and drug addiction during the 1910s, the services and programs which the Health Department has provided have developed in response to changes in federal and provincial legislation and funding, and in response to public opinion. Indeed, until the 1950s, the Department concentrated on establishing its disease control procedures and health education for women and children. But as communicable diseases were replaced as the leading causes of death by chronic diseases, suicide, accidents, and rising morbidity and mortality from self-imposed health risks, the staff had to redefine their approach to mental illness, mental retardation, and substance abuse.

The Mental Health Division was the focal point for the Department's activities. Although its directors shared their colleagues' commitment to prevention, they were drawn into offering treatment and aftercare as a consequence of provincial mental health policies. The situation was compounded by the growing use of recreational drugs in the 1960s and by the arrival of refugees in the 1970s. Underlying all of these changes, however, was continuing conflict between experts who argued that mental illness could be prevented, and those who believed that such diseases had biochemical origins and hence responded only to treatment. Without a straightforward causal explanation, developing educational activities was difficult.

Similar problems beset efforts to deal with substance abuse. Although alcohol use became respectable during the post-war years, drug use remained illegal. The high cost of caring for victims of these problems led federal, provincial and local health authorities to create educational programs and treatment centres. But like the battle against sexually transmitted diseases, the war on substance abuse illustrated the limits of prevention. As a result, the younger generation of health activists argued in favour of reorienting the Division's work culture and focusing on health promotion. This prepared the way for a renewed attack on these challenging problems.

Chapter Twelve

Contemporary Community Concerns: Chronic Diseases and Senior Citizens

"The pendulum of public health effort must eventually swing again in the direction of the adult."[1] When he made this statement in 1934, Gordon Jackson was alerting the local board of health to the demands of contemporary health issues. As the mortality rate from communicable diseases declined, new chronic health threats emerged. Heart disease and cancer quickly acquired the same stigma that tuberculosis once possessed. Since these ailments afflicted middle aged and elderly citizens, they prompted a reassessment of the Department's focus on younger age groups. Dealing with chronic diseases also raised significant questions about the Department's leadership role in the crusade for good health. What strategies would be most effective against these chronic diseases? Should the Department offer treatment facilities, co-ordinate the activities of other parts of the health care system, or stress early detection by using literature prepared by voluntary groups to educate older Torontonians?

Using the Canadian Tuberculosis Association as a model, concerned doctors and their supporters formed the Canadian Cancer Society in 1938, and the Ontario Heart Foundation in 1950. All these voluntary organizations publicized specific chronic health problems, and used fund raising campaigns to generate revenue for medical research and health education material. As John Burnham has argued, this single issue focus fragmented people's perceptions of their bodies as an organic whole, and in conjunction with surgical advances, made them less willing to listen to public health activists who argued in favour of a systematic approach to health maintenance.[2]

From the 1920s to the present, the stress on medical cures has also undercut public interest in prevention. Was there any longer a clear distinction between preventive and curative medicine? In 1929 as his final message to Torontonians, Hastings argued that "Our duty is to turn to practical account the knowledge that has been revealed by those engaged in research, and to present this knowledge to the public in a way that they can properly understand."[3] For his successors, the Department's role in fighting chronic diseases entailed participation in medical and epidemiological research, coordinating educational campaigns with specific voluntary groups, and providing counselling, assessment, and referral for adults who suspected that they had chronic illnesses.

After 1945, the Department pursued this approach vigorously. The federal government's national health grants provided funding for basic and applied research in both curative and preventive techniques for controlling chronic diseases. The province also continued to expand its support for cancer treatment and research. By supporting hospital construction, both levels of government ensured that facilities were available to provide surgical intervention for heart disease victims. During the 1950s and 1960s, the protracted discussions concerning a national health insurance system also affected health departments, because some, like Toronto's, developed services for seniors that became redundant when all Canadians were able to seek private care. Indeed, the propensity of local departments to tackle new programs without assessing their place in the overall administrative structure came under fire from the Canadian Public Health Association in its brief to the Royal Commission on Health Services. The members who prepared the association's submission recommended long-range planning encompassing all components of Canada's health care system. They were ignored in favour of an emphasis on fee-for-service medicine and high tech curative intervention. By the early 1970s, the rising costs of this approach and the galloping inflation of that decade, compelled governments to look at prevention and health education as an alternative to ever more expensive curative services.

By the 1970s, younger staff who had been trained to think in terms of health promotion and behaviour modification strategies were criticizing the Department's approach to chronic diseases and the needs of healthy seniors. From their perspective, the Department's work culture with its hierarchical lines of authority and medical focus, prohibited the type of social activism that contemporary health issues required. Outside the Department, community groups were forming to attack long-standing social disparities, gender roles, and complacent bureaucracies. The clash of worldviews between professional experts and younger activists led to significant changes in the Department's health education techniques for adults and was a factor in the demand to decentralize to meet community needs.

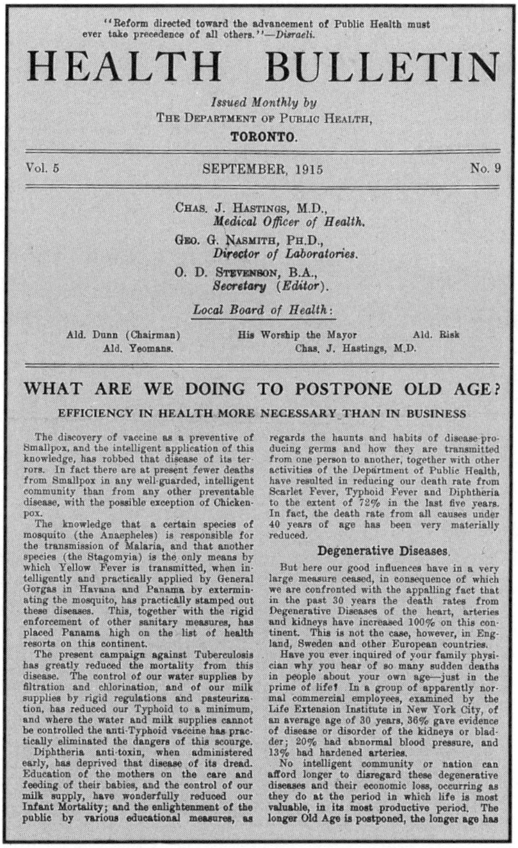

"Reform directed toward the advancement of Public Health must ever take precedence of all others."—*Disraeli.*

HEALTH BULLETIN

Issued Monthly by
THE DEPARTMENT OF PUBLIC HEALTH,
TORONTO.

Vol. 5 SEPTEMBER, 1915 No. 9

CHAS. J. HASTINGS, M.D.,
Medical Officer of Health.
GEO. G. NASMITH, PH.D.,
Director of Laboratories.
O. D. STEVENSON, B.A.,
Secretary (Editor).

Local Board of Health:

Ald. Dunn (Chairman) His Worship the Mayor Ald. Risk
Ald. Yeomans. Chas. J. Hastings, M.D.

WHAT ARE WE DOING TO POSTPONE OLD AGE?

EFFICIENCY IN HEALTH MORE NECESSARY THAN IN BUSINESS

The discovery of vaccine as a preventive of Smallpox, and the intelligent application of this knowledge, has robbed that disease of its terrors. In fact there are at present fewer deaths from Smallpox in any well-guarded, intelligent community than from any other preventable disease, with the possible exception of Chickenpox.

The knowledge that a certain species of mosquito (the Anaepheles) is responsible for the transmission of Malaria, and that another species (the Stagomyia) is the only means by which Yellow Fever is transmitted, when intelligently and practically applied by General Gorgas in Havana and Panama by exterminating the mosquito, has practically stamped out these diseases. This, together with the rigid enforcement of other sanitary measures, has placed Panama high on the list of health resorts on this continent.

The present campaign against Tuberculosis has greatly reduced the mortality from this disease. The control of our water supplies by filtration and chlorination, and of our milk supplies by rigid regulations and pasteurization, has reduced our Typhoid to a minimum, and where the water and milk supplies cannot be controlled the anti-Typhoid vaccine has practically eliminated the dangers of this scourge.

Diphtheria anti-toxin, when administered early, has deprived that disease of its dread. Education of the mothers on the care and feeding of their babies, and the control of our milk supply, have wonderfully reduced our Infant Mortality; and the enlightenment of the public by various educational measures, as regards the haunts and habits of disease-producing germs and how they are transmitted from one person to another, together with other activities of the Department of Public Health, have resulted in reducing our death rate from Scarlet Fever, Typhoid Fever and Diphtheria to the extent of 72% in the last five years. In fact, the death rate from all causes under 40 years of age has been very materially reduced.

Degenerative Diseases.

But here our good influences have in a very large measure ceased, in consequence of which we are confronted with the appalling fact that in the past 30 years the death rates from Degenerative Diseases of the heart, arteries and kidneys have increased 100% on this continent. This is not the case, however, in England, Sweden and other European countries.

Have you ever inquired of your family physician why you hear of so many sudden deaths in people about your own age—just in the prime of life? In a group of apparently normal commercial employees, examined by the Life Extension Institute in New York City, of an average age of 30 years, 36% gave evidence of disease or disorder of the kidneys or bladder; 20% had abnormal blood pressure, and 13% had hardened arteries.

No intelligent community or nation can afford longer to disregard these degenerative diseases and their economic loss, occurring as they do at the period in which life is most valuable, in its most productive period. The longer Old Age is postponed, the longer age has

Charles Hastings alerted Torontonians to the value of periodic physical examinations in 1915.

Fighting Chronic Diseases

"What Can We Do to Extend the Life Line?" When he asked this question in 1920, Hastings was reflecting on nearly a decade of efforts to educate Torontonians about their new enemies: heart disease and cancer. As he and his American contemporaries in the Massachusetts Health Department and the American Society for the Control of Cancer were aware, fear of cancer as a death sentence was widespread in both countries. Heart disease aroused similar fatalism as it became the leading killer of adults over forty. The fear and misunderstanding surrounding these diseases challenged health departments to develop educational material and to publicize preventive measures. They were aided in this work by voluntary organizations and the health education divisions of the federal and provincial health departments. But as the death rates from communicable diseases declined, those from chronic ailments rose, and the public seemed to ignore the common sense advice that Hastings and his successors offered in the *Health Bulletin*.

Throughout the 1920s, Hastings stressed the importance of annual physical examinations to aid in early detection of heart problems and cancer. The push for periodic health examinations was supported by Toronto's Academy of Medicine, but it, like similar American efforts, failed to produce many results because neither doctors nor their patients fully accepted the concept. In contrast to Massachusetts, which established diagnostic clinics for cancer in 1919, the Ontario government moved slowly into this area. Not until 1931 were radio-therapy institutes opened to provide treatment in hospitals in Toronto, London, Kingston and Ottawa. To educate the public, the province's Chief Medical Officer, J.W.S. McCullough, gave nearly 200 speeches on the subject between 1932 and 1934 while his department distributed approximately 100,000 pamphlets

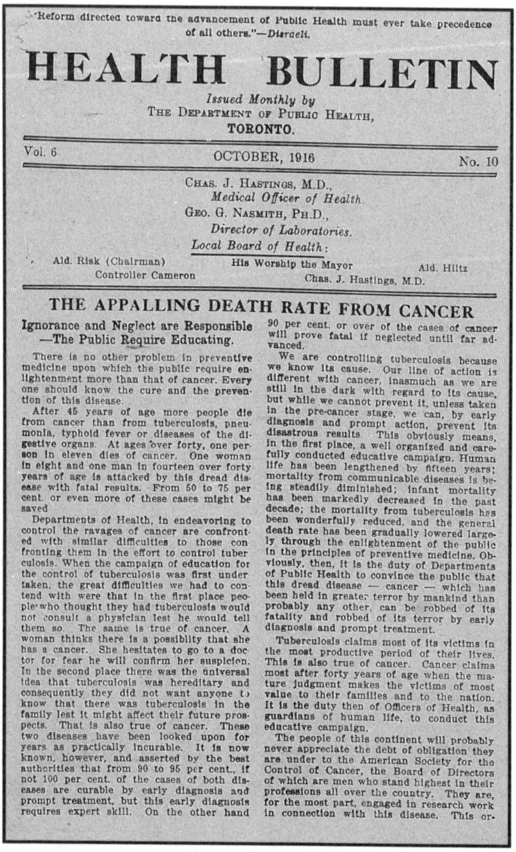

"Reform directed toward the advancement of Public Health must ever take precedence of all others."—*Disraeli.*

HEALTH BULLETIN

Issued Monthly by
THE DEPARTMENT OF PUBLIC HEALTH,
TORONTO.

Vol. 6 OCTOBER, 1916 No. 10

CHAS. J. HASTINGS, M.D.,
Medical Officer of Health.
GEO. G. NASMITH, PH.D.,
Director of Laboratories.
Local Board of Health:
Ald. Risk (Chairman) His Worship the Mayor Ald. Hiltz
Controller Cameron Chas. J. Hastings, M.D.

THE APPALLING DEATH RATE FROM CANCER

Ignorance and Neglect are Responsible —The Public Require Educating.

There is no other problem in preventive medicine upon which the public require enlightenment more than that of cancer. Every one should know the cure and the prevention of this disease.

After 45 years of age more people die from cancer than from tuberculosis, pneumonia, typhoid fever or diseases of the digestive organs. At ages over forty, one person in eleven dies of cancer. One woman in eight and one man in fourteen over forty years of age is attacked by this dread disease with fatal results. From 50 to 75 per cent. or even more of these cases might be saved

Departments of Health, in endeavoring to control the ravages of cancer are confronted with similar difficulties to those confronting them in the effort to control tuberculosis. When the campaign of education for the control of tuberculosis was first undertaken, the great difficulties we had to contend with were that in the first place people who thought they had tuberculosis would not consult a physician lest he would tell them so. The same is true of cancer. A woman thinks there is a possiblity that she has a cancer. She hesitates to go to a doctor for fear he will confirm her suspicion. In the second place there was the universal idea that tuberculosis was hereditary and consequently they did not want anyone to know that there was tuberculosis in the family lest it might affect their future prospects. That is also true of cancer. These two diseases have been looked upon for years as practically incurable. It is now known, however, and asserted by the best authorities that from 90 to 95 per cent., if not 100 per cent. of the cases of both diseases are curable by early diagnosis and prompt treatment, but this early diagnosis requires expert skill. On the other hand 90 per cent. or over of the cases of cancer will prove fatal if neglected until far advanced.

We are controlling tuberculosis because we know its cause. Our line of action is different with cancer, inasmuch as we are still in the dark with regard to its cause, but while we cannot prevent it, unless taken in the pre-cancer stage, we can, by early diagnosis and prompt action, prevent its disastrous results. This obviously means, in the first place, a well organized and carefully conducted educative campaign. Human life has been lengthened by fifteen years; mortality from communicable diseases is being steadily diminished; infant mortality has been markedly decreased in the past decade; the mortality from tuberculosis has been wonderfully reduced, and the general death rate has been gradually lowered largely through the enlightenment of the public in the principles of preventive medicine. Obviously, then, it is the duty of Departments of Public Health to convince the public that this dread disease — cancer — which has been held in greater terror by mankind than probably any other, can be robbed of its fatality and robbed of its terror by early diagnosis and prompt treatment.

Tuberculosis claims most of its victims in the most productive period of their lives. This is also true of cancer. Cancer claims most after forty years of age when the mature judgment makes the victims of most value to their families and to the nation. It is the duty then of Officers of Health, as guardians of human life, to conduct this educative campaign.

The people of this continent will probably never appreciate the debt of obligation they are under to the American Society for the Control of Cancer, the Board of Directors of which are men who stand highest in their professions all over the country. They are, for the most part, engaged in research work in connection with this disease. This or-

In the October 1916 ***Health Bulletin****, Charles Hastings argued that fear of a positive diagnosis made many people ignore the warning symptoms of cancer.*

on the subject. The province defined its role to include education, diagnosis and treatment, control of the use of radium and X-rays, and support for research. Growing public concern about untested cancer cures led to the appointment of an investigating commission in 1938; it concluded that surgery and radium therapy were the only effective cures available.[4]

Hastings, in fact, had made these points using British and American research data a decade earlier. At that time, he also indicated that his Health Department's role was strictly educational. Leaving research to universities around the world, he stated: "It is our duty to broadcast these danger signals, but we cannot force people to protect themselves."[5] His statement highlighted the two variables that would greatly affect the work of his successors: the growing role of the research community and public reluctance to accept and act upon scientific evidence.

By the late 1930s, cancer was the second leading cause of death for Torontonians and indeed for Canadians. On October 12, 1937, the *Globe & Mail* reported that health officials predicted that 11,000 Canadians would die of cancer in 1938, and that 45,000 were suffering from the "dread disease." The news story pointed out that cancer had moved from the fourth to the second leading cause of death because Canada's infant mortality rate and pneumonia death rates had declined significantly. For Toronto's health officers, these national statistics indicated a trend which would require them to shift their attention to adult health concerns.

Two approaches seemed to offer the greatest promise: research and education. During a Labour Day address in 1947, Gordon Jackson told the Toronto Labour Congress that "the throne of King Cancer totters to the attack of our modern Crusader, the Scientist." Overly optimistic as these words were, they reflected the views and hopes of doctors and the public that the various forms of cancer would be conquered by medical science. During the 1950s, the Ontario government expanded its cancer treatment facilities and opened the Princess Margaret Hospital in Toronto to provide "a central facility for cancer treatment and research." The province also funded university fellowships to attract young doctors to the field. But like the bacteriological research of the 1880s, the work of twentieth century cancer researchers has not yet identified a cure. Prevention seems the logical alternative as it did early in the war against communicable diseases.[6]

In December 1947, the first issue of the resurrected *Health Bulletin* informed its readers that the Health Department viewed educating the public about the symptoms of cancer as its principal task because "The first weapon against cancer is knowledge, the second action." Since 70-80% of cancers were treatable if discovered early, the public was urged to consult "regular physicians not the make believe or quack" if the disease was suspected. Well aware that fear of the diagnosis kept many people from seeking medical assistance, the article argued strongly against such fatalism in the modern era. The Department's efforts were seconded by the educational work of the Toronto Branch of the Ontario Division of the Canadian Cancer Society, and the Health League of Canada. Both organizations prepared pamphlets, films, and displays, provided speakers for public ad-

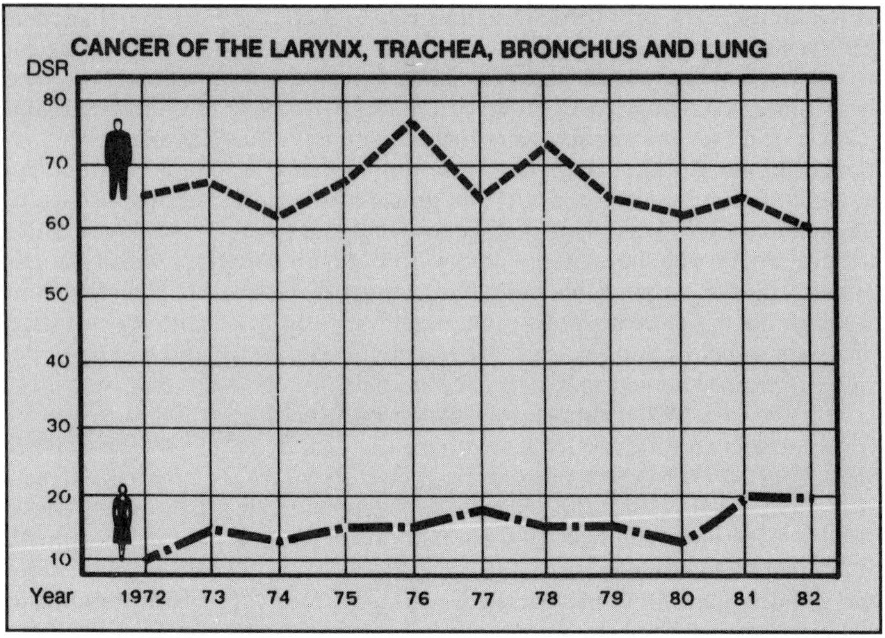

Using directly standardized rates (DSR) to calculate Torontonian's mortality from various forms of cancer, the Department's statisticians showed that lung cancer declined among males but increased among females during the 1970s.

dresses, and cultivated the news media to ensure that accurate information was relayed to anxious citizens. Their efforts were so comprehensive that in 1954, the Health Department abandoned the *Health Bulletin* as a means of educating citizens. As an alternative, the nurses and other staff distributed the material which voluntary groups produced.

Cancer remained a leading killer of adults, and by the 1970s, staff were agitating for a more active role in preventing this cause of premature death. Since breast self-examination aided in uncovering cases of this form of cancer — one of the leading causes of death in women, the nurses, with the assistance of the Canadian Cancer Society, organized a self-examination training session in 1980 for women in the downtown area. Similar shared educational activities were also part of the anti-smoking campaign. All of these efforts were directed at eradicating the stigma which still lingers when cancer is diagnosed.

Heart Disease: The Silent Killer

When general advice about diet, exercise, and annual physical examinations failed to lower death rates from heart disease, medical researchers moved in two directions in the 1950s and 1960s. Canadian surgeons such as William Bigelow and Bill Mustard in Toronto, Arthur Vineberg in Montreal, and J.C. Callaghan in Edmonton, began to experiment with hypothermia, pacemakers, and transplants. During the 1950s as well, the use of hypertensive drugs lowered the death rate from one form of heart trouble. In contrast to this curative focus, the American Surgeon-General, Jacob Mountain, and the Harvard School of Public Health in conjunction with the American National Heart Institute, initiated the Framingham study in 1948–9. This long-term epidemiological project followed a healthy group of male volunteers, aged 30–59, for nearly thirty years, to determine which personal and environmental factors most affected an individual's susceptibility to heart disease. Although the official results of the research were not published in scientific journals until 1966, preliminary findings indicated that heredity, diet, and lack of physical exercise contributed to heart disease.

In 1960, Toronto's local board of health asked its senior administrators to consult the National Heart Foundation of Canada for information on "the latest medical and precautionary measures" because by that date, heart disease was responsible for one-third of the city's mortality.[7] In response to the board's request, the deputy medical officer prepared a report in which he reiterated Hastings's suggestion about the value of periodic health examinations. Moss also observed that evidence concerning the role of cholesterol in clogging the arterial walls was inconclusive and that the causes of heart disease remained unknown, thus limiting the preventive measures against them. In a supplementary report, Dr. Boyd noted that there were no mass screening techniques equivalent to the chest X-ray for tuberculosis, that educational material was lacking, and that the best preventive measure was the reduction of obesity and "scrupulous adherence to sensible dietary and living habits."[8] These conservative responses reflected not only concern about the limits of existing knowledge but also the trepidation which most public health administrators felt about moving beyond their legal obligations. By the early 1970s, inflation made them even less willing to introduce new activities unless they could do so on a cost-shared basis.

During the 1970s, two significant research projects were undertaken in Finland and California to corroborate the Framingham results and to study the effect of health promotion by official health agencies. The North Karelia and Stanford Three (later Five) Cities projects demonstrated convincingly that alterations in diet and effective educational work with communities and individuals, lowered the death rate from heart disease.[9] In 1974, the Ontario Heart Foundation invited the director of the California study to report his findings to Toronto's heart disease experts. The timing was propitious because the federal government had just released its working document and was in the process of organizing public commentary on its proposals for health promotion activities.

All of this activity enabled the authors of *Public Health in the 1980's* to focus on heart disease as a potential area for educational work concerning nutrition, exercise, and stress. Like Charles Hastings, they recommended that people walk rather than drive, and learn to deal with stress effectively. Unlike him, they were able to provide scientific evidence for their suggestions and to create a variety of community-based programs to take that

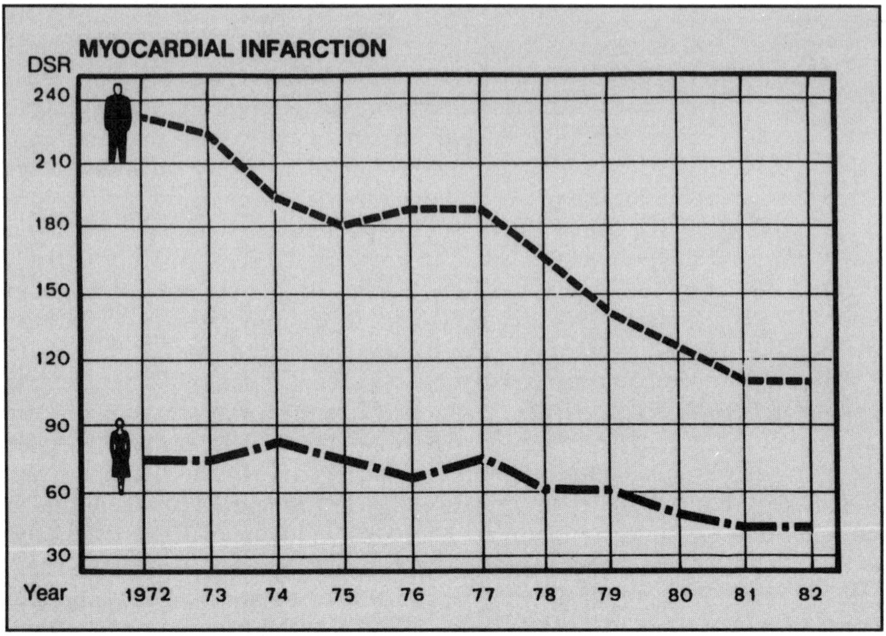

During the 1970s, Toronto's death rate from myocardial infarction (heart attacks) declined as this graph demonstrates.

message to a wide audience. Recent statistics have demonstrated that the death rate from heart disease is declining in Canada and the United States, but cardiovascular and cerebrovascular disease remain significant killers and are now the focus of an international health education campaign.[10]

The Anti-smoking Campaign: Round One, 1960–1974

The anti-smoking campaign illustrates the interplay of research, educational work by government and voluntary agencies, and the gradual switch from individual to community efforts. During the 1950s, American and British researchers demonstrated that smoking caused lung cancer and heart disease. In spite of their findings, Toronto's local board of health continued to give its retiring chairman a lighter to mark his year in office. During the first anti-smoking campaign, one secretary recalled pausing outside Dr. Boyd's office and noticing a small spiral of smoke coming from a desk drawer. These examples show that smoking was socially acceptable, even for health professionals. Combating this health hazard clearly required a change in public opinion.

The Canadian Public Health Association passed its first anti-smoking resolution at the 1960 annual meeting in Halifax. In addition to calling for further research, a ban on advertising, and a strong educational campaign, the resolution also reminded health workers of their duty to set an example.

In Toronto, Alderman Horace Brown, the chairman of the local board, started to educate young adults about the dangers of smoking. Through the creation of a special anti-smoking committee in 1962, the board publicized its proposals, which included restrictions on tobacco advertising and raising taxes on cigarettes to prohibitive levels.[11] That same year, Britain's Royal College of Physicians issued a strong condemnation of smoking and made similar recommendations about the means to eradicate it.

The federal government also got involved and held the First Canadian Conference on Smoking and Health in November 1963. Tobacco industry representatives and the health experts faced each other across the table while Judy LaMarsh, the Minister of National Health and Welfare, announced that the federal government intended to provide funding for education and research to prevent smoking. Early in 1964, Toronto's local board again took the initiative and began to investigate American efforts to assist smokers to break the habit. The proposal for a Department-sponsored smoking withdrawal clinic ran into legal and financial difficulties almost immediately. A letter on this subject to Ontario's Minister of Health received the reply that the city had the right to undertake educational activities, but there was no mention of funding or permitting the use of drugs as was the case in the American clinics.

In April 1964, the Pearson government announced its anti-smoking program; it was targeting teenagers. To ensure that the medical profession was aware of the hazards, the federal government produced a pocket-sized reference book for them and educational kits for the provinces. LaMarsh's ministry also intended to provide $400,000 for education and $200,000 for research. Voluntary groups like the Canadian Cancer Society also undertook education work, focusing on the individual, encouraging him or her not to smoke, or to cut back or quit. The philosophy of the time was that smoking was an individual choice which meant that individuals could choose not to smoke. But federal surveys carried out in Winnipeg and Calgary had demonstrated that some boys started smoking at 5, and some girls at 6, and that they were addicted by 14 or 15. Why then was the problem not treated as addiction and why did the suggestions for raising taxes and limiting advertising fall on deaf ears?

The medical model of preventive and curative work was predicated on research and objective proof of assertions. Both the anti-smoking activists and the tobacco industry carried out research studies which not surprisingly produced conflicting results. Nevertheless, the American Surgeon-General announced his opposition to smoking as a health hazard in January 1964. As research continued, it produced even more damning evidence about smoking as the cause of other forms of heart disease, complications in treating peptic ulcers, low birth weight and prematurity.[12] Translating this knowledge into effective educational programs proved difficult because the medical model presupposed individual treatment in a fee-for-service situation.

What role should the Health Department perform? Members of the local board of health served as liaison with the Board of Education and assisted with the introduction of anti-smoking literature in the schools in an effort to reach students. The Health Department pursued the medical model by coordinating a smoking withdrawal clinic as a pilot project with federal government financing from 1966 to 1969. The clinic was designed to assist adult smokers in quitting and also served as a research project for the University of Toronto's Faculty of Medicine.

After careful psychological and physical assessment, the men selected for the classes were assigned to small groups in which they were shown films and given lectures about the health consequences of smoking. Although the initial results appeared good, some of the students asked for less emphasis on health hazards and more information about behavioural influences. This led the project directors to conclude that "information, if it is to be effectively communicated, must be relevant to the needs of the recipients to whom it is directed." The overall results did not justify making this type of hospital-based clinic a Health Department service, and the responsibility for this type of behaviour modification program devolved on the Canadian Cancer Society's Toronto branch, other service organizations and private companies. In 1978, a survey of Torontonian's attitudes towards smoking revealed that more teenage girls were smoking than had been ten years earlier and that adult smoking had increased as well.[13] Had health educators failed to create an effective program that would appeal to all ages and transform smoking from a socially acceptable, indeed sophisticated adult behaviour, into a socially unacceptable one? Or were they merely experiencing the "long process" necessary to change a deeply entrenched behaviour pattern?

Breakaway for Health: The Second Anti-Smoking Campaign

By the late 1970s, health promoters inside and outside Toronto's Health Department were arguing that a more dynamic, community oriented approach, and a change in target group were necessary. The authors of *Public Health in the 1980's* urged the federal and provincial governments to tax tobacco products more heavily and to use the money to subsidize farmers in converting their land to other crops. That was a feature that had been missing from the 1960s campaign. They also demanded that the province give municipalities the power to regulate smoking in public places. And they pointed out that smoking was an addiction and that current smokers required effective smoking-cessation programs. The report also recommended community activity and more strident advocacy through the creation of an advocacy unit within the Department.

The Health Advocacy Unit was created in 1979 and its director, Gerald Caplan, identified smoking as "probably the major preventable health problem of our age." To create an effective anti-smoking campaign, the Advocacy Unit hired health educators who were to focus their work on combating the socialization of children aged 8–11 to smoke as a result of peer pressure and manipulative advertising. Such a strategy required the active support of the boards of education, parents and the community at large, and was designed to remove the individual emphasis that had dominated earlier efforts.[14] To make these activities effective, the Unit continued to press the local board of health to demand bans on advertising and sports sponsorship by the tobacco companies, and to work for smoke-free facilities in the public and private sector. The motivation for all of this activity was to raise public consciousness and transform smoking from an acceptable stress-relieving, social activity into an anti-social one.

The anti-smoking campaign which the Health Advocacy Unit staff developed was another example of the new public health initiatives of the 1980s. Using "data-based planning, multidisciplinary teamwork, preplanned and on-going evaluation and linking with the community," the Smoking Prevention Program was a marked contrast to its research-oriented predecessors. To reach adults, the campaign focused on smoking in restaurants, work places, and public facilities. As well, the local board of health sponsored a by-law prohibiting smoking in public places, even though inspection staff were aware that they lacked the personnel to enforce it. In February 1983, a Mayor's Task Force on voluntary compliance by restaurant owners was set up to quell public controversy over this by-law. As a result, the legislation was changed to require restaurants to indicate whether they offered non-smoking sections.

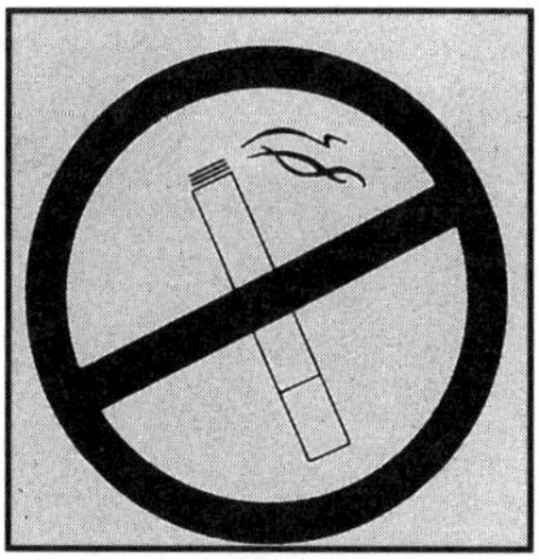

This internationally recognized non-smoking symbol became widespread in Toronto restaurants and businesses during the 1980s as a result of pressure from non-smokers' rights organizations and the Health Department's anti-smoking campaign.

Further publicity resulted from the Stop Smoking Campaign's Cold Turkey contest with Vancouver, held in January 1983. This one day event to mark National Non-Smoker's Week was a victory for Toronto, which got 2,203 pledges to Vancouver's 1,445. It also aroused public awareness of the issue. An evaluation of the activity produced suggestions for change but recommended that the Cold Turkey approach be tried again.[15] The variety of strategies which the Health Advocacy Unit and its successor, the Health Promotion and Advocacy section, used to combat smoking, showed how the campaign against lung cancer developed from a strong medical focus to a community-based prevention program. Like the activities of the family planning division, the recent anti-smoking campaign represents a change in orientation and the recognition that non-medical experts have a role to play in designing the Department's activities.

Living Independent Lives: Seniors' Health

"The Rocking Chair is Not the Answer" was the title of an article which A.R.J. Boyd published in the November/December 1952 issue of *Health*. The deputy medical officer was continuing his discussion of a new public health field by pointing out the importance of providing the nation's growing number of seniors with interesting activities to pursue in retirement. A year later, Toronto's Welfare Council prepared a report on the future needs of the city's elderly which reiterated Boyd's emphasis on keeping seniors "healthy, happy and creatively active." Such views were common throughout the English-speaking world in the post-war era. Since chronic diseases were now the leading killers, the American and Canadian Public Health Associations were urging their members to focus their efforts on this somewhat neglected group.

The Welfare Council's report offered Leon Pequegnat an opportunity to describe what he hoped would be the Health Department's policy toward seniors during the 1950s. Rejecting any involvement in chronic care hospital administration, the medical officer recommended that his staff develop educational programs suitable for "well oldsters" and study "ways and means of ensuring early diagnosis and prompt referral."[16] For Pequegnat and his successors, helping Toronto's seniors to continue living independently was the foundation for all of the Department's initiatives in this field.

Since the 1920s, the Department had been supplying insulin to indigent adult diabetics in their homes. This service aided those who had been diagnosed but what of the population at large? Since the Canadian Diabetic Association feared that the incidence of the disease was increasing, it copied an American innovation and held a "Diabetes Detection Week" during the fall of 1951. The public response to this initiative was disappointing, as fewer people than had been expected were aware of this opportunity for free urine testing. In 1956, Alderman Jean Newman, the board of health's chairman, asked the medical officer to describe the nurses' work with diabetics. In addition to counselling people on the appropriate diet to use to prevent diabetic comas, the staff also arranged for glasses, diet supplements and trips to hospital clinics. Through this activity, the nurses were assisting nearly 1,000 predominantly elderly Torontonians, who generally subsisted on the old age pension and its supplements or on incomes that were barely above the poverty line. Although the responsibility for administering this program was transferred from the Division of Public Health Nursing to the Division of Corporation Medical Services in 1959 (in response to one of the recommendations of the J.D. Woods and Gordon Limited Civic Survey conducted two years earlier), the nurses had seen the plight of poor elderly Torontonians first hand.[17] How could these people and those suffering chronic or terminal diseases best be assisted?

In 1957, the Hillcrest demonstration area was the site of a pilot home care project sponsored by the Health Department with funds from a national health grant. A year later, it was expanded to all the districts. Under Pequegnat's direction, the Pilot Home Care Project demonstrated the Department's ability to co-ordinate the activities of groups such as the Red Cross, the VON, the St. Elizabeth Visiting Nurses, and occupational and physiotherapists on behalf of recently released hospital patients. This was necessary since the city's hospitals were limiting the number of days of convalescence and sending patients home quickly. The chronically and terminally ill who wished to be cared for in their own homes were the other target clientele for this program. In many European cities, similar services were in operation; Oxford, for example, introduced Meals on Wheels in 1955 and added laundry services and personal care a decade later.[18] In Ontario, only four communities provided home care in 1962, but by 1964, Toronto's experiment had proven so successful that the Ontario Hospital Services Commission took over its financing and expanded the program to cover all of Metro.[19] The takeover represented the province's expanding role in service provision in the 1960s.

Providing Personal Advice: The Geriatric Health Centres

In January 1965, the Department opened Geriatric Health Centres for healthy seniors. For $350 and the cost of the district medical officer's time, the East End district office became a weekly advice centre where poor, older women, usually aged 70–80, could have an appointment for a limited physical examination and thirty to ninety minutes of counselling. Dr. J.E.A. Kowalewski, the doctor who pioneered the concept, quickly realized that both the district nurses and the nutritionist were needed because many of these women had social and dietary problems in addition to heart disease and some mental problems. For the first few years of operation, this centre and several others filled a genuine need.

When the deputy officer reported on this pilot project to the first Canadian Conference on Aging in January 1966, his colleagues applauded the innovation. Montreal established similar centres and Vancouver created a

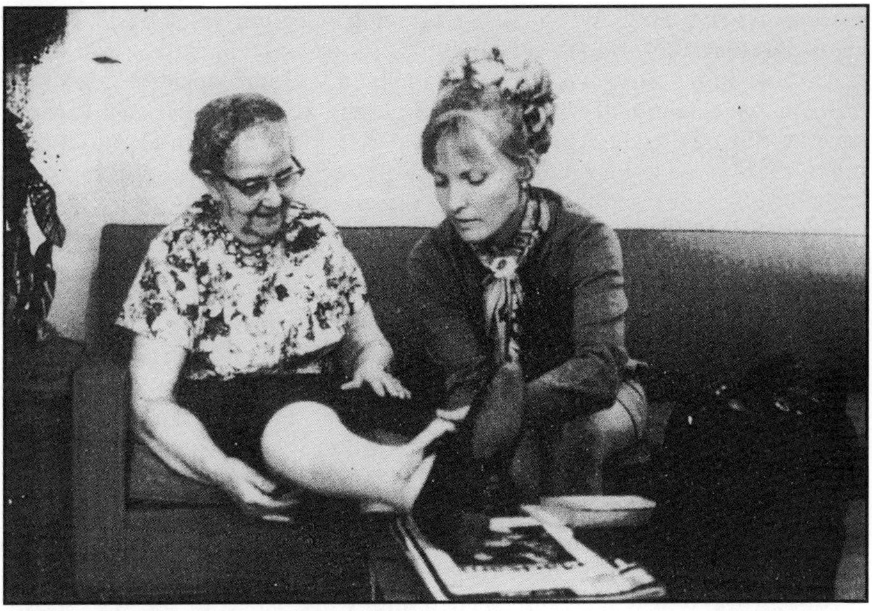

During their home visits, the public health nurses assessed seniors' health and ability to continue living independently.

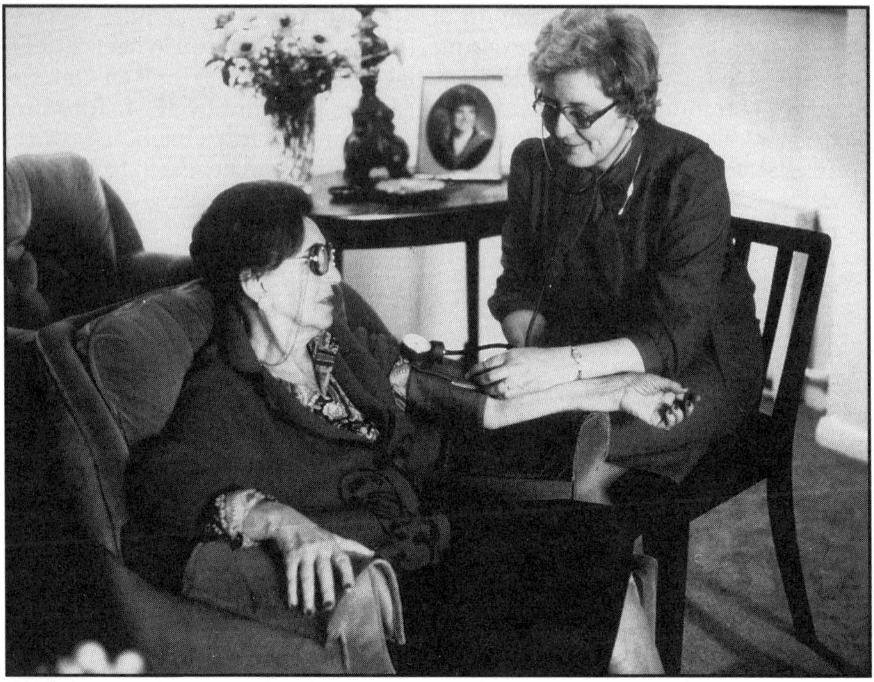

To assist in assessing their clients, public health nurses did blood pressure tests in the home.

more expensive clinic, which also conducted screening tests. By 1972, however, the demand for such services in Toronto and Vancouver had disappeared because "universal medicare" enabled seniors to visit private practitioners. As a result, the medical component of the Department's adult services diminished and the nurses stepped in to give personal guidance on home visits, and to older patients in family practice units, which appeared in large numbers during the 1970s.[20] This rise and decline of the geriatric health centres illustrated the need for evaluation prior to introducing new services, and the impact of external events on the Department's activities.

In 1974, *A New Perspective on Health for Canadians* identified geriatric medicine as one of the least developed aspects of the Canadian health care system. With the proportion of elderly predicted to increase from 8 to 11% of the population between 1965 and 2000, senior citizens' health needs assumed great importance. Four years later, the Health Planning Steering Committee took these concerns one step further when it recommended that the Department provide screening programs for vision defects, hearing, cardiovascular problems, fitness, and nutritional status. One result of these recommendations was the expansion of adult health screening activities through the East End Primary Prevention Project. The project was started in 1978, and the following year, participants were asked to fill out a health questionnaire after they had been tested for their "height, weight, blood pressure, pulse, carbon monoxide inhaled air, stress, fitness, hemoglobin, glucose and albumin (urinalysis), and dental" status. The nurses and medical services physicians who participated in this survey found that although 78% of those surveyed considered themselves to be healthy, only 32% of the 120 people who attended the clinic did not need further assistance. To enable citizens to play a greater role in improving or maintaining their health, the staff prepared a series of talks on lifestyle issues such as heart disease, exercise, nutrition, stress, and addictions.[21] The East End Primary Prevention Project typified modern health education by uniting screening services, self-evaluation, and professional expertise, to promote individual health.

In 1978, the Health Planning Steering Committee also recommended that the board of health "advocate" for income support, and an end to "ghettoizing" seniors in apartment complexes. These suggestions reflected rising public concern about poverty and isolation among seniors. In 1970, the Royal Commission on the Status of Women reported that many single elderly women lived below the poverty line, in spite of the Canada Pension Plan, Old Age Security and various supplements. In 1976, the Senate Report on Poverty confirmed these findings. Although federal pension increases were indexed to the cost of living, studies in the 1980s showed that 55% of Torontonians over 65 had incomes low enough to qualify for the guaranteed income supplement. As the Health Department staff well knew, seniors made sacrifices to maintain their independence and some of these economies, especially food buying restrictions, affected their health.[22]

Isolation from family and friends also took its toll. During the 1960s, the Department's mental health nurses had dealt with the elderly patients who were discharged under the provincial policy of deinstitutionalization, by assisting them in finding accommodation. Neighbours reported other seniors who were facing health problems. During the 1970s, nursing staff in the west end of the city were told about two reclusive elderly men who lived in a house without running water or electricity. With the assistance of the Health Department's community worker, the district nursing supervisor gradually built up sufficient trust that the gentlemen permitted community groups to modernize their plumbing, heating and lighting. Eventually, a local charity provided them with a television, and for the first time, they had contact with the world beyond their front door. As one of them commented: "Somebody cared."[23] For the staff, co-ordinating community support services and assisting seniors' groups to form organizations such as Caring, a telephone contact service for shut-ins, united professional concern with action.

The deaths of several elderly recluses in the late 1970s caused a furor in the Toronto papers and led the Department, in conjunction with Sunnybrook Medical Centre's Psychogeriatric Health Unit and the Queen Elizabeth Hospital (a chronic care facility), to create an interdepartmental task force on the elderly at risk. Few of the staff's assessment and referral activities involved immigrant elderly because for many of these groups allowing a parent to be institutionalized was considered to cause the children to lose face. The fragmentation of the traditional extended family, in fact, had been apparent since the early 1950s, but many families still tried to help the elderly remain at home. As a result, inter-generational conflict grew and the potential for abuse increased. The nursing staff members of the task force recommended that the Department carry out advocacy activities with the provincial health and social service authorities, and argued in favour of better home support services, more relief for primary care givers, and housing options other than nursing homes or chronic care facilities.[24] Since the 1981 Census revealed that 12.5% of Toronto's citizens were seniors, translating these proposals into action would be a priority in most of the health areas.

Conclusion

As Gordon Jackson predicted in 1934, the pendulum has swung towards responding to adult health needs. Since cancer and heart disease threaten all Torontonians, the Health Department has participated in educating them about the signs and symptoms of these degenerative illnesses. During the 1950s and 1960s, the federal and provincial governments both became far more deeply involved in the health care system than they had in the past. Preventive work, however, received a minimal amount of funding, overshadowed as it was by the success of heart surgery and antibiotics. As Canadian and American public health workers sought a new direction, they responded to current problems by co-ordinating community programs for the elderly and the chronically ill. They also tried to link their educational efforts with those of the Cancer and Heart Associations. In contrast to their leadership position in the war on communicable disease, post–1945 health administrators in Canadian and American cities had a less visible presence in the health care spectrum when dealing with the needs of the elderly or with chronic diseases.

Chapter Thirteen

Old Enemies, New Battles: Fluoridation and Air Pollution

During the 1950s and 1960s, public health workers in Britain, the United States and Canada were searching for a new role. Two old enemies — dental decay and air pollution — provided new targets for activism. As scientific research demonstrated the benefits of fluoridating city water supplies and the health risks associated with air pollution and radioactive fall-out, local politicians and citizens began to agitate for action. But Toronto's Health Department could only play a secondary role in these issues because overall responsibility rested with the newly created Metropolitan Toronto government. The province created Metro to rationalize services and to plan effectively for future development. During the 1950s, development meant economic expansion and construction of roads, sewers, schools, hospitals and waterworks. It also contributed to the amalgamation of various municipal services such as the police force and welfare agencies, but resistance from Toronto prevented the unification of local health departments. As a result, no provincial funding was available for new approaches to public health concerns during a decade in which the Department's workload increased markedly as a result of the baby boom and post-war immigration.

Through the 1950s, Metro's health officers, especially Drs. Pequegnat and Boyd, faced strenuous opposition to the proposal to fluoridate the regional water supply. As impartial civil servants, these men were torn between their training and their desire to participate in the public debate on the issue. The conflict demonstrated that the consensus which had been built up over earlier decades had eroded and that professional expertise was vulnerable to attack. Although fluoridation was finally implemented in 1963 after more than ten years of agitation, a new and critical spirit was in evidence. During the 1960s, environmental interest groups were formed and residents' associations began to lobby city council for action on air pollution and other environmental problems. Much of the organizing was an outgrowth of the counter-culture's critique of the flaws in capitalist society. As a result, many of these groups opposed provincial planners and civic administrators who recommended further urban redevelopment, razing homes on the Toronto Islands, and construction of the Spadina Expressway.[1]

For the Health Department, responding to public demands was a long and honourable tradition. Critics in the 1960s and 1970s, however, argued that the crisis response approach to administrative development was ineffective, and urged the Department to modernize by adopting systems management techniques which included planning, evaluation and eliminating obsolete activities and programs. This prepared the way for confrontation between traditionalists and modernizers inside the Health Department and made it a prime candidate for administrative restructuring.

The Fight for Fluoridation

In January 1953, the headline on Toronto's *Health Bulletin*, read "One in a Million." This dramatic title referred to what health authorities around North America believed was the most important advance against one of the commonest diseases known to human beings: "the discovery that one part of fluorine in a million parts of drinking water will prevent tooth decay." Although British researchers had commented on the role of this chemical in preventing cavities as early as 1892, only sporadic research in areas like Colorado, where fluoride occurred naturally in drinking water, was undertaken until the 1930s when the United States Public Health Service started more studies. In 1945, Newburgh, New York, Grand Rapids, Michigan, and Brantford, Ontario, all started adding fluoride to their municipal water supplies in a clinical test of the chemical's effectiveness in preventing tooth decay among children. In Ontario, Stratford which had a natural fluoride in its water, and Sarnia which did not, were used as control cities. Within five years, the results of these experiments demonstrated that children who drank fluoridated water had 60% fewer cavities than those who did not. This evidence and the relatively low cost of the procedure convinced the American Public Health Association to pass a motion supporting the addition to fluoride to municipal water supplies at its 1951 annual meeting in San Francisco. A year later, the Canadian Public Health Association passed a similar resolution. For the first time, Canadian and American dentists and public health administrators believed that they had a primary preventive measure for a costly childhood health problem, and by 1960, twenty-one of the fifty largest American cities had fluoridated their water supplies.[2] Canadian cities were slower to introduce this innovation in spite of the lack of dentists to care for adults and children. Toronto's fight for fluoridation demonstrated many of the factors that prevented immediate implementation.

The battle started in 1952 when the medical officer convinced the local board of health to support the concept. In spite of the board of health's approval, the City's Board of Control refused to grant the request in either 1952 or 1953 because Bill 80 which created Metropolitan Toronto granted that body control of the water supply. As a result, Toronto's board of health passed recommendations favouring fluoridation on an annual basis from 1954 until 1962 in an effort to convince the new agency to implement the measure. In 1955, Metro Council voted 15 to 8 to introduce fluoridation but one member, the Village of Forest Hill, mounted a legal challenge against the by-law which successfully negated that attempt and those of 1956 and 1957.[3]

As a result of this setback, the medical and dental professionals and their supporters, like those in Hamilton and Edmonton, demanded that the city council hold a plebiscite on fluoridation. Many civic politicians in each of these cities did not favour this idea because the opponents of fluoridation were becoming more vocal. Led by CFRB's outspoken broadcaster, Gordon Sinclair, Toronto's opposition advanced two lines of argument: first, that sodium fluoride was "rat poison"; and, second, that the city had no right to infringe on individual liberty by imposing "mass medication." To counter these views, public health administrators turned to the Health League of Canada for publicity and assistance.

Combating "Fluorophobia"

In 1955, the League's magazine, *Health,* published a tongue-in-cheek news report which informed readers that "Fluorophobia Hits Toronto." According to the story's author, "Joe Blow," a new disease was sweeping the city and Gordon Sinclair was its first casualty. He was diagnosed as suffering from "fear of being fluoridated, complicated by an anxiety neurosis inspired by a morbid desire for publicity." Other variations of the malady included individuals who were struck by "myopia fluorophobia (the inability to distinguish truth from fiction), statistical fluorophobia, fluorophobia expensiosis, and Cancer and Heart disease fluorophobia." Each of these imaginary illnesses represented commonly held misconceptions about the consequences of fluoridation.

The Health League tried to counteract these misrepresentations by reprinting the Vancouver Dental Society's careful rebuttal, and by surveying medical and dental experts throughout North America and presenting their views to the public. The League also set up a display at the 1958 Canadian Restaurant Association meeting in Toronto. Visitors were asked to sample fluoridated and unfluoridated water to see if there was a taste difference. Few found any difference and most were amazed by the small amount needed to fluoridate the two sample containers. As one woman remarked: "Is that little bit all you need? Why, I thought from listening to Gordon Sinclair, that it would take shovelfuls. That little bit wouldn't hurt a fly!"[4] Such comments were testimony to the power of radio and they convinced Toronto's new medical officer, A.R.J. Boyd, to take to the airwaves himself.

Continuous conflict between supporters and opponents of fluoridation during the 1950s finally compelled the Frost government to set up an investigating committee in 1959. The Morden Commission attracted opposition groups, like the Christian Scientists and the Canadian Vegetarian Union, and individuals like the American scientist who argued vehemently that fluoridated was "totalitarian." The members also heard testimony from the chief of pediatrics at the Hospital for Sick Children and from a delegation representing the Canadian Public Health Association. The Association's presentation was prepared by Drs. Moss, F.H. Compton, and Pequegnat and represented professionals' concern that Ontario's children grow up without losing teeth and suffering dental decay.[5] When the Morden committee reported in favour of province-wide fluoridation in 1961, the Health League immediately summarized its work in a publicity pamphlet prepared for the next phase of the campaign: convincing the province to pass legislation and the municipalities to implement it.

Entering the Political Arena: Publicizing Prevention

In fact, the Ontario government passed the Fluoridation Act in 1961 and Metro Council faced the task of introducing it unilaterally or holding a plebiscite to let the public decide the matter. The councillors decided to put a question on the 1962 election ballot and the campaigning began in earnest. Toronto's Health Department used a variety of techniques to "sell" the idea of fluoridation. Educational kits were produced to convince aldermen and councillors of the benefits, in spite of the disapproval of some Metro politicians who did not want public funds to finance the pro-fluoridation campaign.[6] To reach the voters, Boyd gave speeches to many civic groups. With the approval of the local board, his staff prepared an exhibit on the topic for the Department's annual display illustrating its services at the CNE.[7] By August, the controversy had reached such heights that Boyd had to get an unlisted phone number to avoid crank calls to his family.[8]

City papers also joined the fray. The *Toronto Star* and the *Telegram* supported fluoridation. In keeping with its sensationalist approach, the *Telegram* headlined one of its articles: "Bad Teeth Can Kill You." The *Star* took a more restrained and factual approach as both papers produced articles and editorials which described the benefits to children from birth to adolescence. Like the Health League, the two dailies also viewed opponents as the type of people who would have opposed chlorination, pasteurization, immunization and vaccination. From their vantage point, progress in prevention clearly required voters to support fluoridation.[9]

In contrast, the *Globe & Mail* opposed fluoridation as "a matter of principle." The editorial writers at the *Globe* did not like the idea that fluoridation would be compulsory for all citizens even though the primary beneficiaries were children. The paper was also not convinced that using the community's water supply was the most efficient or inexpensive way to achieve better dental health. But the *Globe* was careful to distance itself from the fanatics who argued that fluoridation might poison the entire population or that it was a Communist plot "designed to soften our brains and make us an easy prey."[10]

Fluoridation was a key issue in the 1962 municipal election, which also revolved around the issue of Sunday sports and movies and further amalgamation of the municipalities in Metro. All of Toronto's mayoral candidates supported fluoridation although ratepayer resistance still flourished. On December 1, two days before the election, the *Globe & Mail* printed an advertisement which informed readers that all the health officers of Metropolitan Toronto favoured fluoridation. This united front demonstrated the continuing links which had been forged during the joint polio immunization campaign the previous spring. It also indicated that the medical officers believed that their expertise should be the guiding factor in creating public policy. One unforeseen consequence of this unanimity was the provincial government's renewed pressure for amalgamation into a Metropolitan health unit. Although unification did not occur, the senior staff had shed their bureaucratic impartiality in favour of direct intervention in the political realm.

When the votes were counted on December 3, 1962, suburban voters favoured fluoridation while voters in the City of Toronto rejected it by a slim margin. On December 5, 1962, Metro Council announced that fluoridation would begin May 1, 1963. The citizens' groups which opposed the measure threatened further legal action and launched a phone-in protest to the Works Department. Their efforts slowed the implementation of the project until September 4, 1963, but on that day the long years of agitation finally ended.[11]

During their attempts to educate citizens about the benefits of fluoridation, Toronto's medical and dental officers, like supporters everywhere, had always stressed that it would require a generation to demonstrate the

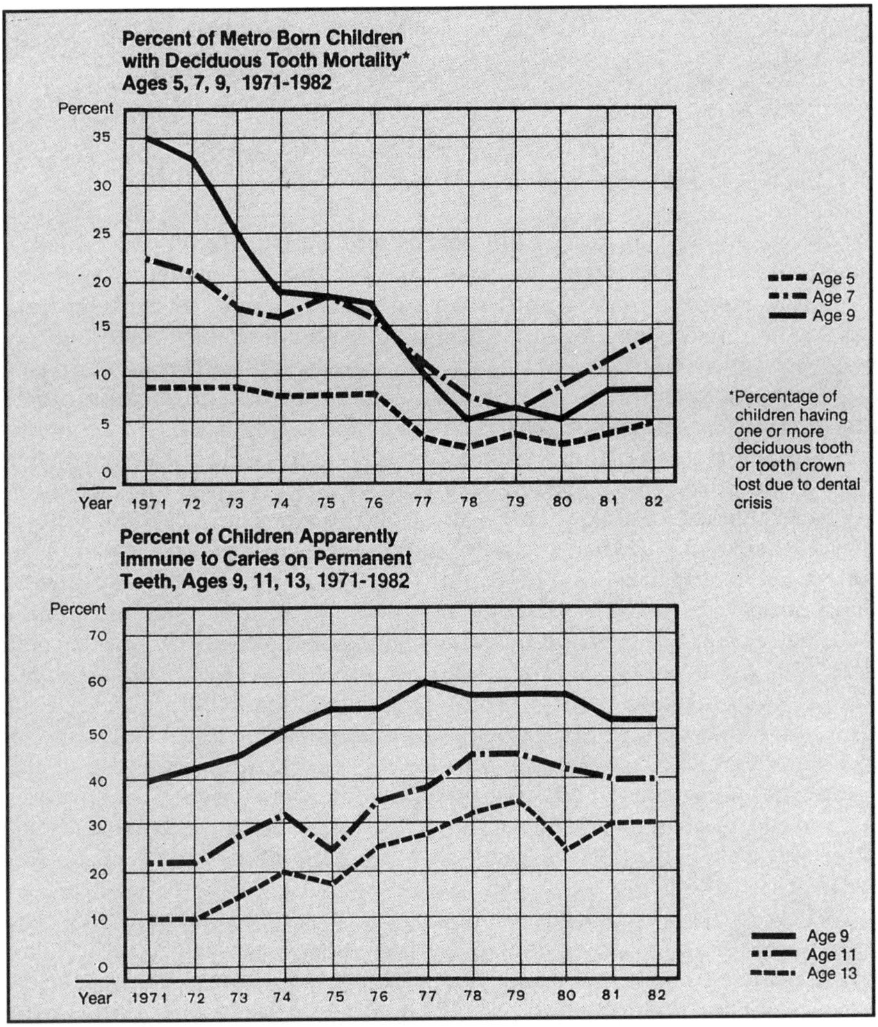

These graphs illustrate the effect of fluoridating Toronto's water supply.

measure's effectiveness. By 1970, however, the Department was reporting that surveys of five year olds born in Metro showed that fluoridation was working already. Even older children had fewer cavities than would be expected.[12] The trend continued, except for immigrant children, many of whom had badly decayed teeth. A comparative study of children's dental health in Toronto and Montreal provided convincing evidence of the effectiveness of fluoridation. From 1963 to 1984, the number of Toronto children aged 9 to 13 who had decayed, missing, or filled teeth had declined by 60%. Montreal, which does not fluoridate its water, saw no decline at all. Of equal importance, opponents' claims that fluoridation would contribute to increasing deaths from cancer or heart disease proved unfounded in Toronto as they had elsewhere.[13]

The fight for fluoridation inaugurated two decades of change for Toronto's Health Department. For Toronto's senior medical and dental staff, the controversy which they and their colleagues in surrounding boroughs experienced as a result of seeking to apply their expertise to a contemporary problem was a harbinger of the greater challenges that lay ahead.

A New Environmental Foe: Air Pollution

By the mid-1930s, the pall of smoke which blanketed most industrial cities in Britain, the United States and Canada no longer merely signified economic progress. British and American researchers demonstrated links between high levels of air pollution and increased mortality from pneumonia, bronchitis, and other respiratory ailments. Rickets also occurred among children who did not receive adequate amounts of sunshine.[14] In addition to these medical reasons for demanding abatement by-laws, the economic costs also warranted consideration as the Mellon Institute in Pittsburgh had proven. In 1938, Hugh Barrett, a young researcher from the School of Hygiene reported Canada's first study of atmospheric pollution. For the previous six years, he had collected data from four stations located in the Junction Triangle, the heart of Toronto's business district, the educational and political centre of the city, and a rural area six miles north of Eglinton Avenue. His analysis showed that when Torontonians lit their morning fires, the city's pollution levels were as bad as the worst British cities. Toronto also matched the five worst American cities — Baltimore, Boston, Chicago, Pittsburgh, and St. Louis — for high pollution levels in the winter but surprisingly, surpassed them in May.[15] Although the purpose of this pioneering study was to establish baseline data for assessing the effectiveness of future abatement efforts, little was done during the Second World War because all efforts were focused on producing the equipment needed for victory.

In 1948, the "Donora Fog", a deadly mixture of pollutants and a temperature inversion in Pennsylvania, alerted North Americans to the dangers of unregulated smoke pollution.[16] Toronto passed a smoke abatement by-law in 1949 and created an advisory committee to educate local industries about the problem. A year later, Hamilton passed its first anti-pollution by-law.[17] Both of these measures became redundant as homeowners and businessmen began to convert to oil heating during the affluent 1950s. The discovery of apparently abundant supplies of oil in Alberta created the postwar petrochemical industry, and with the pent-up demand for consumer goods, spawned the glory years of the North American car industry. Ironically, as it contributed to eliminating one form of air pollution, the oil industry inadvertently created another.

Whose Responsibility?: Air Quality Concerns in the 1950s

When Metro assumed responsibility for air pollution control on January 1, 1956, Toronto's Health Department no longer had an official role to perform. As a result, dealing with air pollution was similar to dealing with water quality concerns: monitoring was the only option available to the Department's staff. This led the retiring medical officer, Dr. Pequegnat, inform his colleagues in the Canadian Public Health Association that "Air pollution control demands teamwork and is an area in which the health officers of many regions can make a substantial contribution."[18] But could they? Did the medical research model really offer the public an effective way to respond to rising fears about the health consequences of air pollution and radioactive fall-out? Should health departments initiate long-term epidemiological studies, or should they confine their efforts to having their inspectors prepare technical reports?

One area of concern during the late 1950s and early 1960s was radioactive fall-out from nuclear tests. In 1962, the medical officer and his deputy reported to the local board of health that although caesium 137, a by-product of nuclear explosions, had a long half-life and contaminated plants and animals, researchers believed that it did not remain in the human body for any length of time. Drs. Boyd and Moss noted that the provincial government radiation laboratory, which monitored contamination levels, was located in Toronto, and stressed that their staff would work with other federal and provincial agencies to protect the quality of the city's food supplies in the event of radioactive fall-out. In their opinion, "man's folly in the atmosphere" or "the accidental malfunction of controlled reactors" were the two potential causes of significant radiation contamination.[19]

For the majority of Torontonians, the local board's concern about nuclear radiation paled in comparison to the 1962 Grey Cup game. The "Fog Bowl" at Exhibition Stadium was called with ten minutes remaining because neither the Hamilton Tiger Cats nor the Winnipeg Blue Bombers could see the end zones or the fans who had come to watch them. A temperature inversion had produced dense smog, which later experts estimated measured 155 on the federal government's air quality scale (introduced in 1970). Since a pollution measurement of 32 on the 1970 scale was the reading at which industries were asked to limit emissions or shut down, conditions in 1962 had been hazardous for people with breathing and heart problems.

In 1963, the medical officer presented several reports to the local board on the role of car emissions in contributing to air pollution. Members of the

Sanitation Division carried out studies on the efforts of car companies and the TTC to reduce pollution from car exhaust. At that point, as the staff regretfully noted "no economically sound" emission control device had been developed.[20] A national air pollution conference held in 1965 prompted an editorial writer for the *Canadian Public Health Journal* to argue that pollution control "requires the talents of many disciplines" and that public health workers had to educate their communities on the issue. He concluded by asking: "Will we accept these challenges now or will we wait until the need is so acute that we must embark on a crash program?"[21]

A New Approach: Public Activism

During the 1960s, environmental activists accepted the challenge. A wide variety of scientists, concerned citizens, and hippies argued that pesticides, acid rain, and suburban development were destroying the environment and endangering people's health by contaminating air, food and water supplies. In 1966, Alderman Harold Menzies, an outspoken member of the board of health, pushed a motion through city council to encourage the local board of health to take an active stance on air pollution. While Menzies recognized that pollution control was a Metro responsibility, he argued that the local board had a duty to protect the health of Torontonians because studies in New York, Philadelphia, and London had "correlated" air pollution with various diseases, eye irritations, reduced visibility, and "pungent odours." Since Toronto was experiencing rapid suburban growth and a significant increase in traffic, he recommended joint study and action against air pollution with federal, provincial, and other local health authorities.[22] Environmental groups also wanted governments to act; they recommended the introduction of scrubbers for industrial smokestacks and emission control devices in cars. To ensure that their suggestions received serious consideration, activists in Toronto formed Pollution Probe in 1969.

One of the consequences of the growing public involvement in environmental issues was the creation of a federal Ministry of the Environment in 1970, and the passage of the Clean Air Act which set air quality standards. Ontario's Ministry of the Environment was founded in 1971,[23] and the new provincial agency quickly adopted federal air pollution measurement standards. Toronto had started using these guidelines to monitor air pollution in 1970. That year the permissible limit was exceeded seventeen times. Through education and control orders where necessary, industry was trained to limit its output during temperature inversions and other health-threatening situations. In 1983, the guidelines were only exceeded three times in Toronto and many experts agreed that the city's air quality had improved as a result of government intervention.[24]

Both *A New Perspective on Health for Canadians* and *Public Health in the 1980's* discussed the health threats associated with environmental pollution. The federal report outlined a Health Field Concept which included environmental factors, human biology, lifestyle, and the health care system, as the four variables which affected Canadians' health. As the federal working document noted, jurisdiction over many sources of contaminants rested with provincial governments, so the senior level intended to lobby them to develop and implement progressive standards. Since Canadians lacked their own pollution impact studies, the federal government also began to offer funds for basic and applied research in this field. In recognition of their lack of legal power, the authors of Toronto's study argued in favour of a monitoring role for the city Health Department, research into the effects of traffic pollution, and advocacy. To achieve such change, however, required a more holistic view of the Health Department's role, and a rejection of the compartmentalization implicit in the medical research model and the current divisional structure. Instead, new types of expertise, new staff and a renewed commitment to activism were required to deal with the increasing number of environmental pollutants that worried health-conscious parents and politicians. As a result, younger staff within the Department began to study for graduate degrees in environmental studies and to encourage re-evaluation of the existing programs and activities. In an age of financial restraint and inflation, new funds were not forthcoming, and the Department had to think about ending obsolete programs, retraining staff and shifting resources to meet these new demands.

Conclusion

From 1950 to 1970, public interest in and understanding of environmental issues developed greatly. For the Health Department, these new concerns added another burden to staff who were working hard to maintain current levels of service to citizens of all ages. What should receive priority? Under existing public health legislation, providing programs for children, adults and environmental sanitation issues were legal obligations. But as Leon Pequegnat noted during his retirement address in 1957, the implied obligations facing health departments indicated the future areas of activity.

But were environmental concerns medical and nursing issues? Certainly the health risks associated with bad teeth, asthma, bronchitis, and lung cancer were well established. But did the Department's mandate cover involvement in eliminating the sources of pollution? Could a single department make a difference or were group action and teamwork essential? The successful campaign for fluoridation demonstrated that unity among local health officers, allied to a strong publicity effort orchestrated by a voluntary group, was an effective strategy for preventive action in a field that had a clear medical component. Public concern about the impact of air pollution and nuclear contamination had a more subtle effect because this prompted the formation of non-governmental organizations, which represented the public, not scientific experts. This development heralded the anti-establishment activism of the late 1960s and 1970s and led to calls to reassess the Health Department's role in fighting old enemies and expanding into new areas.

Chapter Fourteen

Environmental Politics: The Catalyst for Change

> Public health cannot be separated from politics. Although it may be difficult for public health professionals to take social or political action, much of their effort will be irrelevant or inadequate unless this is done.[1]

When this statement was published in 1977, Toronto's Health Department was conducting a searching self-assessment that questioned its philosophical foundation and current activities. The impetus for change came from the social and political upheavals of the 1960s and 1970s. In contrast to the consensus-style politics and respect for professional expertise which had dominated municipal politics in the 1950s, the following two decades saw the rise of participatory democracy and the decline of faith in technocracy. Although this sense of disillusionment was pervasive and threatened teachers and social workers, public health personnel were especially vulnerable because they were the front line in the war against the diseases of both poverty and affluence.[2] All that was necessary was a catalyst, and public unease with the threat of environmental contaminants supplied it. Toronto's experience with lead pollution in the east and west ends, provided a graphic demonstration of the perils of community activism for politicians and the necessity for change in the traditions and structure of the Health Department.

For most Torontonians, the 1950s were notable for rapid economic development under the benign direction of Mayor Nathan Phillips, and the more masterful Metro Chairman, Frederick Gardiner. Both these men expected their senior administrators to provide expert advice, implement policy and maintain an appropriately deferential stand on contentious issues.[3] During the 1960s, critics of both the deferential tradition in Canadian society and the civic boosterism implicit in the stress on economic expansion, began to express their vocal opposition to authority by organizing community groups to protest urban redevelopment projects and business dominance. The reformers scored a victory in 1972 when David Crombie was elected mayor at the head of a small reform contingent.

For the next eight years, the pro- and anti-development forces on city council fought to reshape both municipal institutions and Toronto's future. The Health Department became a rallying point for reformers because for them the lead issue demonstrated the importance of committed activism, not bureaucratic impartiality. As the local board of health became the policy generating force within the Department, its members pushed for structural change. In 1976, to ensure that their initiative outlived their political careers, reformers on the local board organized the Health Planning Steering Committee to develop a new rationale and framework for preventive services. The results of their endeavour were the well-known report, *Public Health in the 1980's*, the creation of the Health Advocacy Unit, and decentralization. These recommendations and the structural changes which they produced were designed to increase community participation and to ensure that health promotion became the foundation for all of the Department's activities.

Citizen Activism and Political Controversy: The Lead Issue

During the 1950s, both Toronto and Metro pursued a growth-oriented strategy that focused on urban redevelopment and expansion. Within the city, slum areas were razed and the affluent began to gentrify homes in the Annex and Cabbagetown. By the mid–1960s, however, sociologists and community organizers were criticizing local politicians' emphasis on growth and their lack of concern about environmental problems, heritage buildings, and the poor. As an alternative to the business-dominated politics which had governed Toronto since the turn of the century, citizen's groups organized neighbourhood associations and sponsored candidates for both city council and the school board. In 1967, New Democratic Party candidates were elected for the first time and Toronto's Board of Education was dominated by reformers who wanted to improve conditions in inner city schools and to deal with racial tension.[4] Such social and political ferment helped to overturn the consensus politics of the past.

The municipal election of December 1972 marked the triumph of an urban reform coalition led by David Crombie, a thirty-six year old lecturer in political science at Ryerson and a former alderman. Determined to respond to community needs, this group found themselves in conflict with old guard politicians and the civic bureaucracy because of their inexperience and focus on social change. One of the newly elected aldermen, Anne Johnston, an occupational therapist at the Queen Street Mental Health Centre, exemplified this trend. Her goal was a seat on the local board of health because she wanted to make it responsive to the health problems of the 1970s, not those of the past.[5]

Her first opportunity arrived on January 16, 1973, when a delegation from the South of King Residents' Association appeared at the board of health's monthly meeting to complain about lead emissions from Toronto Refiners and Smelters Ltd., located at 28 Bathurst Street. In this working class residential neighbourhood, five children had been admitted to the Hospital for Sick Children with lead poisoning between 1960 and 1971. Their concerned parents and other residents appealed to the province for assistance, and in 1971, the Air Management Branch of Ontario's Department of Energy and Resources conducted lead measurements near the plant. The following year, the new Ministry of the Environment provided environmental monitoring and did blood lead level tests. While the province was carrying out these activities, the residents hired a lawyer from the Environmental Law Association to represent them because letters from the Ministry suggested that the factory would be allowed to continue operating. Early in 1973, the citizens turned to the local board of health for support because they had decided that "the buck stops with this committee."[6]

The board listened sympathetically to the delegation and committed the Health Department to research and report on the matter. In February, when the board of health did not provide further information at its regular meeting, Alderman Dan Heap, the residents' council representative, charged that the medical officer and the local board were showing contempt for public concerns. This accusation prompted Johnston and Fiona Nelson, the Board of Education representative, to argue in favour of immediate action in spite of legal difficulties.[7] Like Heap, these politicians believed that confrontation produced more creative and appropriate solutions than the consensus-style politics practiced by older politicians and long-time administrators.

The situation was more complex than the rookie activists recognized. The nuisance provisions of Ontario's Public Health Act had been designed for nineteenth century problems, not twentieth century lead pollution. Although the medical officer and his inspectors could and did investigate complaints made to the local board, abatement orders could not be issued if too great a financial loss or interference with the business would occur. As Moss pointed out to the board in his report, the Haliburton-Pine Ridge-Kawartha Health Unit had just lost a court case on this issue because, according to the judge, its "undue haste" in closing a business had caused the proprietor to go bankrupt. Without adequate proof that Toronto Refiners and Smelters caused a nuisance which was an "immediate dire threat" to the health of residents, the medical officer feared that Toronto would lose any legal battles. This pertinent point failed to sway the board or the residents.

As both the medical officer and the city solicitor pointed out, divided jurisdiction between the city and the Ministry of the Environment was another important factor. If Toronto Refiners and Smelters was creating a nuisance, the Health Department inspectors could issue abatement orders. But, if the company was polluting the air, control notices had to be issued by the ministry. Ideally, both agencies should co-operate to ensure that residents' health was protected, but during the three years that the controversy raged tension flourished between the city and the upper levels of the provincial bureaucracy.

In January and February 1973, the Health Department's inspectors examined Toronto Refiners and Smelters premises and reported to the health officer about the uncovered stockpiles of old batteries which were contributing to dust in the vicinity. As they noted, the company had been in operation since 1945, had expanded several times, and had complied with the Works Department's regulations regarding the disposal of its by-products. When the inspectors made their visits, the battery-crusher had been idle for six months while the owners began to comply with provincial emission control guidelines. The Health Department issued nuisance abatement orders and the company covered its stockpiles and introduced dust control measures to conform to existing public health regulations.

At the end of World War II when Toronto Refiners and Smelters and its competitor, the Canada Metal Company on Eastern Avenue, were opened, both districts were commercial areas. Toronto's insatiable demand for post-war housing meant that as other industries moved to the suburbs, homes were built adjacent to these two factories. Although the city had changed its zoning by-laws to prohibit this type of industry in residential areas, the companies had the right of prior occupancy to justify their presence. They also provided employment for local workers. As a result, residents' demands to close the factories challenged the city's traditional growth ethic and the Health Department's policy of persuasion not coercion in nuisance abatement.

Using Science: Blood Lead Testing

Much of the conflict hinged on the vexing issue of the amount of blood lead that constituted a health hazard. When the issue erupted, relatively little research had been done on the topic although most industrial cities experienced the problem. Unexpectedly, Toronto became a pioneer as the medical staff, inspectors, and public health nurses all contributed to collecting data. As a service and program provider, Toronto's Health Department usually adapted scientific discoveries to suit perceived needs, but the board decided that the staff should contribute to the research process by conducting blood lead level tests on residents to determine acceptable levels. In March 1973, a core working group of six doctors from the Hospital for Sick Children, the Health Department, the School of Hygiene, and the Ministry of Health was formed to establish acceptable testing methods, create a lead testing clinic at HSC, and carry out tests in the Niagara Street district.

Using "hand-picked" nurses familiar with the district, blood tests were conducted from May 14 to June 15 amid mounting public discontent. Some residents objected to what they felt was pressure from the nurses and the Medical Services doctor to donate 100 millilitres of blood rather than having the finger-prick test. Others charged that the lead testing clinic staff had been "off-hand, callous and occasionally incompetent." Such outright complaints had rarely been made in the past and the medical officer responded with the comment that "The staff should not have to accept debasement of their professional qualifications."[8] He compelled the local board to pass a resolution supporting his employees but the gap between his commitment to professional expertise and the board's commitment to community activism was growing.

The preliminary results of the blood lead level tests were not available until late July because Toronto no longer had its own laboratory. The mixed results led the committee to decide to retest people in the 30–39 microgram range and to do physical examinations of those with blood lead levels over 40 micrograms, the then internationally accepted danger level. In light of these contradictory findings, the medical officer urged further investigation and study before the board of health pursued legal action.[9] The delay upset residents, especially since three children from the district were hospitalized during the summer for treatment of excessive lead levels, after Toronto Refiners and Smelters resumed production at the beginning of July. Publicity about the problem led citizens in the east end to ask the University of Toronto's Institute for Environmental Studies to examine the air quality in their neighbourhood. In its report, the institute found lead levels 80 times higher than the city norm. Faced with two environmental pollution problems, the medical officer persuaded the city's executive committee to hire an American lead toxicologist to evaluate the data that now had to be collected from a second area and a control group.[10]

When the results of these tests were reported to the Ministry of the Environment by the city, the Ministry finally imposed a control order on the Canada Metal Company on Friday October 27, 1973. The order was initiated because a Jones Avenue resident had a blood lead level of 200 micrograms per hundred decilitres and two other people tested well above acceptable limits. Three days later, lawyers for the company convinced Judge D.A. Keith to rescind the order because the Ministry had not proven that the company had produced an emergency. Both the *Globe* and the *Star* were critical of the incompetence of the Ministry officials and the resident's groups were furious.

By November, the local board of health was completely disenchanted with the Ministry. The board had been shocked when the Ministry had allowed Toronto Refiners to resume battery crushing and had opposed the construction of an 85 foot smoke stack because there was no guarantee that this would limit soil contamination at homes near the factory. In November then, the board and the city council began to discuss closing the companies and paying them to relocate with funding from the Ministries of Health and the Environment.

The pressure intensified when the medical working group met hostile east end citizens on November 8. Moss and other committee members were shouted down when they tried to argue in favour of more research because residents believed that "nobody gives a damn about us." Moss responded sympathetically: "I feel this is a helluva a way to go about it, that you have to wait for us to prove the direct connection."[11] That observation went to the crux of the matter because the lead companies had hired their own experts who were casting doubt on the city's case by claiming that lead contamination from housepaint, traffic on the Gardiner Expressway, and other sources was the actual cause of residents' high blood lead levels.

Who Decides?: Politicians or Experts?

On November 14 and 16, the local board held marathon meetings at which lead specialists representing the companies and the residents fought to a draw on the issue. Differing opinions on the proper course of action also prevailed among the decision-makers. On one side, the medical officer recommended permitting Canada Metal to build the filters which the Ministry of the Environment had approved. On the other, Alderman Johnston wanted the board of health to issue an order to close the plant. The extreme position which she had taken irritated the vice-president of Canada Metal, who commented that the situation had become too emotional and that his company would welcome visitors to the plant to see the new filters in operation. As a professional administrator, Moss sought to end the conflict through compromise, particularly since he did not believe that the city had a strong case for legal intervention.[12] And Alderman Tom Clifford pointed out that 250 people in his ward would lose their jobs if the board accepted the advice of the Environmental Law Association and closed the plant.

What was at issue here was not only the traditional approach which the Health Department had developed for dealing with environmental issues, but also the relationship of the Health Department and the local board of health. Activists like Anne Johnston were convinced that the Department was lagging in its efforts to respond to community needs. Given the confusion in the scientific community about acceptable standards for lead emissions, the reformers on the board decided that they could not wait for answers and would define their own acceptable levels. They also passed motions urging the Ministry of the Environment to provide monthly reports on the dust fall and ambient air quality near the plants.

The problem with the board's activist stance was that responsibility for carrying out recommendations had been the medical officer's duty since the 1912 amendments to the Public Health Act had made him the chief executive officer of the local board and the administrative head of his department. Although practice had modified his pre-eminence and Toronto's health officers usually consulted their division directors, provincial counterparts, and colleagues at the School of Hygiene when formulating policy, board members such as Anne Johnston, Dan Heap, Dan Leckie and Dr. David Parkinson believed that linking the two functions produced stasis rather than responsiveness to environmental issues. Throughout 1973, Moss was faced with lay people who argued that policy formation was their duty. Sharing or surrendering this role was difficult for someone trained in the traditional medical officer's role and made more trying as it was being carried out in the full glare of publicity.

Redefining Leadership Roles

The politics of the lead issue became more complicated in February 1974, when the lead companies launched court action against Aldermen Johnston and Heap and Dr. David Parkinson of the Hospital for Sick Children, all of whom were members of the local board of health. They were charged with bias and prohibited from discussing the lead issue with their colleagues or journalists, some of whom had also been slapped with injunctions.[13] Since the medical officer was under oath during the court action, he removed himself from the board. Council then passed a by-law to ratify his action. This marked the clear separation of the policy and administrative activities; it also paved the way for expanding community membership on the board.

The separation of political and administrative roles did not go smoothly. After the American experts reported in March 1974, the board spent April and May defining its policy on abatement orders. Confusion over time limits and monitoring duties meant that no orders were issued until May 24. In mid-June, the Minister of the Environment responded to the board's continuing criticisms of his department's lack of action by pointing out that Toronto's chairman had been sent the ministry's controversial interim report on soil contamination in February. Johnston who was chairing the Board in 1974 reacted strongly and threatened to fire Moss if he did not have an acceptable explanation about the missing document. In fact, the report had arrived while he was on sick leave and had been sent through the Department as a technical resource. Although the Sanitation Division staff needed the report for information and guidance, this action was not politic given the strained municipal-provincial relationship. Since the external experts had seen the document before completing their study, the board in fact had not been denied crucial information in the decision-making process. This incident indicated the potential for misunderstanding between the politicians and the administrators.[14]

At the June meeting, the local board also asked the city council for funding for summer lead testing clinics. Alderman Heap was upset that after a year of testing the public still did not know where the children were picking up lead contamination. As the public health inspectors and nurses were aware, young children were quite likely to be eating dirt or playing in it and absorbing the lead that way.[15] Heap's colleague, Dr. Parkinson, pointed out that the Ministry of the Environment had found fourteen potential sources of contamination in its surveys of the two districts. The lead issue was, in fact, much more complex than the reformers wanted to believe. The insistence by Moss and other administrators that further research be undertaken was not simply an attempt to stonewall or ignore the problem. It reflected the experts' desire to find the causes of the problem and an effective resolution.

The scientific method, however, was not exclusively the preserve of the Health Department and its supporters. In June 1974 the lead companies hired Dr. John Horn, a botanist from the University of Western Ontario, to supervise blood lead tests on families living near the Gardiner Expressway to see if automobile exhaust was a factor. Although the researcher asked for the assistance of the Department, he was warned by the deputy health officer that no help could be offered in view of the pending court case. In spite of this, Dr. Horn opted to go ahead on June 28. Moss discussed the matter with the doctors' working group and the members encouraged him to send a telegram to Horn asking for an outline of the proposed research project and indicating concern about the ethics of conducting the experiment. As a result of this, the testing location was changed and few people participated. But was this a genuine attempt to investigate a potential health threat or was it an effort by the lead companies to discredit the Department's expert witnesses?

Whatever the motives, one of the consequences was a slight improvement in the relationship between the chairman of the board of health and the medical officer. Since both of them and Dr. Parkinson were criticized by the lead companies' lawyer for obstructing Horn's research, Alderman Johnston sent him a strong letter rebutting his allegations and threatening to take the matter to the Law Society of Upper Canada. Johnston and Moss also agreed to keep the lines of communication open because they needed to present a united front in the on-going battle to protect the public's interest.

Whose Responsibility?: The Municipal-Provincial Question

Through the fall of 1974, the board continued to monitor the situation. Late in November, the Ministry of the Environment halved permissible lead emission levels and fined the Prestolite Company $2000 for causing air pollution.[16] This evidence of provincial commitment enabled the board of health to rescind its abatement order against the Canada Metal Company on the understanding that the Ministry of the Environment would take responsibility. This confidence proved to be misplaced. In February 1976, after a year of inaction by the ministry, the local board sent a strongly-worded resolution to Premier Davis. One month later, the Ministry of the Environment issued its control order.[17]

One possible reason for the delay was the provincial government's decision to set up an Environmental Hearing Board to investigate lead pollution. In 1975, Anne Johnston presented Toronto's detailed submission because the local board of health could not afford to hire a lawyer. Although the activists hoped to continue to participate in the hearings, lack of money forced the local board to apply to city council and the province for financial assistance. None was forthcoming in spite of the reformers' argument that the hearings would only reflect the views of the lead industry and its supporter, the International Lead Zinc Research Organization. To assist the Environmental Hearing Board with its deliberations, Toronto provided the data tapes which its staff had produced from the one million pieces of information which their research activities produced.[18]

In 1976, the medical officer reported to the board of health on the Environmental Hearing Board's recommendations. He was concerned about the effectiveness of many of the proposals and questioned the reason for limited consultation with municipalities about programs or control orders. Toronto's board endorsed his criticisms and its members added several of their own. The members were shocked that the Environmental Hearing Board could be so naive about industrial polluters and were dismayed that the Report of the Lead Data Task Force had been ignored. And looking back to an offer which Toronto Refiners made in 1973, the board strongly urged the province to support the removal of contaminated soil in polluted areas. The Ministry of the Environment accepted the latter suggestion and set up a committee to discuss soil removal that summer. Agreeing on the amount to be removed and the cost-sharing arrangement to pay for it was a slow process. Not until 1988 would Riverdale residents finally have lead contaminated soil removed from their yards.

For the civic politicians, the final act in the legal drama took place in the summer and fall of 1976. After six days of argument in Divisional Court in June, the case against Johnston, Heap and Parkinson was bound over until October. In the interim, a settlement was worked out. Both sides dropped their charges or orders and agreed to pay their own costs. Since the aldermen and Dr. Parkinson were facing extensive legal fees, they appealed to city council for financial assistance. Mayor Crombie had offered his support in 1974 and the rest of the Executive Committee agreed to the measure on October 1, 1976. The local board of health's activism cost the city $38,600 in legal fees. It also revealed the limitations of many traditional practices and attitudes within the Health Department and served as the catalyst for significant structural changes. When the controversy died down, the Department took on an monitoring role and the city's inspectors used their new found expertise to keep up-to-date on the situation. Fifteen years after the South of King Residents Association asked the local board of health for help, the city bought Toronto Refiners and Smelters and the Ministry of the Environment promised to make the company pay part of the clean-up costs.[19]

Planning for the Future

"Yesterday's successes are today's problems."[20] Public health administrators had been living with the consequences of this truism since the early 1950s. As their old enemies vanished and new ones appeared, health department staff in Canadian, American and British cities adapted slowly to changing circumstances.[21] By 1962, when the Canadian Public Health Association made its presentation to the Royal Commission on Health Services, there was widespread concern about the future of preventive medicine and public health services. The Public Health Association stressed the importance of planning and evaluating current programs and services. As the authors noted: "It cannot be assumed that programs and procedures which have become well established and well accepted are necessarily returning health dividends proportional to the time and effort which they consume."[22] Few health departments heeded this warning during the turbulent 1960s. Instead, they added new duties to existing activities often without assessing either their relevance or cost. Health departments were thus vulnerable to charges that they were rooted in the past and irrelevant to the present.[23]

Neither the Hall Commission nor the Ontario government's 1974 Health Planning Task Force foresaw a significant role for local health departments in a health care system dominated by hospitals, specialists, general practitioners, and government bureaucracy.[24] In 1972, the Ontario Ministry of Health tried to eliminate the remaining local boards of health completely by offering to pay 75% of the costs of preventive services provided by regional health units. But when Toronto and other cities rejected the offer, the province desisted. Four years later, the ministry's own Health Promotion Branch published a background paper in which it described "the unique and indispensable role" which local health departments "fulfil in protecting, maintaining and promoting community health."[25] This turnabout reflected growing interest in prevention rather than "episodic" medicine, the realization that grass roots changes were occurring at the municipal level, and the government's fear of spiralling medical care costs.

A philosophical change was also taking place. In 1974, the federal government's working document, *A New Perspective on Health for Canadians*, introduced the concept of health promotion. In professional circles, health promotion was slowly making inroads as younger staff were trained to see public health problems holistically and to work in multi-disciplinary teams to solve them. For these people, traditional health departments with their discipline-based divisions, multiple layers of bureaucracy and medical orientation were institutions which had "become irrelevant to their society and inadequate to their task."[26] As a result, pressure for structural reform was rising.

In Toronto, the election of the reformers and the lead controversy started the process. As social activists, many of the members of the local board of health no longer accepted medical dominance of public health policy because they believed that "institutions are only artifacts of a society's values and objectives" and hence, must change to suit society's needs. From their perspective, the lead issue had revealed the Department's limited epidemiological capacity, its dependence on classical management structures, and the need for community input in program design and evaluation. In January 1976, the local board created a Health Planning Steering Committee to research the problem, and to suggest appropriate ways to reorganize the department to prepare it for dealing effectively in future with "manmade epidemics" such as smoking and heart disease.

Preparing for Change

The Steering Committee consisted of activists from the local board, the medical officer and his deputy, staff representatives, and external experts from the Ministry of Health, and the city's Management Services and Planning Departments. As part of the reform process, the committee rejected hierarchical organization and introduced the team approach to problem definition and solution. Some progressive members proposed and implemented a three stage reform process similar to the one that had been used to revamp the Board of Education during the late 1960s. The first stage consisted of preparing a provocative *Issue Paper* which summarized the department's shortcomings, current programs and staffing arrangements, outlined potential health hazards, and recommended a "modernized role for Public Health." Next, staff members, interested experts, community agencies, and the public were invited to comment on the *Issue Paper*. Then the Steering Committee set up a series of sub-committees to meet with staff and external groups who wished to have further input into the process. This approach was a marked contrast to previous administrative restructuring which had been imposed from above because the Steering Committee was committed to demonstrating the feasibility of consultative decision-making.

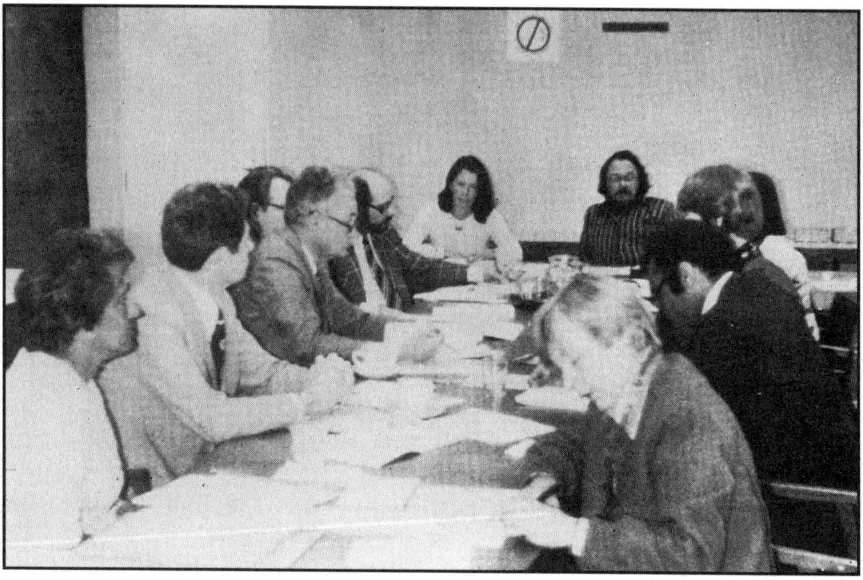

The Health Planning Steering Committee, including Alderman Anne Johnston, seated in the right corner.

While this phase of the work was underway, the committee also hired staff from the University of Toronto's Department of Community Health to prepare a study, which provided an overview of the history of public health in the province, confirmed many of the morale problems which the *Issue Paper* had described, and stated:

> There is no common understanding in the Department or in the community of what is meant by a public health program. It is used in reference to a generic category of services, for a single type of service for a specific health care group, and for internal Department activities. This is not merely a semantic problem but leads to other confusions — it is difficult to distinguish between the relative importance of services; it is hard to identify the target population; objectives may be isolated from or in conflict with each other; lack of differentiation occurs between programs which are regulatory, preventive, diagnostic, or therapeutic; it fails to distinguish services and functions within services.[27]

The university's researchers also argued that the Department needed to clarify its objectives, develop a new sense of mission, and recognize the political component of its activities.[28]

The same themes emerged from staff responses. Many of the nurses and hygienists pointed out that their work was not recognized by the public and that their professional colleagues did not appreciate the benefits of the teamwork approach to district health work. The public health inspectors criticized obsolete legislation, administrative confusion in assigning their duties, and lamented health workers' low profile which they believed occurred because "we are working for an ideal in a society we cannot control." Many of the medical services staff felt that their expertise was undervalued, while the dentists noted that demand for their services was increasing yet facilities were declining. Forty-three percent of the staff contributed individual or group responses, indicating significant dissatisfaction with the hierarchical, discipline-oriented structure of the Department and its traditional approach to public health services.[29]

The community responses were similarly wide-ranging. Many of the 224 community comments indicated that recipients were unaware of the programs which the Department provided, and suggested more effective advertising. Others focused on current and future problems including teen pregnancies, drug and alcohol abuse, cultural conflict in the health care system, the elderly, and environmental issues such as water quality and toxic chemicals. Virtually all of the respondents argued in favour of more community input; some applauded the move to community health centres and family practice units while others expressed their disappointment with such facilities.[30] For the Health Planning Steering Committee, one unexpected benefit of distributing 1,800 copies of the *Issue Paper*, was raising public consciousness about the Department. This strategy also confirmed the reformers' support for community involvement and focused programs.

New Roles, New Structure

The results of these studies were apparent in *Public Health for the 1980's*. As its first goal, the report demanded "a public health system which is self-regulating and responsive to change." To ensure a proper "match" between the Department's policies and programs, the authors stressed the importance of modern planning and evaluation techniques based on extensive, on-going data collection and analysis. They urged the staff to focus on primary prevention and recommended the creation of a special group to provide advocacy on health problems. In contrast to their predecessors, the writers broadened the definition of the Department's role to include involvement in activities which belonged to the federal and provincial governments. They also strongly emphasized the need to dismantle obsolete programs and to develop a more sophisticated approach to environmental issues.

To achieve "flexibility, responsiveness, and innovation," the Steering Committee outlined a new administrative structure. This "mixed model" decentralized services, creating a central office where the medical officer and specialized consultants directed data collection and program support activities, and four new health areas where interdisciplinary teams decided

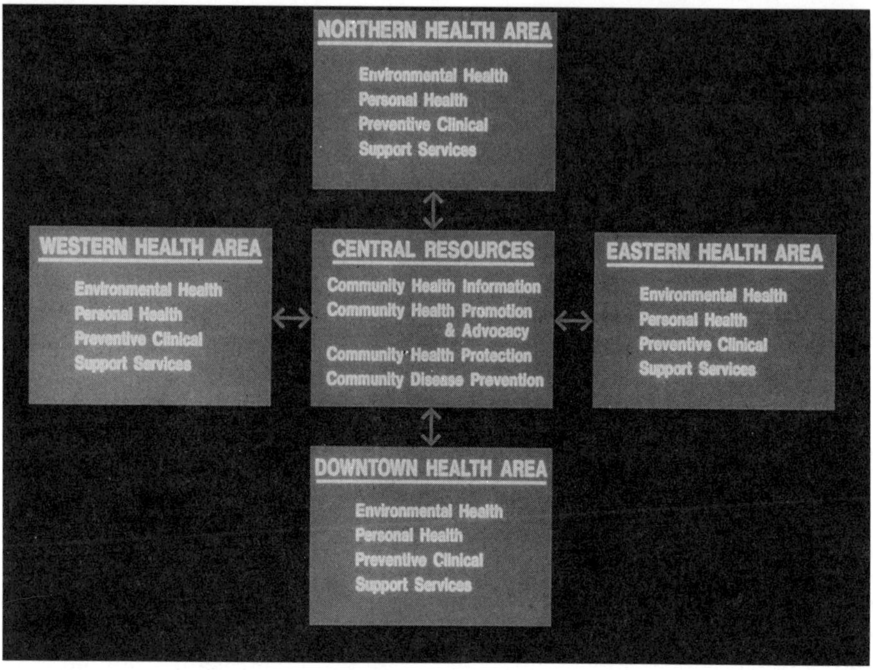

The new administrative structure after decentralization was completed in 1982.

on each area's priorities and programs. The hierarchical model of the past was further eroded by the committee's recommendation for Community Advisory Boards in each health area.[31]

The reformers intended to apply the community model of social development to Toronto's health needs. This theory assumes that local groups can identify problems within their community and, working with experts, devise appropriate solutions to them. The key to this process is understanding the economic and cultural variables which exist in each health area and implementing only the Department's services and programs which best meet these circumstances. To be effective, this approach requires sustained community interest and involvement.

Through its proposal for a complete administrative restructuring, the Steering Committee was consciously breaking with the past. Although it created an Action Team to implement the new system, it ignored the negative connotations of the process. Criticizing one's predecessors for carrying out their legal obligations, and for using the consensus-style policy planning techniques introduced by their British and American colleagues was strategically necessary, but personally destructive. This approach created fear, mistrust, and resistance to change because the reformers were proposing a complete transformation of the Department's work culture. Many older staff felt that their expertise was devalued and were sceptical of the ability of the Community Advisory Boards to maintain public interest in health matters. Only the promise that no one would lose his or her job as a result of decentralization made the new system acceptable to the union and senior staff members. Even those who could accept the need for change were upset by the reformers' casual dismissal of past achievements.[32]

The reformers' proposals were approved by city council in December 1978, and the lengthy process of implementing them was begun with two trial projects: the Health Advocacy Unit and the Eastern Health Area, which was a combination of the East End and Riverdale districts. From 1979 to 1982, the Health Advocacy Unit provided health information and education, conducted some of the Department's public relations activities, and focused on "promotion efforts intended to influence individual and community attitudes towards man-made threats to health." In contrast to their predecessors who had used the medical model of intervention, the unit's members adopted publicity, community organizing, and epidemiological research, as the best methods to attack non-communicable diseases and to remind the public and other levels of government of the importance of prevention. Under the direction of Gerald Caplan, the former director of the New Democratic Party, Toronto's Advocacy Unit earned a reputation as a leader in research and program development for contemporary public health issues. Within the Department, however, the unit was seen as too closely linked to the local board, too politicized, and too prone to publicity stunts. By focusing health promotion activities in one unit, the authors of *Public Health in the 1980's* had been attempting to ensure that their vision was not undermined by bureaucratic inertia; they failed to recognize that the type of ideological and behavioural change that they were recommending required strong support from each staff member.

Some of the pitfalls in this type of reorganization appeared during the first few years of the Eastern Health Area's existence. When the Eastern Health Area office opened in November 1980, organizers intended to use it as a pilot study to limit the trauma of decentralization for the rest of the staff. Factors such as the lack of an associate medical officer and clearly defined core programs meant that the nurses, inspectors, hygienists and support staff generally continued to carry out their previous duties. An Evaluation

The Health Advocacy Unit has the following responsibilities:

- to offer the Department of Public Health and the Local Board of Health skills in the following areas:
  - public advocacy
  - legislative liaison
  - health planning
  - epidemiology and biostatistics
  - public relations
  - health education and promotion
  - community development.

The Health Advocacy Unit.

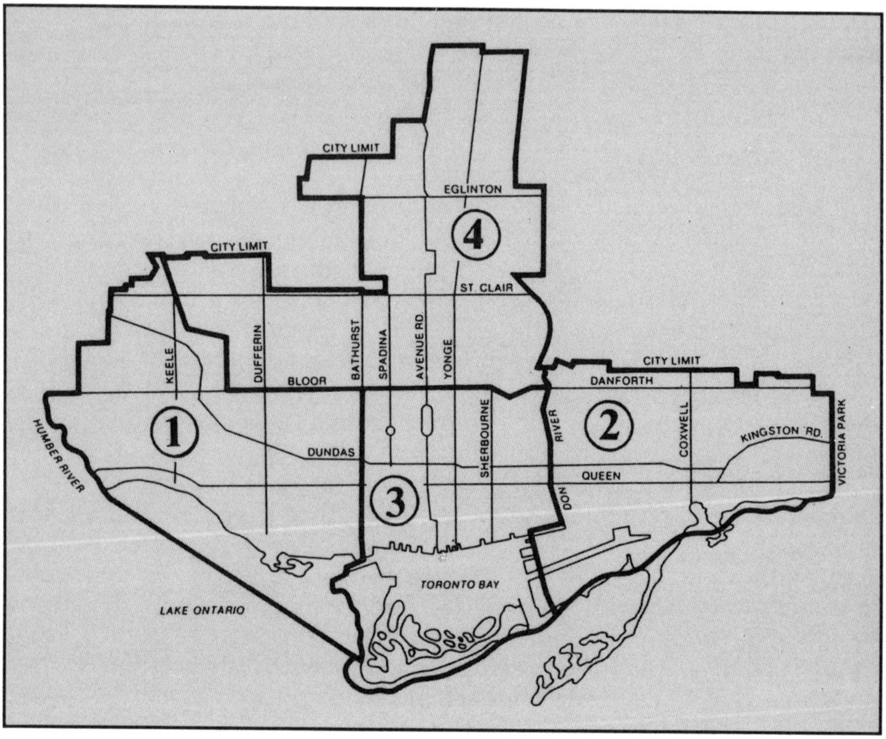

Toronto's eight district offices were amalgamated into four Health Areas between 1979 and 1982.

Task Force set up in 1981, found that the teamwork concept and community involvement were difficult to implement without better understanding of the goals of reorganization and systems management principles. In particular, the unclear relationship between city hall and the health area caused difficulties at the local level. According to the assessment team, the Community Advisory Board's functions also needed further definition, although Department staff had no effective means of ensuring that participants attended the meetings.[33] In the midst of these developments, the medical officer announced his retirement and the local board launched a lengthy search for his successor. The slow process of decentralization ended in 1982 when city council instructed the new medical officer, Dr. A.S. Macpherson, to complete the process by July.

On the eve of its second century, Toronto's Health Department had been restructured to fulfil modern administrative ideals. In each of the four areas, a management team interacted with staff and citizens to focus on specific local needs. The medical officer and his staff carried out general administrative and publicity functions while the four branches of Central Resources — Community Health Protection, Community Health Information, Community Preventive Health, and Community Health Promotion and Advocacy — provided support for all the Department's programs and services. When the province passed its Health Protection and Promotion Act in 1983, Toronto's Department had just completed its reformation and was preparing for a future based on the World Health Organization's definition of health promotion:

> Health promotion is the process of enabling people
> to increase control over, and to improve their health.
> This perspective is derived from a conception of 'health'
> as the extent to which an individual or group is able,
> on the one hand, to change or cope with the environment.
> Health is, therefore, seen as a resource for everyday
> life, not the objective of living; it is a positive
> concept emphasizing social and personal resources, as
> well as physical capabilities.[34]

Conclusion

Between 1950 and 1983, Toronto altered dramatically. So did its Health Department. During these decades, conflict over several different environmental issues tested the Department's ability to respond to contemporary problems and encouraged the transition from medical dominance to public participation in formulating public health policy and implementing public health programs. Unlike cancer, heart disease, mental illness, or addiction, environmental contamination affected everyone. Citizens turned to local governments first during the decade because the federal and provincial governments were only beginning to display interest in these problems. But Toronto's Health Department, like its counterparts elsewhere, was stymied in its attempts to deal with these concerns by lack of power and money. As well, since these issues were not clearly medical, nursing, or inspection problems, the Department had to modify its discipline-based approach to respond to them. By using the methods which had succeeded in the past — investigation, research, and consultation with federal and provincial colleagues — the senior administrators prepared reports which summarized current knowledge and made limited recommendations for action to the local board. In the increasingly confrontational atmosphere of the late 1960s and early 1970s, such efforts did not allay public anxiety.

The lead issue was the catalyst which transformed the Health Department from a service provider to an advocate and innovator. During the controversy, the local board of health opposed both the lead refiners and Ministry of the Environment because the politicians argued that they, not the Department's senior administrators, represented community interests. The switch demonstrated the erosion of professional dominance in policy formation. Restructuring the Department through decentralization and teamwork was intended to complete the transformation. By the 1980s, the federal and provincial governments were also committed to health promotion. Ottawa provided funding for the Health Department's anti-smoking and healthy heart campaigns while the province's revision of its public health legislation introduced "core programs" to ensure that preventive services were widely available. By 1983, the indecision which had racked public health workers about the future of their discipline was gone. Health promotion through community participation had become the foundation for the future.

Conclusion

> Public health is the science and art of preventing disease, prolonging life and promoting physical and mental health and efficiency through organized community efforts.[1]

This definition by the noted American public health expert, Dr. Charles-E.A. Winslow, represented the culmination of decades of public health effort in communities throughout the English-speaking world. With its stress on public health as an art and a science, the definition was acknowledging the complex task facing public health workers: combining service and advocacy. Since 1883 Toronto's Health Department has attempted to fulfil Winslow's definition by responding to the changing political, economic and social developments which have transformed it from a compact, medium-sized centre to a large, multicultural metropolis. These local changes have been paralleled by shifting emphases within the international public health movement, the rise and dominance of curative medicine, and the professionalization of public health practice. The purpose of this study, then, has been to examine the dynamics of the relationship between local factors and long-term trends in preventive medicine and public health.

What lessons does Toronto's experience offer? From the vantage point of more than a century of existence, it is clear that public health activity in the city evolved from a dynamic, socially-conscious reform movement, to a professional bureaucracy which only gradually rediscovered its advocacy role. Toronto's evolution was similar to that of other British, American and Canadian cities but the timing of change was specific to its political and economic circumstances. Like all public institutions, the Health Department had periods of rapid growth and decades of apparent stasis.

Each of these phases corresponded to the evolutionary pattern of the international public health movement. Toronto's health officers and their staffs derived much of their motivation, as well as many of their programs and services, from this source. In the nineteenth century, public health reformers in British, American, and Canadian cities, justified their demands for funding on humanitarian grounds. They argued that unnecessary disease and suffering were too high a price to pay for urban-industrial growth. This viewpoint was widely accepted by other reformers who shared similar religious impulses.[2] Between 1880 and 1920, numerous social reform movements flourished in urban Canada. Temperance, women's rights, "child saving," education reform, and concern about assimilating immigrants, all attracted attention and supporters in Toronto. The common link in all these endeavours was faith in the perfectibility of mankind through expert intervention.[3]

The public health movement formed part of this crusade, which also expressed its belief in the power of science and technology to alleviate the worst of the abuses which were evident in Canada's rapidly growing cities. Public health reformers concentrated their efforts on organizing health departments at the local, provincial, and federal levels. City departments led the way prior to the 1920s, because both senior levels of government were supporting national development schemes. The integration of the reformers' social values with the institutional framework of municipal government, produced conflict between professionals and patronage-oriented politicians because the concept of expertise was an integral component of the reform movement. Professional training was used to legitimize leadership positions and to justify programs and services which required individuals to surrender some of their freedom in return for improvements in the quality of life in the community.

The public health reformers, in particular, debated the issue of public versus private rights. In Toronto, all of the medical officers expressed a preference for "persuasion rather than coercion" and their staff only resorted to prosecution as an extreme measure. Some historians have argued that such activities involved an unacceptable amount of social control, and were a self-serving effort on the part of doctors and other professionals to ensure their economic and political dominance.[4] Such a negative view reflects the 1960s scepticism about all forms of authority and does not do justice to the humanitarian motivations of the majority of public health personnel.

Between 1910 and 1930, the factor which altered the public health movement's ideology was professionalization. During the 1920s, diplomas in public health medicine and nursing became necessary for employment in Toronto's Health Department. Prior to that date, staff had been hired as needed and then encouraged to take further training in their discipline. This shift from amateur to professional health staff took a decade to achieve and was part of the secularisation of the reform movement. Social work concepts and the behavioural sciences, replaced the focus on Christian salvation that had been dominant before 1918. Clients and "distancing" were concepts which fitted into another developing trend in Canadian society at this time: the professional civil servant.

Political neutrality, expertise in a specific field, good management skills, a high tolerance for ambiguity, and anonymity are the characteristics of effective public servants according to modern writers.[5] When Toronto's Health Department was created in 1883, political patronage, not expertise, was the order of the day. As the conflict over the appointment of each of William Canniff's successors demonstrated, city council slowly changed its criteria to focus on professional training. Gordon Jackson's appointment in 1929 signalled the end of the Department's direction by public health reformers and also indicated the council's acceptance of provincially-imposed professional standards. From that point to the 1960s, Toronto's health officers reflected the prevailing emphasis of the international public health movement on research, routine administration, and limited public visibility. Such a change was a marked contrast to the political lobbying and public crusades of their predecessors.

In fact, the seeds of the decline in dynamism were planted by Charles Hastings, whose administration is viewed as the golden age of public health activity in Toronto. When he assumed office in 1910, Hastings decided to reorganize the Department's activities, in keeping with the principles of scientific management that were in operation in Providence, Vancouver, and other North American cities. By dividing the tasks which the inspectors and nurses performed into district and divisional units, Hastings was introducing modern administrative practices. The assumption behind this system was that a highly centralized, hierarchical structure was the most efficient means of ensuring that productivity was maintained.[6] While such systems were successful in the business world, their application to the public service depended on the leadership qualities of the unit supervisors, the medical officer and his deputy, and on external circumstances.

During the 1910s and 1920s, Hastings's genial personality and hands-on management style hid the built-in rigidities of this system. The political and financial support that he received from reform-oriented mayors prior to 1918 also masked potential problems. As a result of Hastings' "flair for health promotion," Toronto earned a well-deserved reputation for innovative services and programs.[7] His successors were faced with the task of coping with structural and personnel problems during depression and war because "public organizations experience constant tension between system building, system transformation, and system decay."[8]

During the 1920s, Toronto's medical profession also began to challenge some of the Health Department's activities. Although the pioneer health officers had been aware of physician opposition to reporting cases of contagious disease, for example, they had assumed that most doctors supported their efforts to improve the environment and control epidemics. The high profile which each of these men had in municipal and medical politics also led them to think that they represented their profession. What they discounted, however, was concern that their efforts would undercut those of young general practitioners, who believed that they could serve the patients who attended the Department's child health clinics and immunization services. This problem intensified in the Great Depression despite the Department's conscious efforts to send patients to their family doctors and dentists and to provide care and medication only for the indigent.

Underlying some of the mainstream doctors' concern was fear of state intervention. Hastings was well-known as an advocate of health insurance, and his successors certainly were affected by discussions on this topic in the 1930s, 1940s, and 1950s. As the old enemies like diphtheria, smallpox and typhoid disappeared, both general practitioners and public health physicians found themselves facing new health threats in the form of chronic and degenerative diseases. As Winslow noted in 1942, these health problems would prove far more intractable than the communicable diseases that they superseded.[9] How could health departments reorganize to meet these needs while continuing to fulfil their statutory obligations in sanitation and disease control? Toronto, like other North American and British cities, grappled with this concern during the 1940s and 1950s.

In contrast to the public attention which had accompanied the introduction of the divisional structure, and the programs and services which developed as the Department expanded its staff to over 500 by 1930, the efforts to refocus on the elderly, immigrants, the mentally ill, and disabled citizens occurred within the Department. What had happened to lessen public interest in preventive services? Improvements in surgical techniques and the introduction of sulphonamides and antibiotics from the late 1930s to the present, enabled the curative approach to dominate public consciousness until the 1960s, when the medical self-help movement emerged. This domination cast public health activities into the shadows and meant that the dichotomy between prevention and cure was never resolved.

Efforts to redefine the Health Department's activities into primary, secondary, and tertiary services were started in the 1950s and 1960s, although they had been implicit since the polio epidemics of the 1930s. These changes evolved very slowly until the 1970s because of the conservatism of senior staff and their adherence to the traditional model of program development. Not until the arrival of younger, activist staff would the Department return to supporting community groups through advocacy.

Further changes also affected public perceptions of the Health Department and its activities. During the 1920s, advertisers used health concerns as a means of selling toothpaste, mouthwash, and other personal hygiene products. Mass circulation magazines and newspapers published these ads while radio broadcast them.[10] How was the Health Department to cope with this flood of information and misinformation? Hastings used his *Health Bulletin*, public addresses, and interviews to combat some of the incorrect information, but his successor was compelled to cease publication as an economy measure during the Depression. As an alternative, the Department turned to material produced by the federal and provincial governments and by voluntary groups like the Canadian Tuberculosis Association, the Canadian Social Hygiene Council, the Canadian Cancer Society, and the Canadian Red Cross. The presence of all these alternate sources of information illustrated the broadening of public health activities and a shift away from control by the city Health Department. Instead of being the leader, Toronto became one player on the team.

By the 1950s and 1960s all preventive agencies were seeking new methods of getting their message to the public. As John Burnham has argued, this task was increasingly difficult as educators and journalists replaced medical scientists in producing and disseminating information. Television further complicated the situation because it stressed the "disease of the week" and the "cure of the week." It also oversimplified complex biological and physiological discoveries for the sake of sensationalism. And even more dangerous in Burnham's estimation, the emphasis on journalistic objectivity and value-free education had robbed health messages of their prescriptive foundation. In contrast to the nineteenth and early twentieth century belief that good health habits based on an understanding of human physiology, would encourage, or perhaps even compel, individuals to live upright lives, the current non-judgmental approach lacks any over-riding imperative to make individuals accept it and act upon it.[11]

The rise of curative medicine, the shift from communicable to lifestyle diseases, and the use of advertising techniques to popularize "health habits" profoundly changed the public's interest in the Health Department. These developments, moreover, were played out against a backdrop of economic, social and political change in Toronto between 1930 and 1983. Although Toronto was not driven into bankruptcy during the Great Depression, spending on public health was cut and the Board of Control used its financial power to bring the Department firmly under control during the Dyke-Bullick incident. As a representative of the second generation of medical officers, Jackson had been trained to administer a large bureaucracy in a period of economic expansion. Like his contemporaries, he found that the cutbacks and lack of hiring accentuated the tendency to inertia which all institutions experience. Even the relative affluence of the war years did not provide relief, as many of the younger staff were serving in the armed forces, and senior staff were looking longingly at retirement.

When the city organized its committee on reconstruction, the Health Department was included in the series of surveys of municipal departments. The Phair Committee reported to the mayor that Toronto's Health Department relied too much on outdated practices, and needed an influx of new blood and an administrative reorganization to deal with post-war problems. This strong condemnation of the Hastings régime reflected the attempts of public health bureaucrats to find a way to reanimate the dynamic reform tradition of the early twentieth century. In fact, the future of the Health Department, like other civic concerns, was ignored in the controversy over the creation of a metropolitan government for Toronto and the surrounding region.

The introduction of Metropolitan Toronto in 1953–54 did not have an immediate impact on the Health Department because most of the Department's accepted duties remained its responsibility. But control over the quality of the city's water supply, sewage treatment, and garbage disposal became Metro's tasks. The most obvious result of this change was the long fight for fluoridation.

By 1957, the creation of Metro had prompted the city to undertake a survey of all its administrative practices. In their report, J.D. Woods and Gordon Limited recommended decentralization of the Health Department. Although this suggestion was not implemented, three years later, the Metro Chairman was arguing in favour of amalgamating all of the health departments within the region.[12] Both of these threats to the structure and services offered by Toronto's Health Department were turned back and the Department continued its incremental approach to dealing with current health problems.

From its dominant leadership role in the nineteenth and early twentieth century, the Department became one voice among many by the 1950s. With the expansion of federal and provincial involvement and funding after 1945, the department became a partner in a series of pilot projects intended to demonstrate the effectiveness of specific activities and intervention. The slow progress toward a national system of health insurance also affected the

Department. What duties would remain if such a system were implemented? Should the senior staff have been able to predict that implementing OHIP would lessen attendance at child welfare and geriatric clinics? And, during the 1970s, should the Department have been lobbying more effectively to modify provincial public health legislation? The 1960s and 1970s were tumultuous decades for health care professionals in Canada and Toronto's Health Department was greatly affected by the changes occurring outside its jurisdiction.

The 1960s, like the 1930s, were a watershed decade. Toronto had started several slum clearance projects in the 1950s and some came to completion in the following decade. The rapid growth of the surrounding regions had encouraged substantial redevelopment in the downtown core. Famous landmarks fell before the wreckers as skyscrapers and highrise apartment buildings altered the city's streets. Optimism about the continuation of the boom was so great that a new city hall was constructed. When it opened in 1965, Health Department staff were thrilled to have more space, even if the building leaked!

The staff were less enthusiastic about some other aspects of the 1960s. Aldermanic critics, like Harold Menzies, held the Department's inspection procedures up to ridicule. The hepatitis outbreak in 1968 demonstrated the lack of public relations skills within the Department. And women's groups protested the lack of city-sponsored birth control clinics, even though counselling on this matter was illegal until the Criminal Code was amended in 1969. The combination of all these factors brought the organizational values of senior management under attack by the junior staff. Medical and nursing education during this decade and the 1970s became increasingly client-oriented. The previous deference to authority was challenged both inside and outside the Department, much to the chagrin of older staff whose sense of professional identity had become an entrenched norm in the organization's work culture.

An urban reform movement, which looked to the early twentieth century for inspiration, also arose in the late 1960s to promote neighbourhood interests and to challenge the development-oriented aldermen who had dominated Toronto's politics during the boom era. In 1972 the reformers won a small majority. One of the first targets of their reforming zeal was the Health Department, which they claimed was unresponsive to community needs because it was still fighting nineteenth century problems. What the reformers failed to recognize, was that much of the Department's activity was defined by the seventeen provincial statutes which applied to it,[13] by the conditions of federal and provincial grants, and by the traditions which formed its organizational culture.

For the next ten years, the reformers struggled to shift the Department, from a classical management structure and an incremental approach to policy development, to systems management and a focus on district needs. They were aided in this by changes in the national and international public health movements. Both groups found a renewed interest in prevention as the cost of curative measures sky-rocketed. Similarly, the recognition that environmental factors and culturally conditioned behaviour affected individual's health shifted the focus away from individual behaviour and onto society as a whole. Clearly, a new advocacy role was unfolding. As the preventive group closest to most Torontonians, the Health Department had to respond to changing needs, to the new theories advanced by public health agencies, and to the old problems that had assumed new guises.

Looking back over the Toronto Health Department's first century is a salutary activity. The historical record reveals the complex interaction of local politics with international ideas, health reformers with health professionals, tradition with innovation, and continuity with change.

Abbreviations

A E H O O	Association of Executive Health Officers of Ontario
A J P H	*American Journal of Public Health*
A P H A	American Public Health Association
A O	Archives of Ontario
B M R	Bureau of Municipal Research
C J P H	*Canadian Journal of Public Health*
C P H A	Canadian Public Health Association
C T A	City of Toronto Archives
D P H	Department of Public Health
L B H	Local Board of Health
M H O	Medical Health Officer (1883–1912)
M O H	Medical Officer of Health (1912–present)
O D H	Ontario Department of Health (1924–1972)
P B H	Provincial Board of Health (1882–1927)
R G	Record Group
T C C	Toronto City Council

Notes

Introduction

1. Heather MacDougall," 'Health is Wealth:' The Development of Public Health Activities in Toronto, 1834–1890," Ph.D. thesis, University of Toronto, 1982.
2. J.M.S. Careless, *Toronto to 1918: An Illustrated History* (Toronto, 1984) 109–48.
3. See Paul Adolphus Bator, " 'Saving Lives on the Wholesale Plan:' Public Health Reform in the City of Toronto, 1900–1930," Ph.D. thesis, University of Toronto, 1979, Jeanne L. Brand, *Doctors and the State: The British Medical Profession and Government Action in Public Health, 1870-1912* (Baltimore, 1965) and Barbara G. Rosenkrantz,*Public Health and the State: Changing Views in Massachusetts, 1842–1936* (Cambridge, Mass., 1972).
4. J.W.S. McCullough, "Early History of Public Health in Upper and Lower Canada," *National Hygiene and Public Welfare*, 58 (Jan. 1922): 17–31; Heather MacDougall, "'Enlightening the Public:' The Views and Values of the Association of Executive Health Officers of Ontario, 1886–1903" in Charles G. Roland, (ed.) *Health, Disease and Medicine: Essays in Canadian History* (Toronto, 1984): 437–8.
5. See R.A. Lewis, *Edwin Chadwick and the Public Health Movement, 1832–1854*(London, 1952), and A.S. Wohl, *Endangered Lives: Public Health in Victorian Britain* (London, 1983).
6. See John M. Eyler, *Victorian Social Medicine: The Ideas and Methods of William Farr* (Baltimore, 1979), M.W. Flinn, *Public Health Reform in Britain* (London, 1968) and R.J. Lambert,*Sir John Simon (1816–1904) and English Social Administration*(London, 1963).
7. There is a controversy over the relative contribution which health officers and the medical profession made to improving health prior to the chemotherapeutic discoveries of the 1930s. Thomas McKeown initiated the discussion in McKeown and R.G. Brown, "Medical Evidence Related to English Population Changes in the Eighteenth Century," *Population Studies*, ix (1955): 119–41 and in his book, *The Modern Rise of Population* (London, 1976). He responded to his critics in *The Origins of Human Disease* (Oxford, 1988). For the most recent and perceptive critique of the McKeown thesis, see Simon Szreter, "The Importance of Social Intervention in Britain's Mortality Decline c.1850-1914: a Re-interpretation of the Role of Public Health," *Social History of Medicine*, 1 (April, 1988): 1–37.
8. See John Duffy, *A History of Public Health in New York City, 1866–1966*, Vol. II, (New York, 1974); Judith Walzer Leavitt, *The Healthiest City: Milwaukee and the Politics of Health Reform* (Princeton, 1982); and Stuart Galishoff's two books, *Safeguarding the Public Health: Newark, 1895–1918* (Westport, Conn.,1975) and *The Nation's Unhealthiest City: Newark 1855–1895* (New Brunswick, 1988). For Canadian developments, see Caroline Gray, *Historical Records of the City of Hamilton, 1847–1973* (Hamilton, 1986); John Taylor, *Ottawa: An Illustrated History* (Toronto, 1986) and Terry Copp, *The Anatomy of Poverty* (Toronto, 1974).
9. See Frederick P. Gorham, "History of Bacteriology and Its Contribution to Public Health Work," and Hugh S. Cumming, "The United States Quarantine System During the Past Fifty Years," in Mazcyk P. Ravenel, (ed.) *A Half Century of Public Health: Jubilee Historical Volume of the American Public Health Association* (New York, 1921, reprinted 1970).
10. R.D. Defries, *The First Forty Years 1914–1955: The Connaught Medical Research Laboratories* (Toronto, 1968).
11. See Charles Chapin, "History of State and Municipal Control of Disease," in Ravenel, op. cit., for a discussion of the evolution of modern public health practices.

Chapter One

1. Canada. Department of National Health and Welfare, *A New Perspective on Health for Canadians: A Working Document* (Ottawa, 1974): 5.
2. *Canadian Practitioner*, 8 (1883): 52.
3. Heather MacDougall, "The Limitations of Public Health in Toronto's Municipal Politics: The Canniff Years, 1883–1890," *Bulletin of the History of Medicine*, 55 (1981): 186–202.
4. Heather MacDougall, "'Health is Wealth': The Development of Public Health Activities in Toronto, 1834–1890," Ph.D. thesis, University of Toronto, 1982, p. 222–46.
5. William Canniff, "Sanitary Education of the Masses, as Conducted in the City of Toronto During a Period of Four Months," *Health and Home*, 1884, p. 34–5.
6. "The City's Health," *News*, January 30, 1884.
7. Heather MacDougall, "'Enlightening the Public': The Views and Values of the Association of Executive Health Officers of Ontario, 1886–1903," in Charles G. Roland, (ed.) *Health, Disease and Medicine: Essays in Canadian History* (Toronto, 1984): 436–40.
8. MacDougall, "Limitations of Public Health Activity," p. 196–7.
9. TCC, *Minutes*, 1890, Appendix, p. 1960–1, 2467.
10. For the British example see Jane Lewis, *What Price Community Medicine?* (Brighton, 1986), and Jessie Parfit, *The Health of a City: Oxford 1770–1974* (Oxford, 1987). For the American model see John Duffy, *A History of Public Health in New York City, 1866–1966* (New York, 1972); Judith Walzer Leavitt, *The Healthiest City: Milwaukee and the Politics of Health Reform* (Princeton, 1982); Stuart Galishoff, *Safeguarding the Public Health: Newark, 1895–1918* (Westport, Conn., 1975), and Galishoff, *Newark: The Nation's Unhealthiest City* (New Brunswick, 1988).
11. *Toronto World*, March 17, 1891, announces Allen's appointment. For his dismissal see TCC, *Minutes*, February 20, 27, 1893, and *Toronto Mail*, February 20, 21, 1893. Allen's obituaries, in the *Globe* and the *Mail & Empire* on October 5, 1922, indicate that he was a surgeon at St. Michael's Hospital, an ardent imperialist and a Conservative party member.
12. Association of Executive Health Officers, *Annual Report* (Toronto, 1897): 35.
13. Undated clipping circa 1905, from Dr. Charles Sheard of Stamford, Connecticut.
14. Maureen Riddell, *The Edmonton Local Board of Health 1871–1980* (Edmonton, 1980): 24–6.
15. Margaret W. Andrews, "The Emergence of Bureaucracy: The Vancouver Health Department, 1886–1914," *Journal of Urban History* (Feb., 1986): 144.
16. Andrews, p. 145–7.
17. City of Toronto Archives, Bator Collection, SC, 215, Communication from Charles Sheard, Esq., M.D., resigning his position as Medical Health Officer of the City of Toronto, September 22, 1910. After his retirement, Sheard was elected as a member of Parliament and lobbied strongly for the creation of a national health department. He and other supporters were successful in 1919.
18. Interview with Mrs. Audrey Williams, Charles Hastings's daughter, June, 1984.
19. Charles J. Hastings, "Democracy and Public Health Administration," *AJPH*, 9 (Feb. and Mar., 1919): 4.
20. Mary Powell, "Public Health Litigation in Ontario, 1884–1920," in Roland op. cit., p. 412–35. See also Charles Humphries, *'Honest Enough to be Bold': The Life and Times of James Pliny Whitney* (Toronto, 1985).
21. Bureau of Municipal Research, *Administrative Study of the Toronto Department of Public Health as of March 1st, 1915* (Toronto, 1915): 1–53 (Hereafter BMR).
22. LBH, Minutes, #24, March 26, 1926.
23. Henry F. Vaughan, "Local Health Services in the United States: The Story of the CAP," *AJPH*, 60 (Jan. 1972): 96–103.
24. LBH, Correspondence, Letters from the City Solicitor, July 21, 27, 1926.
25. For a discussion of the change in attitude see Ramsay Cook, *The Regenerators* (Toronto, 1985), Richard Allen, *The Social Passion* (Toronto, 1971) and Don S. Kirschner, *The Paradox of Professionalism* (New York, 1986).
26. Kirschner, p. 141.
27. *Health Bulletin*, June, 1929.

28. University of Toronto School of Hygiene, *Calendar for 1972–3* (Toronto, 1972) Appendix A: "Historical Developments Influencing Graduate Teaching and Research in Public Health," p. 90. See also Paul Bator and Dr. Andrew J. Rhodes, *Within Reach of Everyone: A History of the University of Toronto School of Hygiene and the Connaught Laboratories*, Vol. 1, 1927–1955 (Ottawa, 1990).
29. See University of Toronto, *Calendar*, 1925–6, p. 407–8; School of Hygiene, *Calendar*, 1940–41, p. 10–11.
30. Charles Hastings, *Report Outlining the Activities of the Medical, Dental and Nursing Services of the Department of Public Health* (Toronto, 1927): 4.
31. Ibid.
32. Frank Denton, "Toronto Leads the World in Public Health Service," *Toronto Star Weekly*, September 27, 1924, p. 18.

Chapter Two

1. Gordon P. Jackson, *City Health Services: An outline of a municipal health programme, as developed by the Department of Public Health, Toronto, Canada.* Reprinted from the Academy of Medicine *Bulletin* (Toronto, 1930): 1.
2. George Rosen, *Preventive Medicine in the United States 1900–1975: Trends and Interpretations* (New York, 1977): 51.
3. See University of Toronto, School of Hygiene, *Calendar*, 1965–6, p. 58–9.
4. Gordon P. Jackson, *City Health Services.*
5. For the Dyke-Bullick incident see Marion Royce, *Eunice Dyke: Health Care Pioneer* (Toronto, 1983): 135–54; *Canada Lancet*, 73 (January, 1933): 45.
6. *Toronto Star*, December 1, 1942, p. 4.
7. See Ira V. Hiscock, *Community Health Organization*, (New York, 1939): 28–41.
8. Ontario Department of Health, *Report of a survey of the Services extended by the Health Department of the City of Toronto with appropriate Recommendations* (Toronto, December 4, 1943): 7. (Hereafter *Phair Report*).
9. CTA, RG 36, A1, Box 2, File: Classification Questionnaires — Health: Leon A. Pequegnat, Deputy Medical Officer of Health, completed January 23, 1946. Interview with Dr. G.W.O. Moss, August, 1986.
10. "Dr. G.P. Jackson Toronto M.O.H. Dies Suddenly," *Toronto Daily Star*, August 14, 1951.
11. Rosen, *Preventive Medicine*, p. 61.
12. LBH, Minutes, #122, May 5, 1947.
13. *Globe & Mail*, Tuesday, September 18, 1951; *Telegram*, September 18, 1951.
14. L.A. Pequegnat, "Changing Responsibilities in Public Health," *CJPH*, 48 (July, 1957): 267–75.
15. Nathan Phillips, Q. C., *Mayor of All the People* (Toronto, 1967): 86.
16. J.D. Woods and Gordon Limited, *Civic Survey* (Toronto, 1957): 267–87.
17. DPH, Correspondence, Letter A.R.J. Boyd to Carl E. Brannan, Executive Assistant, Committee of Implementation, April 30, 1958.
18. Daniel M. Fox, *Health Policies, Health Politics: The British and American Experience 1911–1965* (Princeton, 1986): 114, 168–9.
19. "A Submission to the Royal Commission on Health Services," by the Canadian Public Health Association, *CJPH*, 53 (June, 1962): 229–40.
20. CPHA, Committee on Salaries and Qualifications of Public Health Personnel, *Recommended Qualification Requirements and Minimum Salaries for Public Health Personnel in Canada*, Fifth Revision (Toronto, 1965): 5–6.
21. *Toronto Star*, Saturday, August 17, 1968, p. 11.
22. United States Department of Health, Education and Welfare Public Health Service, *Medical Care in Transition* Vol. III. Reprints from the *American Journal of Public Health*, 1962–66 (U.S. Government Printing Office, 1967): 104–5.
23. LBH, Minutes, April 27, 1971.
24. Interview with Dr. G.W.O. Moss, August, 1986.
25. Ibid.
26. Canadian Public Health Association, *Annual Report*, 1967–8, p. 5–6; 1968–9, p. 10.
27. LBH, Minutes, #102, August 8, 1972.

Chapter Three

1. Theresa George and Jenniece Larsen, "The Culture of Nursing," in Alice Baumgart and J. Larsen, (eds.) *Canadian Nursing Faces the Future: Development and Change* (Toronto, 1988): 63.
2. Robert Wilson, *A Retrospect: A Short review of the steps taken in Sanitation to transform the Town of Muddy York into the Queen City of the West* (Toronto, 1934): 31.
3. *News*, June 6, 1884.
4. William Canniff, "Sanitary Education of the Masses, as Conducted in the City of Toronto During a Period of Four Months," *Health and Home*, 1884, p. 35.
5. Wilson, *A Retrospect*, p. 24.
6. Ibid., 30; Terry Copp, *The Anatomy of Poverty* (Toronto, 1974): 91; Caroline Gray, *Historical Records of the City of Hamilton, 1847–1973* (Hamilton, 1986): 58.
7. W.S. Walton, "The History of the Society of Medical Officers of Health, 1856–1956," *Public Health* (May, 1956): 183–4.
8. BMR, *Report*, 1915, p. 7–8.
9. Ernest W.J. Hague, "Some Modern Tendencies in Public Health Work," *CJPH*, 15 (1924): 526.
10. The Sanitary Inspectors' Association of Canada, Ontario Branch, *CJPH*, 15 (1924): 576–7.
11. W.M. Frazer, *A History of English Public Health, 1834–1939* (London, 1950): 232–3.
12. See "The 1941 Examinations for the Certificate in Sanitary Inspection (Canada)," *CJPH*, 32 (1941): 581–3, for a sample examination paper and a summary of the results of the nation-wide test.
13. CPHA, *Annual Report*, 1954–5, p. 16.
14. J.T. Phair, "The Sanitary Inspector in an Approved Public Health Service," *CJPH*, 36 (June, 1945): 250–2.
15. Interviews with W.D. Connery, June, 1986, and James Flaherty, July, 1986. Ontario Ministry of Health, *Annual Report*, 1981–2, "A Century of Caring, 1881–1982," p. 75.
16. BMR, p. 41.
17. Interview with former inspector Alex McDonald, September, 1986.
18. *Phair Report* (Toronto, 1943): 51; see also G.P. Jackson, "Summary of a study with related comments and recommendations Re: Survey of the Toronto Department of Public Health," June 26, 1944, p. 21–3.
19. Melville F. Matthews, "The Sanitary Inspector and Public Relations," *CJPH*, 34 (1943): 80.
20. Veronica Strong-Boag, *The New Day Recalled* (Toronto, 1988): 203–4.
21. Ontario Department of Health, *Report of the Ontario Health Survey Committee* (Toronto, 1952): 399.
22. CPHA, Annual Report, Part IV, *CJPH*, 55 (September, 1964): 402–3.
23. LBH, Minutes, #302, 1974.
24. University of Toronto Faculty of Medicine, Department of Community Health, *Public Health in the City of Toronto* (Toronto, 1977): 62.
25. Barbara Melosh, *"The Physician's Hand:" Work Culture and Conflict in American Nursing* (Philadelphia, 1982): 114–18.
26. Charles Hastings, "An Outline of Public Health Administration in Toronto." Reprint from the *Medical Journal and Record* (October 26, 1926): 10–11. This paper had originally been presented to the Institute of Hygiene in London, England, June 29, 1926.
27. Marion Royce, *Eunice Dyke: Health Care Pioneer* (Toronto, 1983): 37–40.
28. City of Toronto Archives, RG 11, F1, Nursing Division Historical Files, Dyke's Brown Book. This ledger contains Dyke's version of the early history of her division.
29. Charles J. Hastings, "Nursing Organization as Developed in Toronto," *The Nation's Health* (Feb. 15, 1923): 62. Dyke's Brown Book, p. 312.
30. Eunice H. Dyke, *The Public Health Nurse*, Illinois State Department of Public Health Educational Circular No. 35. Address given before Conference of Illinois Health Officers, Chicago, October 15, 1928, p. 3.

31. Dyke's Brown Book, p. 148.
32. Eunice H. Dyke, *The Public Health Nurse* (Chicago, 1928): 7–8.
33. George M. Weir, *Survey of Nursing Education in Canada* (Toronto, 1932): 141-2. Florence Emory published *Public Health Nursing in Canada: Principles and Practice* (Toronto, 1945) in response to Weir's recommendation.
34. Esther M. Beith, "Supply and Demand of Public Health Nurses," *Canadian Nurse,* 28 (1932): 665.
35. Interview with Mary Willett, July, 1986; material from Madeline Smillie's 1979 retirement address given to researcher in August, 1986.
36. *Phair Report,* p. 37–40; Jackson's response, 1944, p. 29–31; G.P. Jackson, *City Health Services* (Toronto, 1930): 8.
37. A.M. Jeffrey, "How the Private Physician Looks at Public Health Nursing," *Canadian Nurse,* 29 (Jan., 1933): 31–4.
38. Interview with Mary Willett, July, 1986.
39. CTA, RG11, F1, Department of Public Health Nursing Files, Director of Public Health Nursing, *Report,* 1958, p. 2–3. See also Royce, p. 107–8, 117–8 and Dyke's Brown Book.
40. Jean Leask, "The Public Health Nursing Assistant in the Toronto Department of Public Health," *CJPH,* 59 (May, 1960): 194–8.
41. Myrna Clark-Slater and Edna Walsh, "Official and Voluntary Agencies — The Generalist Role," in Miriam Stewart, Jean Innes, Sarah Searl and Carol Smillie, (eds.) *Community Health Nursing in Canada* (Toronto, 1985): 169.
42. Educational consultants' submission to the Department's Health Planning Steering Committee, 1976, p. 1–10.

Chapter Four

1. *Toronto Telegram,* January 16, 1971.
2. *Globe,* November 6, 1884.
3. Edwin Chadwick, *The Sanitary Condition of the Labouring Poor* (London, 1842); R. Lambert, *Sir John Simon (1816–1904) and English Social Administration* (London, 1963); A.S. Wohl, *Endangered Lives* (Cambridge, Mass., 1983).
4. PBH, Fourth Annual Report, *Ontario Sessional Papers,* Vol. 17, Part VII, No. 70, Appendix, 1885, p. 96.
5. William Canniff, "Sanitary Education of the Masses, as Conducted in the City of Toronto During A Period of Four Months," *Health and Home,* 1884, p. 34–36.
6. John Taylor, *Ottawa: An Illustrated History* (Toronto, 1986): 106–08; Carolyn Gray, *Historical Records of the City of Hamilton, 1847–1973* (Hamilton, 1986): 58.
7. *News,* September 11, 1884.
8. PBH, Eighth Annual Report, *Ontario Sessional Papers,* Vol. 22, Part VII, No. 72, 1890, p. 25.
9. Taylor, p. 108; Rosemary Ruth Gagan, "Disease Mortality and Public Health, Hamilton, Ontario, 1900–1914," M.A. thesis, McMaster University, 1981, p. 143, 184.
10. TCC, *Minutes,* LBH, Annual Report, 1904, p. 16–18.
11. Ira V. Hiscock, *Community Health Organization* (New York, 1939): 197–204.
12. *Phair Report,* p. 20–1.
13. CPHA, Study Committee on Public Health Practice, *Report of the Study Committee on Public Health Practice in Canada* (Toronto, 1950): 49.
14. MOH, Monthly Report, January 1933, p. 7; DPH, *Annual Statement,* 1980, p. 96, 98–100.
15. Ibid.
16. LBH, Report No. 3, Monthly Report of the Medical Officer of Health, February 1925, p. 1.
17. Ad. Groulx, *Le Service de Santé de la Ville de Montréal* (Montréal, 1954): 39–40.
18. Interview with Inspector James Flaherty, July, 1986.
19. DPH, *Annual Statement,* 1970, p.132; 1980, p. 99.
20. Interviews with Inspector W.D. Connery, June, 1986, and Inspector James Flaherty, July, 1986.

21. J.M.S. Careless, *Toronto to 1918* (Toronto, 1984): Appendix; James Lemon, *Toronto Since 1918* (Toronto, 1985): Appendix.
22. See Terry Copp, *The Anatomy of Poverty* (Toronto, 1974): 70–87; John Weaver, *Hamilton: An Illustrated History* (Toronto, 1984); Maureen Riddell, *Edmonton Local Board of Health, 1871–1980* (Edmonton, 1980); John Duffy, *A History of Public Health in New York City, 1866–1966* (New York, 1974); Stuart Galishoff, *Newark: The Nation's Unhealthiest City* (New Brunswick, 1988); Judith W. Leavitt, *The Healthiest City* (Princeton, 1982).
23. Shirley Spragge, "A Confluence of Interests: Housing Reform in Toronto, 1900–1920," in A.F.J. Artibise and G. Stelter, (eds.) *The Usable Urban Past* (Toronto, 1979): 247-67.
24. PBH, Tenth Annual Report, 1891, *Ontario Sessional Papers,* Vol. 24, Part V, No. 26, 1892, p. 101–05.
25. Charles Hastings, *Report on Slum Conditions in Toronto* (Toronto, 1911): 19.
26. LBH, Report No. 3, February 1925, p. 2.
27. Riddell, p. 37–8.
28. J.S. Schoales, "Importance of Housing and Lodging-House Inspection," *The Canadian Practitioner and Review,* 62 (March, 1917): 103.
29. MOH, *Monthly Report,* May 1925.
30. Advisory Committee, *Report of the Lieutenant-Governor's Committee on Housing Conditions in Toronto* (Toronto, 1934): 55, 68. (Hereafter *Bruce Report.*)
31. *Bruce Report,* 68.
32. LBH, Correspondence, Mayor Day to the Local Board of Health, June 18, 1934.
33. Riddell, p. 42–3.
34. CTA, RG 36, A1, Box 2, File: Classification Questionnaires — Health A–H. This questionnaire was completed by Herbert James Armitage, a full-time health inspector with the Sanitation Division on September 24, 1945. Armitage had completed the Public Health Certificate of the Royal Sanitary Institute to qualify for his position.
35. Hiscock, 198.
36. CPHA, Study Committee on Public Health Practice, *Report of the Study Committee on Public Health Practice* (Toronto, 1950): 50.
37. Albert Rose, *Regent Park* (Toronto, 1958): 144–46.
38. The creation of the Metropolitan Toronto Housing Authority in 1955 also played a role, as Frederick Gardiner, the first Metro Chairman, did not believe in slum clearance and wanted to build homes in the suburbs. See T. Colton, *Big Daddy: Frederick G. Gardiner and the Building of Metropolitan Toronto* (Toronto, 1980): 161-2.
39. *Telegram,* "Ghetto of Poverty," March 4, 1965, p. 33; interview with Inspector James Flaherty, July, 1986.
40. Flaherty interview.
41. DPH, *Annual Statement,* 1965, p. 102–3; 1967, p. 108.
42. DPH, *Annual Statement,* 1968, p. 126–7; 1971, p. 129–30.
43. Henry Mietkiewicz and Bob Mackowycz, *Dream Tower: The Life and Legacy of Rochdale College* (Toronto, 1988): 29.
44. Mietkiewicz and Mackowycz, p. 29, 71; interview with James Flaherty, July, 1986.
45. *News,* October 5, 1886.
46. Charles M. Sheard, "City of Toronto Disposal of Sewage and Water Filtration," *Empire Club Speeches, 1907–08* (Toronto, 1910): 77.
47. ODH, Fifteenth Annual Report, for the Year 1939, *Ontario Sessional Papers,* Vol. 72, Part IV, No. 14, 1940, p. 144.
48. MOH, *Monthly Report,* June, 1938, p. 3; LBH, Minutes, 1942.
49. In *Big Daddy,* Colton points out that as the first chairman of Metro, Gardiner stated that five modernized water filtration plants, almost 200 miles of trunk sewers and watermains, two new sewage treatment plants and six remodelled ones had been brought into operation by 1961, p. 160; *Toronto Daily Star* August 18, 1959, p. 1; *Globe & Mail* April 13, 1967, p. 6.
50. City of Toronto, DPH, *Toronto's Drinking Water: A Chemical Assessment* (April, 1984): 19, in fact says that more sophisticated testing methods, used in the early 1980s, had doubled the number of contaminants discovered to 800.
51. City of Toronto, LBH, Report of the Health Planning Steering Committee, *Public Health in the 1980's* (Toronto, 1978): 55.

52. *News*, December 31, 1886.
53. K.M. Yorke, "Saving Lives on the Wholesale Plan: How Toronto Has Been Made the Healthiest of Large Cities," *Maclean's Magazine*, 28 (July, 1915): 20–2, 93–6.
54. Frederick P. Gorham, "The History of Bacteriology and Its Contribution to Public Health Work," in M.P. Ravenel, (ed.) *A Half Century of Public Health* (New York, 1921, reprinted 1970): 81–2; *Toronto Daily Star*, March 21, 1910; Wilson G. Smellie, *Public Health: Its Promise for the Future* (New York, 1955): 345–6, 350.
55. Yorke, 21; F. Adams, "Water Chlorination Experience at Toronto, Canada," *American Journal of Public Health*, 6 (1916): 867–69.
56. N.J. Howard, "Observations in the Toronto Filtration Laboratories During the Past 25 Years." Reprinted from *Journal of the American Waterworks Association*, 29 (February, 1937): 173–87; see also ODH, Tenth Annual Report for 1934, *Ontario Sessional Papers*, Vol. 67, Part IV, No. 14, 1935, p. 64.
57. MOH, *Monthly Report*, February 12, 1934, p. 15.
58. *CJPH*, 33 (1942): 49–50.
59. LBH, Minutes, February 20, 1963.
60. *Toronto's Drinking Water: A Chemical Assessment*, p. 2–15.

Chapter Five

1. "Don't All Apply At Once," *News*, February 7, 1883.
2. MHO, *Annual Report*, 1886.
3. See MHO, *Annual Reports*, 1896, 1897, 1904.
4. MacDougall, "Health is Wealth," Ph.D. thesis, University of Toronto, 1982, p. 282–326; Bureau of Municipal Research *Administrative Study of the Toronto Department of Public Health as of March 1st, 1915* (Toronto, 1915): 40–42. (Hereafter BMR).
5. A.R.B. Richmond, "Food Control in Toronto," *CJPH*, 26 (1935): 422–27.
6. *Globe & Mail*, Oct. 9, 1957, p. 4; Oct. 16, 1957, p. 4; Jan. 17, 1958, p. 5.
7. *Globe & Mail*, March 3, 1960, p. 31; March 4, 1960, p. 1; March 10, 1960, p. 5.
8. LBH, Special Meeting January 31, 1962, Minutes, #19; Ibid., Special Meeting, November 14, 1962, Minutes, #148.
9. *Toronto Telegram*, December 7, 1962, p. 47.
10. Maureen Riddell, *Edmonton Local Board of Health, 1871–1980* (Edmonton, 1980): 114–5.
11. PBH, Eighth Annual Report, *Ontario Sessional Papers*, Vol. 22, Part VII, No. 72, 1890, p. 24.
12. Mary Powell, "Public Health Litigation in Ontario, 1884–1920," in C.G. Roland, (ed.) *Health, Disease and Medicine: Essays in Canadian History* (Toronto, 1984): 412–35. In fact, the Council *Minutes* indicate that the City Solicitor wanted the Council to pay the fine since the legal principle had been established.
13. MHO, *Annual Reports*, 1893, 1896, 1897, 1899; see also, AEHOO, *Annual Report*, 1900, p. 8.
14. TCC, *Minutes*, 1909, LBH, Report No. 1, p. 126–7.
15. Paul Adolphus Bator, "'Saving Lives on the Wholesale Plan': Public Health Reform in the City of Toronto, 1900–1930," Ph.D. thesis, University of Toronto, 1979, and Cynthia Abeele, "'Nations are made of Babies': Maternal and Child Welfare in Ontario, 1914–1940," Ph.D. thesis, University of Guelph, 1987.
16. Interview with Mrs. Audrey Williams, Hastings's daughter, June, 1984; *Toronto Star*, January 20, 1931.
17. TCC, *Minutes*, 1910, LBH, Report No. 9, Nov. 2, 1910.
18. *Health Bulletin*, November, 1912.
19. *News*, July 5, 1911; Abeele thesis, p. 92.
20. BMR, p. 10–11.
21. Charles E. North, "Milk and Its Relation to Public Health," in M.P. Ravenel, (ed.), *A Half Century of Public Health* (New York, 1921 reprinted 1970): 236–89; Riddell, p. 14–15, 58, 115–6. In fact, Edmonton did not make pasteurization compulsory until 1974.
22. Interview with Nancy Laing, August, 1986; letter from Mrs. Mary Sheen, Charles Sheard's niece, August 7, 1986.

23. *Health Bulletin*, June, 1911, April, May, September, October, November, December, 1912, February, April, May, July, 1913; Medical Officer of Health, *Monthly Report*, July, August, 1913.
24. Charles E. North, "Milk and Its Relation to Public Health," in Ravenel, p. 236-89.
25. Geddes Smith, "Health Un-Ltd.", *The Survey*, October, 1924, p. 44.
26. "Toronto's Milk Campaign," *Public Health Journal*, 12 (1921): 183-4.
27. Charles Hastings, *Report of the Medical Officer of Health on the Safeguarding of Toronto's Milk Supply with special reference to Pasteurization* (Toronto, 1915, revised 1926); *Health Bulletin*, September 7, 1929, p. 2.
28. Charles J. Hastings, *How Can We Best Safeguard Our Milk Supply?* (Washington: Government Printing Office, 1924).
29. LBH, Report No. 3, Monthly Report of the Medical Officer of Health, February 1934, p. 12. The Department's interest in the quality of milk supplies remained high as the following articles demonstrate: A.B. Moffat and J. MacKay, Division of Laboratories, Department of Public Health, City of Toronto, "The Coliform Test in Pasteurized Milk," *CJPH*, 29 (June, 1938): 283–87; A.R.B. Richmond, "The Production of Clean Milk," *CJPH*, 32 (April, 1941): 163–68.
30. MOH, *Monthly Report*, February, 1934, p. 11, 13.
31. *Phair Report*, 1943, p. 31.
32. DPH, *Annual Statement*, 1975, p. 104.
33. BMR, p. 42–3.
34. LBH, Minutes, October 13, 1923.
35. *Health Bulletin*, September 7, 1929, p. 4.
36. Richmond, "Food Control in Toronto," p. 426.
37. LBH, Minutes, September 30, 1943.
38. LBH, Minutes, 1945.
39. Interview with Inspector W.D. Connery, June, 1986.
40. *Globe & Mail*, Saturday, November 22, 1986, A1, A15. Edmonton experienced similar concerns, and in 1974 its Environmental Health section staff argued that publicizing the names of restaurants that were closed would succeed only if equal publicity was given to those who were allowed to re-open after they had complied with the Department's requirements.
41. *Telegram*, November 7, 1956, p. 13.
42. DPH, *Annual Statement*, 1967, p. 126–7.
43. DPH, *Annual Statement*, 1980, p. 95.
44. Ira V. Hiscock, *Community Health Organization* (New York, 1939): 192.
45. LBH, Minutes, December 30, 1944.
46. LBH, Minutes, February 14, 1944.
47. *Health*, October, 1964, p. 18–19, 29; see also *Globe & Mail*, August 15, 1963.
48. CPHA, Study Committee on Public Health Practice, *Report of the Study Committee on Public Health Practice* (Toronto, 1950): 49.
49. Interview with W.D. Connery who served as a restaurant inspector from 1948 to 1958.
50. *Globe & Mail*, June 9, 1960, p. 5.
51. DPH, *Annual Statement*, 1964, p. 91–3.
52. DPH, *Annual Statement*, 1965, p. 113–115.
53. Interview with W.D. Connery, June, 1986.
54. DPH, *Annual Statement*, 1977, p. 5.
55. DPH, *Annual Statement*, 1980, p. 87.
56. Health Department Correspondence, L.A. Pequegnat to W.S. Dunfield, May 17, 1956; copy Dunfield to Pequegnat same day.
57. Interview with former inspector Alex McDonald, September, 1986.
58. In his interview, Bud Connery recollected how patrons had responded to one restaurateur's efforts to conform to Health Department orders to improve the cleanliness of his restrooms; someone broke the toilet and put paper towels all over the newly painted walls.
59. *Telegram*, October 15, 1971.
60. John Last, *Public Health and Human Ecology* (East Norwalk, Conn., 1987): 122-3. Accord-

ing to recent newspaper reports, a third strain, Hepatitis C, which is non-A and non-B has just been identified.

61. *Globe & Mail,* August 8, 9, 10, 13, 14, 15, 16, 17, 1968; *Telegram,* August 3, 6, 13, 1968; *Toronto Star,* August 17, 1968.
62. DPH, *Annual Statement,* 1968, p. 125–6.
63. DPH, *Annual Statement,* 1965, p. 116–7.
64. DPH, *Annual Statement,* 1973, p. 124–5.
65. DPH, *Annual Statement,* 1976, p. 7–8.
66. DPH, *Annual Statement,* 1975, p. 81, 104.
67. DPH, *Annual Statement,* 1976, p. 7–8.

Chapter Six

1. MOH, *Monthly Report,* November, 1919, p. 1.
2. American Public Health Association, *Communicable Diseases in Man* (Washington, 1981): 315–6.
3. City of Toronto, Medical Health Department, *Annual Report,* 1888, p. 59–62.
4. *News,* August 18, 19, 1885.
5. Ad. Groulx, *Le Service de Santé de la Ville de Montréal* (Montréal, 1954): 8.
6. MacDougall, "'Health is Wealth': The Development of Public Health Activity in Toronto, 1834–1890," p. 222–281.
7. This horse drawn ambulance was the first vehicle in what became the Division of Morgue and Ambulances in 1912. During World War I, the first motorized ambulance was purchased and in 1933, the Police Department turned the responsibility for assisting accident victims over to the Health Department. Labour and parts shortages in World War II led the board of health to contract with private ambulance companies to ensure citizens speedy transportation to medical facilities. Although the various health departments in Metropolitan Toronto did not unite in 1953, Metro's interest in co-ordinating regional services led it to create the Metropolitan Ambulance Service in 1967 to provide prompt responses to emergency situations throughout the rapidly growing suburbs.
8. LBH, Minutes, April 24, 1944; MOH, *Monthly Report,* August, 1931, p. 2.
9. Department of Health, *Annual Report,* 1893, p. 7.
10. CTA, RG 11, Department of Public Health, Shutt Scrapbook, newspaper clipping dated 1910.
11. AEHOO, *Annual Report,* 1897 (Toronto, 1898): 4–10.
12. *News,* September 14, 26, 1885.
13. LBH, *Annual Report,* 1886, p. 9; *Annual Report,* 1888, Appendix, p. 58.
14. Barbara Craig, "Smallpox in Ontario: Perception of Disease, 1884-1885," in C.G. Roland, (ed.) *Health, Disease and Medicine: Essays in Canadian History* (Toronto, 1984): 245. In her note, Dr. Craig states that Ross was stopped on the Montreal-Toronto train by Provincial Board of Health inspectors who discovered a recent vaccination mark. While this may have affected his credibility in 1885, it evidently did not deter him from creating his organization in 1888.
15. *News,* October 20, 1888.
16. Craig, op. cit., p. 227, 229; Paul Adolphus Bator, "The Health Reformers versus the Common Canadian: The Controversy over Compulsory Vaccination Against Smallpox in Toronto and Ontario, 1900-1920," *Ontario History,* 74, no. 4 (December, 1983): 348-73.
17. MHO, *Annual Report,* 1899, p. 6-10.
18. AEHOO, *Annual Report,* 1900 (Toronto, 1901): 10-13.
19. Ibid.; MHO, *Annual Report,* 1904, p. 14.
20. *Toronto Daily Star,* March 2, 1906, p. 7; *World,* March 14, 1906, p. 10.
21. Maureen Riddell, *Edmonton Local Board of Health, 1871-1980* (Edmonton, 1980): 15, 21.
22. Bator, "The Health Reformers...," p. 355; Katharine Arnup, "The Struggle over Compulsory Vaccination in the City of Toronto 1900–1920," unpublished paper presented to the Canadian Historical Association, June 1985.

23. *World*, November 20, 1919.
24. *World*, November 7, 10, 20, December 11, 1919; *Telegram*, November 27, 1919; *Toronto Daily Star*, December 6, 8, 1919; *Mail & Empire*, December 11, 1919.
25. J.G. FitzGerald, *An Introduction to the Practice of Preventive Medicine* (St. Louis, 1926): 208–9.
26. MOH, *Monthly Report*, February, 1924, p. 1–2; *Mail & Empire*, February 8, 1928.
27. A similar, but more violent and deadly public opposition to smallpox vaccination in 1894 is analyzed in Judith Walzer Leavitt, "Politics and Public Health: Smallpox in Milwaukee, 1894–1895," in J.W. Leavitt and R.L. Numbers, (eds.) *Sickness & Health in America* (Madison, 1978): 403–414.
28. *Phair Report*, p. 15–6.
29. Interview with Dr. G.W.O. Moss, August, 1986. Dr. Moss stated that the family had stopped in New York City to give lectures and when the news of the disease was passed on to the American authorities great concern arose. New York's Health Department undertook a mass vaccination campaign to combat a potential outbreak.
30. Katherine McCuaig, "'From Social Reform to Social Service.' The Changing Role of Volunteers: The Anti-tuberculosis Campaign, 1900–1930," *Canadian Historical Review*, 61 (December, 1980): 480–1.
31. LBH, *Annual Report*, 1899.
32. M.L. Meiklejohn, "Anti-tuberculosis Work in Canada," *Canadian Nurse*, 3 (November, 1907): 581–2, 585.
33. *Health Bulletin*, December, 1911, p. 1–2.
34. E.H. Dyke, "Report of the Tuberculosis Visiting Nurses in Toronto," *Canadian Nurse*, 8 (July, 1912): 379–80.
35. Dr. Howard Seiden, "Tuberculosis still problem disease," *Toronto Star*, May 3, 1984; *Communicable Diseases in Man*, p. 372–78. The occurrence rate according to the APHA is 30% for contacts.
36. Ira V. Hiscock, *Community Health Organization* (New York, 1939): 100.
37. R.D. Defries, (ed.) *The Development of Public Health in Canada* (Toronto, 1940): 84–5.
38. Ibid., p. 84; LBH, Minutes, August 9, 1938.
39. Hiscock, p. 99–121.
40. *Phair Report* (Toronto, 1943): 18–20; City of Toronto Department of Public Health, Summary of a study, with related comments and recommendations Re: Survey of Toronto Department of Health. Submitted to the Local Board of Health by Gordon Park Jackson, Medical Officer of Health, June 26, 1944, p. 9–11.
41. LBH, Minutes, September 11, 17, 19, 21, 25, 1945.
42. DPH, *Annual Statement*, 1967, p. 72–3.
43. DPH, *Annual Statement*, 1980, p. 26–28.
44. DPH, *Annual Statement*, 1981, p. 5, 23.
45. MOH, *Monthly Report*, November, 1919, p. 5.

Chapter Seven

1. University of Toronto, Faculty of Medicine, Department of Community Health, *Public Health in the City of Toronto* (Toronto, 1977): 135.
2. George Rosen, *Preventive Medicine in the United States 1900–1975: Trends and Interpretations* (New York, 1977): 63.
3. Harry F. Dowling, *Fighting Infection* (Cambridge, Mass., 1977): 18–19.
4. PBH, Nineteenth Annual Report, *Ontario Sessional Papers*, Vol. 33, Part VI, No. 33, 1901, p. 30.
5. AEHOO, *Annual Report*, 1897, p. 35.
6. Allan Chase, *Magic Shots* (New York, 1982): 183.
7. John Ferguson, *The Ontario Medical Association, 1880–1930* (Toronto, 1930): 45.
8. Letter dated August 7, 1986 from Mrs. Mary Sheen, Charles Sheard's niece, describing her childhood experience with the city's disease control measures.
9. Chase, p. 184–7; Dowling, p. 29–30.

10. R.D. Defries, *The First Forty Years, 1914–1955: Connaught Medical Research Laboratories* (Toronto, 1968): 1.
11. *Health Bulletin*, May, 1916, p. 3.
12. *Health Bulletin*, September, 1915, p. 3.
13. Interview with Alex McDonald, September, 1986.
14. *Health Bulletin*, April, 1913.
15. Chase, p. 188–90, 199–201; Maureen Riddell, *Edmonton Local Board of Health, 1871–1980* (Edmonton, 1980): p. 22, 32.
16. Defries, *The First Forty Years*, p. 79. Ramon's toxoid produced less reaction and serum sickness than Park's product. See also C.E. Dolman, "Landmarks and Pioneers in the Control of Diphtheria," *CJPH*, 64 (July-August, 1973): 319–20.
17. "City's Health Board Not Told Inoculation Permitted to Lapse," *Toronto Star*, January 19, 1931.
18. Health Department Correspondence, G.P. Jackson to Mayor William Stewart and the Board of Control, June 30, 1931.
19. On page 320 of his article, Dolman says that Hamilton had only one reported case of diphtheria in 1932 and no deaths in either 1931 or 1932.
20. *Globe & Mail*, November 14, 1987, C3.
21. Sidney M. Katz, "A City Without Diphtheria," *Health*, March 1941, p. 8, 17; Mabel Ferris, "Toronto's Toxoid Week," *Health*, Spring Issue 1944, p. 16, 27, 29; Jane Lewis, "The Prevention of Diphtheria in Canada and Britain 1914–1945," *Journal of Social History* (Fall, 1986): 163–76.
22. Academy of Medicine, *Bulletin* (June, 1942): 176–7.
23. CPHA, Study Committee on Public Health Practice, *Report of the Study Committee on Public Health Practice in Canada* (Toronto, 1950): 41–2.
24. G.W.O. Moss, "Use of Antigens," *CJPH*, 51 (April, 1960): 129–30.
25. *Telegram*, November 16, 1962, p. 1–2.
26. *Globe & Mail*, December 7, 1963.
27. Frances L. Perkins, *Summary of Staff Submissions* (May, 1978): 13; interview with Dr. Mavis Rampersaud, former director of the Medical Services Division, July, 1986.
28. Dowling, p. 204.
29. Dowling, p. 205–6, 209–10.
30. *Health Bulletin*, September, 1926; MOH, *Monthly Report*, July, 1929.
31. *Toronto Star*, August 12, 18, 19, 30, September 11, October 28, 1930.
32. Dowling, p. 106.
33. MOH, *Monthly Report*, September, 1934; interview with Nancy Laing, September, 1986.
34. Dowling, p. 206–7, 211–12.
35. TCC, *Minutes*, Appendix, Report of the Medical Officer of Health Dealing with the Infantile Paralysis Situation, September 20, 1937, p. 13.
36. Veronica Strong-Boag, *A New Day Recalled* (Toronto, 1988): 10.
37 F.F. Tisdall, Alan Brown, R.D. Defries, M.A. Ross and A.H. Sellers, "Zinc-Sulphate Nasal Spray in the Prophylaxis of Poliomyelitis," *CJPH*, 27 (November, 1937): 523–543.
38. Scott Young, *Neil and Me* (Toronto, 1988): 34–6.
39. DPH, *Annual Statement*, 1953, p.19.
40. Dowling, p. 212–15; J.W.K. Ferguson, "The Story of Poliomyelitis Vaccines," *CJPH*, 55 (May, 1964): 183–90.
41. Dowling, p. 215.
42. Paul Martin, *A Very Public Life*, Vol. 2 (Toronto, 1982): 72–5. Both Paul Martin and his son, Paul Martin Jr., suffered from polio as children and part of his decision was based on his determination to prevent other families from suffering the fear that his family had experienced. He also consulted widely with Canadian medical experts and had great confidence in the quality of the vaccine produced in this country.
43. C.S. Anglin and N.L. Silverthorne, "Where do we stand on Polio Immunization?," *Health*, July-August, 1956, p. 10–11, 22.
44. LBH, Minutes, #117, #118, August 25, 1959.
45. DPH, *Annual Statement*, 1959, p. 107–8; LBH, Minutes, #125, September 2, 1959.
46. "Polio a Threat to Everyone!-MOH," *Toronto Telegram*, April 24, 1961, p. 1.

47. The Salk vaccine produced antibodies in the blood and nasal secretions but not in the intestines. Many immunologists saw the Sabin vaccine as a booster for those already immunized by the Salk vaccine. Toronto area health officers had been prominent in assessing the effectiveness of the Salk vaccine. For example, see G.W.O. Moss and W.M. Mosley, "Immunization: Equipment and Technique," *CJPH*, 46 (March, 1955): 128–9; C.W.J. Armstrong, G.W.O. Moss, F.C. Potter, "The Antibody Response to Poliomyelitis Vaccine in School-Children at the Time of Initial Vaccination and One Year Later," *CJPH*, 48 (March, 1957): 96–100; D.R.E. MacLeod, C.W.J. Armstrong, G.W.O. Moss, F.C. Potter, R.J. Wilson, "Poliovirus Antibody Response After Various Vaccination Schedules and at Different Ages," *Canadian Medical Association Journal*, 81 (September, 1959): 443–9; G.W.O. Moss, "Observations on the Use of Antigens," *CJPH*, 51 (April, 1960): 129-34; R.J. Wilson, G.W.O. Moss, J.P. Jacobs, D.R.E. MacLeod, "Persistence of Antibody Following Booster Dose of Poliomyelitis Vaccine," *CJPH*, 53 (January, 1962): 17–21.
48. A.R.J. Boyd and W. Mosley, "The Use of Poliovirus Vaccine Live, Oral (Sabin), Trivalent, in Metropolitan Toronto, 1962," *CJPH*, 53 (August, 1962): 326–9; G.W.O. Moss, "Immunization Procedures-National and International," Panel Presentation to a joint meeting of the Canadian and Ontario Medical Associations, June 14, 1963.
49. *Toronto Star*, March 6, May 1, 5, 1962; *Telegram*, May 16, 1962.
50. John Duffy, *A History of Public Health in New York City, 1866–1966* (New York, 1974): 332; Riddell, p. 46–7.
51. Moss, "Observations on the Use of Antigens," *CJPH*, 51 (April, 1960): 134.

Chapter Eight

1. MOH, *Monthly Report*, November, 1914, p. 261.
2. Cynthia Abeele, "'Nations are Built of Babies': Maternal and Child Welfare in Ontario, 1914–1940," Ph.D. thesis, University of Guelph, 1987, p. 93; R.E. Mills, "Birth Registration and the Public Health Department," City of Toronto Archives, RG 11, Public Health Historical Files, c. 1915, p. 3.
3. Ann Oakley, *The Captured Womb* (Oxford, 1986): 37–44; Judith W. Leavitt, *The Healthiest City* (Princeton, 1982): 216–27.
4. CTA, RG 11, Nursing Division Historical Files, Dyke's Brown Book, p. 386-82. Dyke used several portions of this ledger book to record aspects of the early years of the Division of Public Health nursing and as a result the pagination is reversed.
5. Dyke's Brown Book, p. 382–1.
6. Abeele, op. cit., Ch. 2. See also Veronica Strong-Boag, *The New Day Recalled* (Toronto, 1988): 150–2, 162–4, 168.
7. J.G. FitzGerald, *An Introduction to the Practice of Preventive Medicine* (St. Louis, 1926): 522–44.
8. Toronto Academy of Medicine, *Bulletin* (February, 1929): 7–8.
9. E. Dyke, "Team Play for Health," *Canadian Nurse*, 15 (December, 1919): 2175–9; "A Day with the District Nurse," *Toronto Sunday World*, Magazine Section, October 26, 1924, p. 18.
10. Dyke's Brown Book, 1914, 1915, 1917; TCC, *Minutes*, #324, 1925.
11. Strong-Boag, p. 164-68; see also John Burnham, *How Science Lost and Superstition Won* (New Brunswick and London, 1987): Ch. 2.
12. CTA, RG 11, F1, Box 1, Nursing Historical Files, undated speech entitled, "Changing Practices in Infant Hygiene." Internal evidence commenting on the impact of the Depression suggests that this was written in 1936 or 1937. In the same file, see also the Department's well-known pamphlet, *The Care of the Baby*, dated June 24, 1935.
13. Academy of Medicine, *Bulletin* (February, 1929): 7–8; (April, 1929): 17–8; George Rosen, *Preventive Medicine in the United States 1900–1975: Trends and Interpretations* (New York, 1975): 45–6, 53–4.
14. MOH, *Monthly Report*, April, 1924.
15. LBH, Minutes, November 8, 1933.

16. LBH Correspondence, G.P. Jackson to the Local Board of Health, November 28, 1933.
17. Jane Lewis, *What Price Community Medicine?* (Brighton, 1986): 30–1; Rosen, op. cit.
18. Summary of a Study with related comments and recommendations Re: Survey of Toronto Department of Public Health Submitted to the Local Board of Health by G.P. Jackson, June 26, 1944, p. 16.
19. Pre-School Examinations for Hillcrest District, a one page announcement in the Academy of Medicine, *Bulletin*, 25 (July, 1952): 135–6; L.A. Pequegnat, "Plans of the Toronto Department of Public Health," Ibid., 26 (December, 1952): 41–6.
20. G.K. Martin and K.B. Ladd, "Maternal and Child Health Services in Ontario, 1958," *CJPH*, 52 (March, 1961): 111–19.
21. R.B. Freeman, in *Nursing Outlook*, 9, (1961): 605–7.
22. CTA, RG 11, F1, Box 1, Nursing Historical Files, Reports on the Child Health Centres, 1961, and Maternal and Child Health: the Program of Visiting Based on Developmental Aspects of Growth and Maturation, March 14, 1962.
23. DPH, *Annual Statement*, 1961, p. 67-9.
24. Jessie Parfit, *The Health of a City: Oxford, 1774–1974* (Oxford, 1987): 113.
25. University of Toronto, Faculty of Medicine, Department of Community Health, *Public Health in the City of Toronto* (Toronto, 1977): 135.
26. Charles Hastings, "The Value of the Public Health Nurse in Health and Welfare Administration," *AJPH* (1920): 712–16.
27. Oakley, p. 44–5, 54–6.
28. Charles Hastings, *A Report on the Medical, Dental and Nursing Services in the City of Toronto* (Toronto, 1927): 7.
29. BMR, p. 27.
30. Marion Royce, *Eunice Dyke: Health Care Pioneer* (Toronto, 1983): 93–4.
31. Daphne Read, (ed.) *The Great War and Canadian Society: An Oral History* (Toronto, 1978): 62–3; Strong-Boag, p. 150–3, 157–61.
32. Abeele, p. 136–140.
33. MOH, *Monthly Report*, February, 1936, p. 8.
34. Alice Thomson, "The City of Toronto Maternal Welfare Service," *The Trained Nurse and Hospital Review*, October 1, 1940, p. 1–5.
35. Thomson, op. cit.
36. Maud Stapley, "An Experiment in Prenatal Education," *Canadian Nurse* (February, 1948), p. 1–3.
37. Maureen Riddell, *Edmonton's Local Board of Health 1871–1980* (Edmonton, 1980): 98.
38. "Father's Classes — What Next?," *Health* (May-June, 1953): 24.
39. City of Toronto, LBH, Report of the Health Planning Steering Committee, *Public Health in the 1980's* (Toronto, 1978): 55.
40. DPH, *Annual Statement*, 1980, p. 153; May Yoshida and Mary Davies, "Contemporary Canadian Investigations 1 An Innovative Project - Childbearing and Childrearing: Recent Immigrant Families in the Urban Toronto Setting," in Miriam Stewart et. al. (eds.)*Community Health Nursing in Canada* (Toronto, 1985): 662–78.
41. L.M. Latchford, H. Milne, M. Vaughan, E.P. McClinton and J.A. Harris, "Food Intake Study of Expectant Mothers Attending Prenatal Classes in Metropolitan Toronto," *CJPH*, 61 (1970): 525–33; J. Hendry and J. Shea, "Pre and Postnatal Care Sought by Adolescent Mothers," *CJPH*, 71 (1980): 112–115.
42. Oakley, p. 132, 215.
43. Judith Walzer Leavitt, *Brought to Bed: Childbirth in America, 1750– 1950* (New York, 1986): 171.
44. Suzann Buckley, "The Search for the Decline of Maternal Mortality: The Place of Hospital Records," in W. Mitchinson and J.D. McGinnis, (eds.) *Essays in the History of Canadian Medicine* (Toronto, 1988): 148–63.
45. W.G. Cosbie, "The Effect of Better Obstetrics on Maternal Mortality," Academy of Medicine, *Bulletin*, 20 (July, 1947): 211.
46. *Globe & Mail*, May 11, 1960, p. 5.
47. Oakley, p. 254; Leavitt, *Brought to Bed*, p. 212–18.

48. *Toronto Star,* December 1, 1979.
49. DPH, *Annual Statement,* 1980, p. 153; P.E. Jones and D.M. Craig, "Nursing practice in the community: primary health care," in A. Baumgart and J. Larsen, (eds.) *Canadian Nursing Faces the Future: Development and Change* (Toronto, 1988): 138.

Chapter Nine

1. Charles Hastings, "An Outline of Public Health Service in Toronto Schools," World Federation of Education Associations, *Conference Proceedings,* 1927, p. 432.
2. See Neil Sutherland, "'To Create A Strong and Healthy Race': School Children in the Public Health Movement," in S.E.D. Shortt, (ed.) *Medicine in Canadian Society: Historical Perspectives* (Montreal, 1981): 361–94.
3. Lina L. Rogers, "School Nursing," *Canadian Nurse,* 8 (July, 1912): 366–9; Rogers, "School Nursing in Toronto, Canada," *Canadian Nurse,* 8 (October, 1912): 539–44; E.M. Paul, "School Nursing," *Canadian Nurse,* 10 (October, 1914): 586–93; Lina R. Struthers, *The School Nurse* (New York, 1917).
4. Toronto Board of Education Archives, Press Clippings, Reel #2, Loose Leaf Scrapbook, 1916–17–18. See *Toronto Telegram,* January 29, 1916, April 19, 1916, June 1, 1916. Also *Toronto Star,* December 29, 30, 1916.
5. Struthers, *The School Nurse,* p. 94–102.
6. Board of Education, *Minutes,* 1916, p. 26–27, 76 and scrapbook.
7. *Toronto Telegram,* March 2, 1917.
8. Maureen Riddell, *Edmonton Local Board of Health, 1871–1980* (Edmonton, 1980): 49–51, 65–6.
9. TCC, *Minutes,* 1917, Appendix A, p. 748–50.
10. Charles J. Hastings, *Report Outlining the Activities of the Medical, Dental and Nursing Services of the Department of Public Health* (Toronto, 1922): 4–5.
11. "Department of Public Health Height and Weight Tables of Toronto School Children," *CJPH* , 15 (1924): 391–403; Grant Fleming, "Child Hygiene," *CJPH* , 14 (July, 1923): 293–4; F.S. Burke, "A System of School Medical Inspection," *CJPH,* 30 (January, 1929): 7–17.
12. LBH, Minutes, November 8, 1933; LBH Correspondence, G.P.Jackson to Local Board of Health, November 28, 1933.
13. Lina Rogers, "School Nursing in Toronto, Canada," *Canadian Nurse,* 8 (October, 1912): 539-44; Eunice Dyke, "Health Service in Schools," *CJPH,* 13 (February, 1922): 49-57. For the American model see John Burnham, *How Science Lost and Superstition Won* (New Brunswick and London, 1987): 58–62; Don S. Kirschner, *The Paradox of Professionalism* (New York, 1986): 66–73.
14. Eunice H. Dyke, "Team Play for Health," *Canadian Nurse,* 15 (December, 1919): 2175–79.
15. Annie G. Dove, "Health Teaching in School Fêtes," *Canadian Nurse,* 24 (October, 1928): 534.
16. Barbara Ross, "Trends in School Health Supervision," *Canadian Nurse,* 27 (January, 1931): 32–3.
17. "Forest Schools," *CJPH,* 3 (June, 1912): 350.
18. Rogers, "School Nursing," *Canadian Nurse* (June, 1912): 369; Robert Stamp, *The Schools of Ontario, 1876–1976* (Toronto, 1982): 68.
19. MOH, *Monthly Report,* September, 1924, p. 3.
20. *Health Bulletin,* April, 1921, p. 2.
21. *CJPH,* 12 (1921): 563 and Eric Clarke, "Mental Hygiene in Toronto Schools," *CJPH,* 14 (1923): 127-33. The commentators also noted that truancy had been reduced and that the manual training and domestic arts courses which the students in these classes received fitted them for future employment.
22. Emma Clarke, "The Problem Child and the School Nurse," *Canadian Nurse,* 24 (January, 1928): 28–34; Emma Clarke, "Mental Health in the School," *Canadian Nurse,* 25 (August, 1929): 422–5.
23. MOH, *Monthly Report,* October, 1932; C.G. Stogdill, "Problem Children, their Parents and Teachers," *CJPH,* 27 (February, 1936): 74.

24. MOH, *Monthly Report*, February, 1933.
25. MOH, *Monthly Report*, October, 1932, October, 1935.
26. *Phair Report* (Toronto, 1943): 25-8.
27. J.G. Hall, R.E. Francey and M.L. Girvin, "A Program for the Ineducable-Trainable Child," *CJPH*, 47 (September, 1956): 388–94; Ruth E. Francey, "Psychological Test Changes in Mentally Retarded Children During Training," *CJPH*, 51 (February, 1960): 69–74.
28. Stamp, p. 233–5.
29. *Globe & Mail*, July 23, 1971.
30. TCC, *Minutes*, 1977, Appendix A, p. 1803–5; DPH, *Annual Statement*, 1977, p. 75; 1978, p. 60; 1980, p. 113.
31. DPH, *Annual Statement*, 1980, p. 146–7.
32. Hugh Garner, *Cabbagetown* (Toronto, 1968): 304–5.
33. W.H. Doherty, "A Brief History of Dental Inspection and School Dental Clinics in Toronto," *CJPH*, 5 (March, 1914): 139–40; *Mail*, November 15, 1911; *Health Bulletin*, March, 1913; Bureau of Municipal Research, *Report* (1915): 37–8.
34. Fleming, p. 293; Dyke, 1922, p. 53.
35. Dyke, 1922, p. 53-4; Hastings, *Report*, 1927, p. 8; Division of Dental Services, *Annual Report*, 1932; *Phair Report*, p. 40–2; DPH, *Annual Statement*, 1950, p. 59–60.
36. MOH, *Monthly Report*, April, 1931; Dental Division, *Annual Report*, 1932, p. 1.
37. MOH, *Monthly Report*, April, 1933, p. 1–2; Dental Division, *Annual Report*, 1934; LBH Correspondence, G.P. Jackson to Local Board of Health, April 10, 1935.
38. Summary of a Study with related comments and recommendations Re: Survey of Toronto Department of Health Submitted to the Local Board of Health by G.P. Jackson, June 26, 1944, p. 40.
39. DPH, *Annual Statement*, 1955, p. 71–2; Dental Division, *Annual Report*, 1957, p. 6–7; CTA, RG 11, F1, Box 1, Dental Health Care 1956–64; F.H. Compton, "How a dental service works to protect children's health," *Health* (September-October, 1959): 12–3, 27–8.
40. Dental Division, *Annual Report*, 1957, p. 1–11; DPH, *Annual Statement*, 1960, p. 87–89.
41. Dr. A.S. Macpherson, Letter to the Editor, *Globe & Mail*, August 7, 1987, A6.
42. *Health Bulletin*, August, 1916, 1917, 1919.
43. J.G. FitzGerald, *An Introduction to the Practice of Preventive Medicine* (St. Louis, 1926): 560–3; B.A. Ross, "Distribution of Milk in Toronto Schools," *Canadian Nurse*, 18 (April, 1922): 291–21; *Health Bulletin*, March 9, 23, 1929; George Rosen, *Preventive Medicine in the United States 1900–1975: Trends and Interpretations* (New York, 1977): 5, 35.
44. E.W. McHenry, "Nutrition in Toronto," *CJPH*, 30 (January, 1939): 4–11; McHenry, "Toronto Poor Families Get Too Little Food," *Health* (April, 1939): 5, 23; CTA, RG 11, F1, Box 1, Nutrition Services 1940–1961, Correspondence, E. Hickey to G.P. Jackson, October 2, 1940; Alan Brown, "What Can Be Done to Improve Child Health?," *Toronto Star*, December 26, 1941; LBH, Minutes, March 12, 1942.
45. Oakley, p. 122–3.
46. CTA, RG 11, F1, Box 1, Nutrition Services, Correspondence L.A. Pequegnat to R.G. Struthers, Ontario Division of Health Administration, concerning the work of the Department's nutritionist, October 10, 1947; 1947 Salary Brief from the Nursing Division; Director of Public Health Nursing, *Report*, 1958, p. 16–7; interview with Linda Latchford, July, 1986.
47. McHenry, *CJPH*, 40 (June, 1949): 271–4.
48. Janet M. Wardlaw, "Food Facts and Fallacies," *Health*, (Jan.–Feb., Mar.–Apr., 1955):12, 15, 28; 13, 27.
49. CTA, RG 11, F1, Box 1, Nursing Division Historical Files, Director of Public Health Nursing, *Report*, 1958, and interview with Linda Latchford, July, 1986.
50. Interview with Linda Latchford, July, 1986.
51. CTA, RG 11, F1, Box 1, Nutrition Services 1940–1961; H. Milne, G.H. Beaton, L.M. Latchford, M. Vaughan and G.W.O. Moss, "Hemoglobin levels and iron intakes of infants attending selected child health centres in the City of Toronto," *CMAJ*, 105 (August 7, 1971): 279–82.
52. Burnham, p. 78–84.

53. LBH, Minutes, June 15, 1979; DPH, *Annual Statement*, 1980, p. 161–4.

Chapter Ten

1. C.S. Clark, *Of Toronto the Good: The Queen City of Canada As It Is* (Montreal, 1898, reprinted 1970): 81–136.
2. Jay Cassel, *The Secret Plague: Venereal Disease in Canada 1838-1939* (Toronto, 1987): 116–121, 122–30, 141–44, 147–75. For the American experience see Allan M. Brandt, *No Magic Bullet: A Social History of Venereal Disease in the United States Since 1880* (New York, 1985): 32–5, 38–51, 92–3.
3. Harry F. Dowling, *Fighting Infection* (Cambridge, Mass., 1977): 91–5.
4. Ontario Statutes, An Act for the Prevention of Venereal Disease, Chapter 42, March 26, 1918.
5. Cassel, p. 166–70, 176–7, 215–19; G.D.W. Cameron, "The Department of National Health and Welfare," in R.D. Defries, (ed.) *Federal and Provincial Health Services in Canada* (Toronto, 1959): 2–3.
6. Francis E. Brown, "Public Health Nurses in Venereal Disease Clinics," *CJPH*, 14 (1923): 76–81; Brown, "The Social Aspects of Venereal Disease Control," *CJPH*, 15 (1924): 72–82.
7. Charles Hastings, "Nursing Organization as Developed in Toronto," *The Nation's Health*, February 15, 1923, p. 62, 64–5.
8. Edna L. Moore, "VD Control in Ontario," *CJPH*, 14 (1923): 74.
9. Dowling, p. 100–03; Ira V. Hiscock, *Community Health Organization* (New York, 1939): 88–98.
10. Dowling, p. 98–9.
11. Robert Stamp, *The Schools of Ontario, 1876–1976* (Toronto, 1982): 69; Michael Bliss, "'Pure Books on Avoided Subjects': Pre-Freudian Sexual Ideas in Canada," in S.E.D. Shortt, (ed.) *Medicine in Canadian Society* (Montreal, 1981): 255–84; W.E. Struthers, "Medical Inspection of Schools in Toronto," *CJPH*, 5 (February, 1914): 75; J.G. FitzGerald, *An Introduction to the Practice of Preventive Medicine* (St. Louis, 1926): 565–7; Veronica Strong-Boag, *The New Day Recalled* (Toronto, 1988): 15; Brown, "Social Aspects of Venereal Disease Control," *CJPH*, 15 (1924): 80–2.
12. *CJPH*, 15 (1924): 54, 92.
13. Cassel, p. 176–245.
14. Janice Dickin McGinnis, "From Salvarsan to Penicillin: Medical Science and VD Control in Canada," in W. Mitchinson and J. McGinnis, (eds.) *Essays in the History of Canadian Medicine* (Toronto, 1988): 133–43.
15. L.A. Pequegnat, "The Applied Aspects of the Venereal Disease Legislation of Ontario," *CJPH*, 27 (May, 1936): 228–35.
16. L.A. Pequegnat, "Points of Interest to the General Practitioner in the Control of Venereal Disease in Urban Centres," Academy of Medicine, *Bulletin*, 14 (March, 1941): 125–23.
17. Brandt, *No Magic Bullet*, p. 42–5, 150–60.
18. John C. Scott, "Toronto's VD Fight," *Health*, Autumn 1944, p. 27; interview with Nancy Laing, August, 1986.
19. LBH, Minutes, October 23, October 25, November 25, December 6, 20, 1944.
20. Interview with former nurse, Nancy Cuyler, September, 1986.
21. Interviews with Nancy Cuyler, Michael Davis and James Flaherty in July, August and September, 1986.
22. LBH, Minutes, September 11, 1945.
23. DPH, *Annual Statement*, 1948, p. 45–6.
24. Brandt, p. 171–2, 177–8.
25. *Globe & Mail*, Tuesday, September 12, 1961, p. 5; DPH, *Annual Statement*, 1961, p. 61–3.
26. DPH, *Annual Statement*, 1968, p. 75. In 1963, 497 cases of syphilis and 1,483 of gonorrhea were reported in Toronto. By 1968, syphilis had declined to 366 cases but gonorrhea had risen to 1,945 cases. See also *Telegram*, July 7, December 22, 1967. For the American experience see Dowling, *Fighting Infection*, p. 148.

27. "Yorkville: Danger for runaway girls, tears and anger for parents," *Globe & Mail*, November 2, 1967, p. 1, 9.
28. Henry Mietkiewicz and Bob Mackowycz, *Dream Tower: The Life and Legacy of Rochdale College* (Toronto, 1988): 72–4.
29. Interview with James Flaherty, July, 1986.
30. LBH, Minutes, November 16, 1976; City of Toronto, LBH, Report of the Health Planning Steering Committee, *Public Health in the 1980's* (Toronto, 1978): 40–2; DPH, *Annual Statement*, 1980, p.19–23.
31. DPH, *Annual Statement*, 1982, p. 59.
32. *Toronto Star*, April 28, 1927, p. 17.
33. Angus McLaren, "The First Campaigns for Birth Control Clinics in British Columbia," *Journal of Canadian Studies*, 19 (Fall, 1984): 50–64.
34. Angus McLaren and Arlene Tigar McLaren, *The Bedroom and the State: The Changing Practices and Politics of Contraception and Abortion in Canada, 1880-1980* (Toronto, 1986): 54–70, 92–123, 170.
35. Interviews with former public health nurses Nancy Cuyler, Madeline Smillie and Mary Willett in July, August and September, 1986.
36. McLaren and McLaren, *Bedroom*, p. 132-3.
37. *Globe & Mail*, January 21, 27, March 4, 6, 1965. See *Toronto Daily Star*, February 27, 1968 for an article describing the arrangements which the local board of health made for paying staff at Toronto General Hospital's birth control clinic.
38. CTA, RG 11, F1, Nursing Historical Division Files, Department of Health memo, January, 1965.
39. R. Wilson, G.W.O. Moss, E.G. Laugharne, E.M. Read, "Family Planning in a Co-ordinated Hospital and Community Setting," *CJPH*, 58 (December, 1967): 527-534.
40. Maureen Riddell, *Edmonton's Local Board of Health, 1871–1980* (Edmonton, 1980): 103.
41. City of Toronto, DPH, *Health is a Cultural Affair* (Toronto, 1985).
42. LBH, Minutes, #42, May 25, 1971.
43. TCC, *Minutes*, 1971, Appendix A, p. 384–91.
44. See the annual reports of the Family Planning Services Division in the *Annual Statements*, 1976–1984. Interviews with Anne Johnston and Elizabeth Parker in July, 1986.

Chapter Eleven

1. Canada, Department of Health, *Achieving Health for All: A Framework for Health Promotion* (Ottawa, 1986): 5.
2. Sidney Katz, "The Amazing Career of Clare Hincks," *Maclean's Magazine*, August 1, 1954, p. 10, 32–4.
3. MOH, Report to the LBH, February 7, 1933.
4. LBH, Correspondence, G.P. Jackson to Mayor H.E. McCallum, September 25, 1950.
5. John Burnham, *How Science Lost and Superstition Won* (New Brunswick and London, 1987): 66–7; *Saturday Night*, editorial, October 3, 1950.
6. See TCC, *Minutes*, 1951, Appendix, p. 1951–1970; DPH, *Annual Statement*, 1951, p. 65–6; *Toronto Star*, June 21, 1950; January 18, 19, 22, 23, 24, February 23, 1951; *Globe & Mail*, January 19, 23, 24, 1951.
7. Harvey G. Simmons, *Unbalanced: Mental Health Policy in Ontario, 1930–1989* (Toronto, 1990): 55, 58–61.
8. Simmons, p.59–60.
10. Interview with Nancy Cuyler, September, 1986. She switched from the VD Division to mental health nursing in the early 1960s.
10. DPH, *Annual Statement*, 1966, p. 66; 1971, p. 85.
11. DPH, *Annual Statement*, 1959, p. 58–60; DPH, *Health is a Cultural Affair* (Toronto, 1985): 14, 28, 38–42, 57–8, 73–4.
12. Interview with Dr. Edgar Wong, the former director of Mental Health, June, 1986; DPH, *Annual Statement*, 1980, p. 142.

13 Clarence Robinson, "Changing Patterns in Mental Health," *CJPH*, 54 (November, 1963): 502.
14. DPH, *Annual Statement*, 1960, p. 82.
15. LBH, Minutes, #132, 1966; DPH, *Annual Statement*, 1971, p .84.
16. DPH, *Annual Statement*, 1963, p. 49.
17. Simmons, p. 61.
18. LBH, Report No. 3, *The Unequal Society: A Challenge to Public Health*, prepared by Earl Miller and Joey Edwardh (March, 1983): 3927.
19. City of Toronto, LBH, Report of the Health Planning Steering Committee, *Public Health in the 1980's* (Toronto, 1978): 47–9.
20. L. Elinson, F. Goettler and D. Kuhl, "Epidemiologic Characteristics of Suicide in Toronto," *CJPH*, 74 (Nov./Dec., 1983): 422–27.
21. Lily Contento, "Addiction groups toast 40-year campaign," *Toronto Star*, August 1, 1989, N7.
22. Canada, Department of National Health and Welfare, *A New Perspective on Health for Canadians: A Working Document* (Ottawa, 1974): 16, 22, 66–72.
23. The Addiction Research Foundation had been created as the Alcoholism Addiction Research Foundation under provincial legislation passed in 1948.
24. Interview with Anne Johnston, July, 1986.
25. Maureen Murphy, "Why Won't They Shape Up? Resistance to the Promotion of Health," *CJPH*, 73 (Nov./Dec., 1982): 429.
26. "The National Curse of the Drug Traffic," *Health Bulletin*, February, 1923.
27. A.K. Haywood, "Vice and Drugs in Montreal," *CJPH*, 14 (January, 1923): 19.
28. *Health Bulletin*, February, 1923.
29. Henry Mietkiewicz and Bob Mackowycz, *Dream Tower: The Life and Legacy of Rochdale College* (Toronto, 1988): 72–6.
30. Maureen Riddell, *Edmonton Local Board of Health, 1871–1980* (Edmonton, 1980): 105–6.
31. DPH, *Annual Statement*, 1983, p. 12, 15.

Chapter Twelve

1. MOH, *Monthly Report*, February, 1934.
2. John Burnham, *How Science Lost and Superstition Won* (New Brunswick, 1987): 83.
3. *Health Bulletin*, June 29, 1929, p. 2.
4. Ontario Department of Health, 10th Annual Report, 1934, *Ontario Sessional Papers*, Vol. 67, Part IV, No. 14, 1935, p. 98–100; J.T. Phair, "Public Health in Ontario," in R.D. Defries, (ed.) *The Development of Public Health in Canada* (Toronto, 1940): 73–4.
5. *Health Bulletin*, May, 1929, p. 4.
6. George Rosen, *Preventive Medicine in the United States 1900–1975: Trends and Interpretations* (New York, 1977): 65–7.
7. LBH, Minutes, Jan. 20, Apr. 27, 1960.
8. TCC, *Minutes*, 1960, Appendix A, p. 873–8, 2656–8.
9. J.T. Salonen et al., "Changes in morbidity and mortality during comprehensive community programs to control cardiovascular disease during 1972–77 in North Karelia," *British Medical Journal*, 2 (1979): 1178–83; M.P. Stein et al., "Results of a two-year health education campaign on dietary behaviour: The Stanford Three Community Study," *Circulation*, 54 (November, 1976): 826–32.
10. Rosen, *Preventive Medicine*, p. 64, 68. DPH, Working Group on Cardiovascular Disease, September, 1986.
11. LBH, Minutes, #70, 1962; *Telegram*, "Health Bd Opens War on Smoking," Sept. 26, 1962, p. 13.
12. G.W.O. Moss, "Smoking and Health — The Association and You," *CJPH*, 56 (January, 1965): 34–6.
13. Norman C. Delarue, "A Study in Smoking Withdrawal," *CJPH*, 64 (March/April, 1973) Smoking and Health Supplement S5–S19; Delarue, "The anti-smoking clinic: is it a potential community service?," *CMAJ*, 108 (May 5, 1973): 1164–73; Roy J. Shephard and

Robert LaBarre, "Current Attitudes Towards Smoking in Toronto," *CJPH,* 69 (March/April, 1978): 121–6.
14. DPH, *Annual Statement,* 1980, p. 104–5.
15. DPH, *Annual Statement,* 1983, p. 20, 23.
16. The Welfare Council of Toronto, *A Coordinated Program of Community Services for Older People in Toronto,* May 8, 1953; *Report of the Commissioner of Public Welfare and the Medical Officer of Health on the Foregoing Suggestions of the Welfare Council of Toronto,* September 3, 1953, p. 15–6, 27–8.
17. CTA, RG 11 F1 Box 1 Diabetes & Insulin, 1955–60; LBH, Minutes, #141, September 18, 1951; #28, January 22, 1952.
18. Jessie Parfit, *The Health of a City: Oxford 1770-1974* (Oxford, 1987): 121–4.
19. See *CJPH,* 49 (August, 1958): 359; Marion I. Barter, "The Pilot Home Care Project of Toronto," *CJPH,* 54 (February, 1963): 55-62; DPH, *Annual Statement,* 1959, p. 112; 1960, p. 63; 1962, p. 64–5; 1963, p. 135; *CJPH,* 55 (May, 1964): 227.
20. LBH, Minutes, #80, May 4, 1966; Deputy Medical Officer, Report to the local board of health on the subject of Geriatric Health Centres, November 27, 1968; G.W.O. Moss, "Changing Patterns in Services for Senior Citizens: A Public Health Viewpoint," OPHA presentation October 20, 1972; DPH, *Annual Statement,* 1971, p. 111–16.
21. DPH, *Annual Statement,* 1979, p. 83.
22. LBH, Report No. 3, *The Unequal Society: A Challenge to Public Health* (March, 1983): 3298.
23. Interview with Betty Davidson, former Director of Public Health Nursing, August, 1986.
24. DPH, *Annual Statement,* 1980, p. 157.

Chapter Thirteen

1. James Lemon, *Toronto since 1918* (Toronto, 1985): 158–72.
2. George Rosen, *Preventive Medicine in the United States 1900–1975: Trends and Interpretations* (New York, 1977): 65.
3. Toronto City Council, *Minutes,* 1953, Appendix A, p. 604–07; LBH, Minutes, February 17, 1953; January 18, February 15, 1955; DPH, *Annual Statement,* 1954, p. 68; 1956, p. 74; 1957, p. 83; see also *Toronto Star,* May 18, November 11, 1955.
4. *Health,* Jan./Feb., 1953, July/Aug., Nov./Dec., 1954; Mar./Apr., Sept./Oct., 1955, Mar./Apr., Sept./Oct., 1965; Health League of Canada Summary of Conclusions and Recommendations, from the Report of the Ontario Fluoridation Investigation Committee, 1961.
5. G.W.O. Moss, "The Canadian Public Health Association Annual Report, Part 1, 1959–60," *CJPH,* 51 (June, 1960): 246.
6. *Toronto Star,* May 2, 1962.
7. CTA, RG 11, Health Department Records, Speech by A.R.J. Boyd to Canadian Progress Club, West Toronto, March 13, 1962; Statement prepared for radio broadcast, November 9, 1962.
8. Interview with Dr. G.W.O. Moss, August, 1986.
9. *Toronto Star,* May 18, November 11, 1955; November 23, 1962; *Toronto Telegram,* March 23, October 21, 1960; November 27, 28, December 4, 1962.
10. *Globe & Mail,* November 27, 1962, p. 6.
11. *Globe & Mail,* "Metro Sets May 1 Date for Start of Fluoridation," December 5, 1962; *Toronto Telegram,* "Our Water Fluoridated," September 4, 1963.
12. LBH, Minutes, March 3, 1970.
13. *Toronto Star,* Saturday, January 28, 1989, H2.
14. Rosen, *Preventive Medicine,* p. 5–6; Hugh M. Barrett, "Atmospheric Pollution in Toronto, Canada," *CJPH,* 29 (January, 1938): 1–2.
15. Barrett, p. 3–11.
16. Open University, *Caring for Health: History and Diversity* (Milton Keynes, 1985): 79. London's great killer fog of December 1952 apparently raised mortality from respiratory diseases by over 3,500 deaths. This tragedy prompted the National Society for Smoke Abatement, concerned members of Parliament, and a few committed medical officers to

lobby for legislation. Their efforts were successful and the Clean Air Act was passed in 1956.

17. Carolyn Gray, *Historical Records of the City of Hamilton, 1847–1973* (Hamilton, 1986): 61.
18. L.A. Pequegnat, "Changing Responsibilities in Public Health," *CJPH*, 48 (July, 1957): 273.
19. LBH, Minutes, August 29, 1967, 33.
20. LBH, Minutes, February 20, 1963; DPH, *Annual Statement*, 1963, p. 85; Patricia Orwen, "AIR — Without it we die, yet we pollute it", *Toronto Star*, Saturday, May 26, 1984, B4.
21. *CJPH*, 56 (1965): 350.
22. LBH, Minutes, March 2, 1966.
23. Dixon Thompson, "Environmental Agencies"; Robert T. Franson, "Environmental Law," *The Canadian Encyclopedia*, 1 (Edmonton, 1985): 585–7.
24. Orwen, B4.

Chapter Fourteen

1. University of Toronto, Faculty of Medicine, Department of Community Health, *Public Health in the City of Toronto* (Toronto, 1977): 145.
2. Howard Buchbinder, "Social Planning or Social Control: An Account of a Confrontation with the Social Welfare Establishment," in Alan Powell, (ed.) *The City: Attacking Modern Myths* (Toronto, 1972): 132–60.
3. Nathan Phillips, Q.C., *Mayor of All the People* (Toronto, 1967): 78; Timothy Colton, *Big Daddy: Frederick G. Gardiner and the Building of Metropolitan Toronto* (Toronto, 1980): 80, 88–92.
4. James Lemon, *Toronto Since 1918* (Toronto, 1985): 151–2.
5. Interview with Anne Johnston, July, 1986.
6 LBH, Minutes, #52, #53, March 7, 1973; TCC, *Minutes*, 1971, Appendix A, LBH Report No. 7, p. 3013–20; *Globe & Mail*, February 28, March 8, 22, 1973.
7. Anne Parsons, "Children near lead refinery will be examined," *Globe & Mail*, February 18, 1973.
8. Alden Baker, "MOH demands full backing for staff following lead study complaints," *Globe & Mail*, June 14, 1973.
9. TCC, *Minutes*, 1973, Appendix A, p. 3260.
10. "East End Smelter," *Globe & Mail*, September 13, 1973. See also *Globe & Mail*, September 15, 18, October 5, 1973.
11. Joan Hollobon, "Anti-pollution officials shouted down at smelter protest," *Globe & Mail*, November 9, 1973.
12. "Plant closing cut lead levels sharply, scientists say," *Toronto Star*, November 15, 1973.
13. Interview with Anne Johnston, July, 1986; Deborah Wilson, "Niagara Street residents convinced smelter poisoned their lives," *Globe & Mail*, December 20, 1988, A16.
14. *Globe & Mail*, June 26, July 12, 1973.
15. Interviews with W.D. Connery, James Flaherty and Mary Willett in June and July, 1986.
16. *Globe & Mail*, November 16, 27, 1974.
17. TCC, *Minutes*, 1976, Appendix A, LBH, Report No. 2, p. 1409.
18. LBH, Minutes, #56, #56A, February 26, 1975; interview with Dr. G.W.O. Moss, August, 1986.
19. "Toronto backs scheme to acquire lead smelter and shut it next June," *Globe & Mail*, July 12, 1988, A14; Wilson, *Globe & Mail*, December 20, 1988, A16.
20. DPH, *Reorganization — Phase One*, May 5, 1980, p. 7.
21. George Rosen, *Preventive Medicine in the United States 1900–1975: Trends and Interpretations* (New York, 1977): p. 62–3, 69–77; Jane Lewis, *What Price Community Medicine?* (Brighton, 1986): 57–69.
22. "A Submission to the Royal Commission on Health Services by the Canadian Public Health Association," *CJPH*, 53 (June, 1962): 229, 238.
23. Ian McIntosh, "On Having Been a Medical Officer of Health," *CJPH*, 69 (September/October, 1978): 375–8.

24. University of Toronto, Department of Community Health, *Public Health in the City of Toronto* (Toronto, 1977): 126, 148.
25. Ontario Ministry of Health, Health Promotion Branch, *The Local Official Health Agency: A Background Paper* (Toronto, 1976): 1.
26. City of Toronto, LBH, Report of the Health Planning Steering Committee, *Public Health in the 1980's* (Toronto, 1978): 34.
27. University of Toronto, Department of Community Health, *Public Health in the City of Toronto* (Toronto, 1977): xxxviii.
28. Ibid., p. 65, 145.
29. Frances L. Perkins, *Summary of Staff Submissions,* May, 1978, p. 1–19.
30. L.A. Cass, *Summary of Community Responses,* May, 1978, p. 1–48.
31. *Public Health in the 1980's,* p. 67–71.
32. Interviews with Michael Davis, Dr. Bill Frank, and Dr. Arthur Steurmann in July and August, 1986.
33. DPH, *Reorganization — Phase One,* May 5, 1980 and DPH, *Evaluation Task Force,* December, 1981.
34. World Health Organization (WHO), *Health Promotion: A discussion document of the concept and principles* (Copenhagen, 1984).

Conclusion

1. "Here's what Public Health means to you," *Health,* Mar./Apr., 1956, p. 16.
2. See Ramsay Cook, *The Regenerators: Social Criticism in late Victorian Canada* (Toronto, 1985); Richard Allen, *The Social Passion: Religion and Social Reform in Canada, 1914–28* (Toronto, 1971).
3. See R.C. Brown and R. Cook, *Canada 1896–1921: A Nation Transformed* (Toronto, 1974); P. Rutherford, (ed.) *Saving the Canadian City, 1880–1920* (Toronto, 1974); Neil Sutherland, *Children in English-Canadian Society* (Toronto, 1976).
4. See Ronald Hamowy, *Canadian Medicine: A Study in Restricted Entry* (Vancouver, 1984) for a Canadian example of this predominantly American phenomenon.
5. Timothy W. Plumptre, *Beyond the Bottom Line: Management in Government* (Canada, 1988): 93–96.
6. See Plumptre; Michael J. White, Ross Clayton, Robert Myrtle, Gilbert Siegel and Aaron Rose, *Managing Public Systems: Analytic Techniques for Public Administration* (North Scituate, Mass., 1980).
7. J.T. Phair, *Report of a Survey of the Services Extended by the Health Department of the City of Toronto with appropriate Recommendations* (Toronto, December 4, 1943): 2.
8. White et al., p. 4.
9. John C. Burnham, *How Superstition Won and Science Lost. Popularizing Science and Health in the United States* (New Brunswick and London, 1987): 70–1.
10. Burnham, p. 58, 65.
11. Burnham, p. 66–83.
12. Timothy Colton, *Big Daddy: Frederick G. Gardiner and the Building of Metropolitan Toronto* (Toronto, 1980).
13. K.D. Jaffray and S.M. Makuch, *Local Decision-making and Administration: A Study for the Royal Commission on Metropolitan Toronto* (Toronto, 1977), Appendix B.

Note on Sources

Official records provide the foundation for this study. From 1883 to the present, Toronto's Department of Public Health has produced an annual report which documented the staff's activities. The reports are complete for the Canniff regime from 1883–1890 but only scattered ones are available for the Sheard administration. Under Charles Hastings, monthly reports were presented to the local board of health and these provide an excellent source of information concerning the work of the progressive reformers. His successors continued this practice and their reports were printed in the minutes of the local board of health. The board's minutes were a significant source of information about citizen concerns and the politician's response to the these problems. Contentious issues such as the takeover of school medical inspection, the Dyke-Bullick incident, fluoridation, and the lead problem were discussed by the city council as well as the local board, and the city council minutes and Board of Control records were consulted to establish a broader context. All of these records are available in the Health Department or in the City of Toronto Archives.

Provincial and federal authorities also played a role in the development of health services in the city. During the 1880s and 1890s, the Provincial Board of Health published a detailed annual report which included extracts of local boards of health's reports, in the *Ontario Sessional Papers*. The federal Department of Agriculture published the national mortality statistics that had been reported to it, from 1883 to 1893 when the responsibility shifted to the provinces. In general, Canadian mortality statistics were questionable until the Dominion Bureau of Statistics was established in 1922. Although Toronto published annual compilations of its leading causes of death, there are no century-long charts or graphs in this study because the international disease classification system was updated every ten years with the result that reclassifying diseases from one category to another makes meaningful comparisons difficult. Furthermore, the standard international system of comparing morbidity and mortality rates for various diseases by cases per 1,000 or per 100,000 only produced gross statistics. Such data often masked the socio-economic variables making some sections of the city appear significantly less healthy than others

Ottawa and Queen's Park became much more active in health matters after 1945. The national health grants paid for the Ontario Health Survey, conducted between 1948 and 1952. This overview of the province's health care personnel, their training and some of their activities provided a snapshot of Toronto's Health Department at the end of Gordon Jackson's period in office. Slightly more than a decade later, the Royal Commission on Health Services again examined Toronto's Department of Public Health and noted the large number of projects and staff education opportunities which federal funds had supported. Through the 1970s and 1980s, changes in federal and provincial health policy and funding had a significant impact on the Health Department, and thus various task force reports and *A New Perspective on Health for Canadians* were consulted to uncover the context in which the staff were working in the modern period.

With the exception of William Canniff, none of the city's medical officers left personal papers. To overcome this lack of information, medical journals and other periodicals were examined. In the nineteenth century, the leading Canadian medical journals such as the *Canadian Practitioner* and the *Canada Lancet* covered public health matters but with the creation of the Canadian Public Health Association and the establishment of its journal, the mainstream medical periodicals published less information. From 1910 onward, the *Canadian Journal of Public Health* was a mine of information about the programs and services which Toronto and other Canadian cities provided. Tracking the Department's staff as they took positions throughout the country, demonstrated the extent of the city's influence. The increasingly scientific content of the journal articles also paralleled the changes in attitudes among public health professionals, as Canadians adopted each of the phases of the international public health movement.

For more than a century, Toronto's newspapers have reported on the work of the Health Department. During the 1880s and 1890s, political considerations determined the type of reporting because strong Liberal papers such as the *Globe* contended with Conservative papers such as the *World* and the *Mail and Empire* to influence civic policy. After 1900, a more popular orientation developed in papers such as the *Toronto Star* and the *Toronto Telegram*; as a result, the Health Department's activities were described in greater detail. The city's papers contributed to educating citizens about health matters and generally applauded the work of the Hastings administration. During the period from 1930 to the end of the 1950s, press interest declined as larger national and international concerns attracted its attention. In the 1960s, local topics re-emerged and reporters began to highlight social issues such as family planning and sexually transmitted diseases. News stories and editorials started to criticize the Department for its slow response to changing attitudes and to arouse public interest in environmental problems. Like all sources, newspaper accounts of controversial matters must be used with care but they do provide the human element so often missing in official records.

In addition to written records, a series of interviews was conducted with current and former staff, former members of local board of health, and relatives of former health officers. These discussions fleshed out the sometimes bland annual reports and added the "human touch" which was, and is, an integral part of the Department's work culture.

And finally, the visual record adds a vital element to this study. Photographs, signs, and sample record forms vividly illustrate the staff's daily activities. Most of the photographs in this book are drawn from two well-known collections in the City of Toronto Archives — the Department of Public Works Collection and the James Collection. From 1911 to the mid-1940s, the city's photographers created a splendid historical resource which was supplemented with further material from the Metropolitan Toronto Library and the Archives of Ontario. Unfortunately, few photographs of activities in the 1950s and 1960s have survived. Although local newspapers and city staff began to take more pictures during the 1970s, many of the originals have already been lost. As a result, later chapters have fewer illustrations and many contemporary photographs are copies of material in the Department's *Annual Statements*.

Selected Bibiliography

Allen, Richard. *The Social Passion: Religion and Social Reform in Canada, 1914–28.* Toronto: University of Toronto Press, 1971.

Andrews, Margaret W., "The Emergence of Bureaucracy: The Vancouver Health Department, 1886–1914," *Journal of Urban History,* 12 (Feb. 1986): 131–55.

Artibise, A.F.J. and Stelter, Gilbert, eds. *The Usable Urban Past: Planning and Politics in the Modern Canadian City.* Ottawa: Carleton University Press, 1979.

Bator, Paul and Dr. Andrew J. Rhodes. *Within Reach of Everyone: A History of the University of Toronto School of Hygiene and the Connaught Laboratories,* Vol. 1, 1927–55. Ottawa: CPHA, 1990.

Baumgart, Alice and Jenniece Larsen, eds. *Canadian Nursing Faces the Future.* St. Louis: C.V. Mosby, 1988.

Brandt, Allan M. *No Magic Bullet: A Social History of Venereal Disease in the United States Since 1880.* New York: Oxford University Press, 1985.

Brown, R.C. and G.R. Cook, *Canada 1896–1921: A Nation Transformed* . Toronto: McClelland & Stewart, 1974.

Bureau of Municipal Research. *Administrative Study of the Toronto Department of Public Health as of March 1st, 1915.* Toronto, 1915.

Burnham, John. *How Science Lost and Superstition Won. Popularizing Science and Health in the United States.* New Brunswick and London: Rutgers University Press, 1987.

Canada. Department of National Health and Welfare. *A New Perspective on Health for Canadians: A Working Document.* Ottawa, 1974.

Canada. Department of National Health and Welfare. *Achieving Health for All: A Framework for Health Promotion.* Ottawa, 1986.

Canada. Statistics Canada. *Toronto 150: Portrait of a Changing City.* Ottawa, 1984.

CPHA. Committee on Salaries and Qualifications of Public Health Personnel. *Recommended Qualification Requirements and Minimum Salaries for Public Health Personnel in Canada.* Fifth Revision, 1965. Toronto, 1965.

CPHA. Study Committee on Public Health Practice in Canada. *Report of the Study Committee on Public Health Practice in Canada.* Toronto, 1950.

CPHA. *Ontario Public Health: Some Current Issues,* Ottawa: CPHA, 1977.

Cassel, Jay. *The Secret Plague: Venereal Disease in Canada 1838–1939.* Toronto: University of Toronto Press, 1987.

Careless, J.M.S. *Toronto to 1918: An Illustrated History.* Toronto: James Lorimer and Company, 1984.

Chase, Allan. *Magic Shots.* New York: William Morrow & Company, Inc., 1982.

Colton, Timothy. *Big Daddy: Frederick G. Gardiner and the Building of Metropolitan Toronto.* Toronto: University of Toronto Press, 1980.

Copp, Terry. *The Anatomy of Poverty: The Condition of the Working Class in Montreal, 1897–1929.* Toronto: McClelland and Stewart, 1974.

Defries, R.D., ed. *The Development of Public Health in Canada.* Toronto: CPHA, 1940.

Defries, R.D., ed. *Federal and Provincial Health Services in Canada.* Toronto: CPHA, 1959.

Defries, R.D. "Dr. Edward Playter—A Vision Fulfilled," *CJPH,* 50 (September, 1959): 368–77.

Defries, R.D. *The First Forty Years 1914–1955: Connaught Medical Research Laboratories, University of Toronto.* Toronto: University of Toronto Press, 1968.

Dowling, Harry F. *Fighting Infection*. Cambridge, Mass.: Harvard University Press, 1977.
Duffy, John. *A History of Public Health in New York City, 1866–1966*. Vol. II, New York: Russell Sage Foundation, 1974.
Eyler, John M. *Victorian Social Medicine: The Ideas and Methods of William Farr*. Baltimore and London: Johns Hopkins University Press, 1979.
Ferguson, John. *The Ontario Medical Association, 1880–1930*. Toronto: Murray Printing Co. Ltd., 1930.
FitzGerald, J.G. *An Introduction to the Practice of Preventive Medicine*. St. Louis: C.V. Mosby, 1922, 2nd edition, 1926.
Fox, Daniel. *Health Policies, Health Politics: The British and American Experience, 1911–1965*. Princeton: Princeton University Press, 1986.
Galishoff, Stuart. *Safeguarding the Public Health: Newark, 1895–1918*. Westport, Conn.: Greenwood Press, 1975.
Galishoff, Stuart. *Newark: The Nation's Unhealthiest City*. New Brunswick: Rutgers University Press, 1988.
Garner, Hugh. *Cabbagetown*. Toronto: McGraw-Hill Ryerson Limited, 1950, reprinted 1968.
Gray, Caroline. *Historical Records of the City of Hamilton, 1847–1973*. Hamilton: McMaster University, 1986.
Groulx, Ad. *Le Service de Santé de la Ville de Montréal: Evolution et Organisation Actuelle*. Montréal, 1954.
Hamowy, Ronald. *Canadian Medicine: A Study in Restricted Entry*. Vancouver: The Fraser Institute, 1984.
Haskell, Thomas L., ed. *The Authority of Experts: Studies in History and Theory*. Bloomington: Indiana University Press, 1984.
Hastings, John E., Mindell, William R., Browne, John W. and Barnsley, Janet M., "Canadian Health Administrator Study," *CJPH*, 72 Supplement One, (March/April, 1981): 1–61.
Hiscock, Ira V. *Community Health Organization: A Manual of Administration and Procedure Primarily for Urban Areas*. New York: The Commonwealth Fund, 1939.
Howell, James M., ed. *Think Prevention!: Report of the Joint Committee on Preventive Medicine*. Edmonton: Alberta Hospital Association and Health Units Association of Alberta, 1987.
Kirschner, Don S. *The Paradox of Professionalism: Reform and Public Service in Urban America*, 1900–1940. New York: Greenwood, 1986.
Lambert, R.J. *Sir John Simon (1816–1904) and English Social Administration*. London: MacGibbon and Kee, 1963.
Last, John. *Public Health and Human Ecology*. East Norwalk, Conn.: Appleton and Lange, 1987.
Leavitt, Judith Walzer. *The Healthiest City: Milwaukee and the Politics of Health Reform*. Princeton: Princeton University Press, 1982.
Leavitt, Judith Walzer. *Brought to Bed: Childbirth in America, 1750–1950*. New York: Oxford University Press, 1986.
Lemon, James. *Toronto Since 1918: An Illustrated History*. Toronto: James Lorimer and Company, 1985.
Lewis, Jane. *What Price Community Medicine?* Brighton: Wheatsheaf Press, 1986.
MacDougall, Heather, "The Limitations of Public Health in Toronto's Municipal Politics: The Canniff Years, 1883–1890," *Bulletin of the History of Medicine*, 55

(1981): 186–202.
MacDougall, Heather, "'Enlightening the Public:' The Views and Values of the Association of Executive Health Officers of Ontario, 1886–1903," in Charles G. Roland, ed. *Health, Disease and Medicine: Essays in Canadian History*. Toronto: Copp Clark Ltd., 1984: 436–464.
MacDougall, Heather, "Public Health and the 'Sanitary Idea' in Toronto, 1866–1890," in Wendy Mitchinson and Janice McGinnis, eds. *Essays in the History of Canadian Medicine*. Toronto: McClelland & Stewart, 1988: 62–87.
McLaren, Angus and Arlene Tigar McLaren. *The Bedroom and the State: The Changing Practices and Politics of Contraception and Abortion in Canada, 1880–1980*. Toronto: McClelland & Stewart, 1986.
McKeown, Thomas. *The Modern Rise of Population*. New York: Academic Press, 1976.
McKeown, Thomas. *Origins of Human Disease*. Oxford: Basil Blackwell, 1988.
Melosh, Barbara. *"The Physician's Hand:" Work Culture and Conflict in American Nursing*. Philadelphia: Temple University Press, 1982.
Oakley, Ann. *The Captured Womb: A History of the Medical Care of Pregnant Women*. Oxford: Basil Blackwell, 1986.
Ontario. Department of Health. *Report of a Survey of the Services Extended by the Health Department of the City of Toronto with appropriate Recommendations*. Toronto, 1943.
Ontario. Department of Health. *Report of the Ontario Health Survey Committee*. Vol. I–III. Toronto, 1952.
Ontario. Ministry of Health. Health Promotion Branch. *The Local Official Health Agency in Ontario: A Background Paper*. Toronto, 1976.
Ontario. Ministry of Health. *Annual Report for 1981–82*. "A Century of Caring." Toronto, 1982.
Parfit, Jessie. *The Health of a City: Oxford, 1770–1974*. Oxford: Amate Press, 1987.
Paul, John R. *A History of Poliomyelitis*. New Haven and London: Yale University Press, 1971.
Pettigrew, Eileen. *The Silent Enemy: Canada and the Deadly Flu of 1918*. Saskatoon: Western Producer Prairie Books, 1983.
Petroff, Lillian. "Macedonians in Toronto: From Encampment to Settlement," *Urban History Review*, 2 (1978): 58–73.
Phillips, Nathan, Q.C. *Mayor of the All the People*. Toronto: McClelland & Stewart, 1967.
Piva, Michael. *The Condition of the Working Class in Toronto, 1900–1921*. Ottawa: University of Ottawa Press, 1979.
Plumptre, Timothy. *Beyond the Bottom Line: Management in Government*. Canada: Institute for Research on Public Policy, 1988.
Powell, Alan, ed. *The City: Attacking Modern Myths*. Toronto: McClelland & Stewart, 1972.
Ravenel, Mazyck P., ed. *A Half Century of Public Health: Jubilee Historical Volume of the American Public Health Association*. New York: APHA, 1921, reprinted 1970.
Riddell, Maureen. *Edmonton Local Board of Health, 1871–1980*. Edmonton: 1980.
Risk, Margaret McNeill. "The Origins and Development of Public Health Nursing in Toronto from 1890–1918," M.A. thesis, University of Toronto, 1973.
Rogers, Lina S. *The School Nurse*. New York: G.P. Putnam & Son, 1917.
Rose, Albert. *Regent Park*. Toronto: University of Toronto Press, 1958.
Rosen, George. *A History of Public Health*. New York: M.D. Publications, Inc., 1958.
Rosen, George. *From Medical Police to Social Medicine: Essays on the History of Health*

Care. New York: Science History Publications, 1974.
Rosen, George. *Preventive Medicine in the United States 1900–1975: Trends and Interpretations*. New York: Prodist, 1977.
Rosenkrantz, Barbara Gutmann. *Public Health and the State: Changing Views in Massachusetts, 1842–1936*. Cambridge, Mass.: Harvard University Press, 1972.
Royce, Marion. *Eunice H. Dyke: Health Care Pioneer*. Toronto: Dundurn Press, 1983.
Rutherford, Paul, ed. *Saving the Canadian City: The First Phase, 1880–1920*. Toronto: University of Toronto Press, 1974.
Shortt, S.E.D., ed. *Medicine in Canadian Society: Historical Perspectives*. Montreal: McGill-Queens University Press, 1981.
Simmons, Harvey G. *Unbalanced: Mental Health Policy in Ontario, 1930–1989*. Toronto: Wall & Thompson, 1990.
Stamp, Robert. *The Schools of Ontario, 1876–1976*. Toronto: University of Toronto Press, 1982.
Starr, Paul. *The Social Transformation of American Medicine*. New York: Basic Books, Inc., 1982.
Stewart, Miriam, Jean Innes, Sarah Searl, and Carol Smillie, eds. *Community Health Nursing in Canada*. Toronto: Gage Educational, 1985.
Strong-Boag, Veronica. *The New Day Recalled: Lives of Girls and Women in English Canada, 1919–1939*. Toronto: Penguin Books, 1988.
Sutherland, Neil. *Children in English-Canadian Society: Framing the Twentieth Century Consensus*. Toronto: University of Toronto Press, 1976.
Taylor, John. *Ottawa: An Illustrated History*. Toronto: James Lorimer and Company, 1986.
Toronto. Local Board of Health. Report of the Health Planning Steering Committee. *Public Health in the 1980's*. Toronto, May, 1980.
Walton, W.S., "The History of the Society of Medical Officers of Health, 1856–1956," *Public Health* (May, 1956): 160–226.
Weaver, John. *Hamilton: An Illustrated History*. Toronto: James Lorimer and Company, 1984.
Weir, George M. *Survey of Nursing Education in Canada*. Toronto: University of Toronto Press, 1932.
White, Michael J., Clayton, Ross, Myrtle, Robert, Siegel, Gilbert and Rose, Aaron. *Managing Public Systems: Analytic Techniques for Public Administration*. North Sciutate, Mass.: Duxbury Press, 1980.
Winslow, C.-E. A. *The Conquest of Epidemic Disease: A Chapter in the History of Ideas*. Madison: University of Wisconsin Press, 1980, reprint of 1938 edition.
Wohl, Anthony S. *Endangered Lives: Public Health in Victorian Britain*. Cambridge, Mass.: Harvard University Press, 1983.

Illustration Credits

Archives of Ontario: p. 88 lower.
Author: p. 101, 191, 213, 243, 251, 252.
Bureau of Municipal Research: p. 163.
City of Toronto Archives: p. 28, 58, 60, 61, 62, 63, 67, 68, 74, 75, 76, 77, 78, 79, 89, 90, 98, 99, 100, 104, 105 upper, 108, 109, 124, 126, 129 upper and lower, 130, 141, 142, 143, 161, 164, 165, 166 upper and lower, 171, 175, 178, 187, 190, 192, 194, 195, 199, 200, 201, 202 upper and lower, 205, 228 upper, 229.
Canadian Journal of Public Health: p. 54 and 55.
Department of Public Health: p. 91, 95, 96, 105 lower, 106, 107, 112, 113, 133, 144, 146, 153, 155, 169, 172, 173, 177, 197, 206, 207, 208 upper and lower, 262, 286.
Department of Public Health, *Annual Statement*: p. 39, 40, 42, 43, 47, 48, 49, 111, 114, 115, 134 upper and lower, 145, 174, 180, 183, 203, 221, 222, 223, 228 lower, 237, 239, 240, 241, 254, 256, 259, 261, 269, 284, 287, 288.
Department of Public Health, Scrapbook #2: p. 120 upper and lower.
Department of Public Health, Statistical Services Division: p. 150, 151, 182.
Metropolitan Toronto Library: p. 18, 22, 25, 88 upper, 94, 103 lower, 127, 128, 193.
Dr. George W.O. Moss: p. 45.
News : p. 72.
Dr. Charles Sheard, III: p. 23.
Toronto Fire Department: p. 44.
Toronto Star: p. 35, 103 upper, 172.
Toronto Telegram: p. 153.
York University Archives, *Toronto Telegram Collection*: p. 82, 83, 156.
Cover credit, front: City of Toronto Archives
back: Department of Public Health, Janet Saylor, City of Toronto Archives.

Index

Printed in Canada